Preventing Childhood Obesity
Health in the Balance

Committee on Prevention of Obesity in Children and Youth

Food and Nutrition Board
Board on Health Promotion and Disease Prevention

Jeffrey P. Koplan, Catharyn T. Liverman, Vivica I. Kraak, *Editors*

INSTITUTE OF MEDICINE
OF THE NATIONAL ACADEMIES

THE NATIONAL ACADEMIES PRESS
Washington, D.C.
www.nap.edu

THE NATIONAL ACADEMIES PRESS 500 Fifth Street, N.W. Washington, DC 20001

NOTICE: The project that is the subject of this report was approved by the Governing Board of the National Research Council, whose members are drawn from the councils of the National Academy of Sciences, the National Academy of Engineering, and the Institute of Medicine. The members of the committee responsible for the report were chosen for their special competences and with regard for appropriate balance.

The study was supported by Contract No. 200-2000-00629, T.O. #14 between the National Academy of Sciences and the Centers for Disease Control and Prevention; by Contract No. N01-OD-4-2139, T.O. #126 with the National Institutes of Health; and by Grant No. 047513 with The Robert Wood Johnson Foundation. The contracts were supported by funds from the U.S. Department of Health and Human Services' Office of Disease Prevention and Health Promotion; Centers for Disease Control and Prevention; National Institute of Diabetes and Digestive and Kidney Diseases; National Heart, Lung, and Blood Institute; National Institute of Child Health and Human Development; and the Division of Nutrition Research Coordination of the National Institutes of Health. Any opinions, findings, conclusions, or recommendations expressed in this publication are those of the authors and do not necessarily reflect the views of the organizations or agencies that provided support for the project.

Library of Congress Cataloging-in-Publication Data

Institute of Medicine (U.S.). Committee on Prevention of Obesity in Children and Youth.
  Preventing childhood obesity : health in the balance / Committee on Prevention of Obesity in Children and Youth, Food and Nutrition Board, Board on Health Promotion and Disease Prevention ; Jeffrey P. Koplan, Catharyn T. Liverman, Vivica I. Kraak, editors.
     p. ; cm.
  Includes bibliographical references and index.
  ISBN 0-309-09196-9 (hardcover) — ISBN 0-309-09315-5
  1. Obesity in children—United States—Prevention. 2. Child health services—United States. 3. Nutrition policy—United States. 4. Health promotion—United States.
  [DNLM: 1. Obesity—prevention & control—Adolescent. 2. Obesity—prevention & control—Child. 3. Health Policy—Adolescent. 4. Health Policy—Child. 5. Health Promotion—methods. 6. Social Environment. WD 210 I604p 2005] I. Koplan, Jeffrey. II. Liverman, Catharyn T. III. Kraak, Vivica I. IV. Institute of Medicine (U.S.). Board on Health Promotion and Disease Prevention. V. Title.
  RJ399.C6I575 2005
  618.92'398—dc22

                                2004026241

Additional copies of this report are available from the National Academies Press, 500 Fifth Street, N.W., Box 285, Washington, DC 20055. Call (800) 624-6242 or (202) 334-3313 (in the Washington metropolitan area), Internet, http://www.nap.edu.

For more information about the Institute of Medicine, visit the IOM home page at: www.iom.edu.

Illustration by Becky Heavner.

Printed in the United States of America.

The serpent has been a symbol of long life, healing, and knowledge among almost all cultures and religions since the beginning of recorded history. The serpent adopted as a logotype by the Institute of Medicine is a relief carving from ancient Greece, now held by the Staatliche Museen in Berlin.

First Printing, January 2005
Second Printing, November 2005

"Knowing is not enough; we must apply.
Willing is not enough; we must do."
—Goethe

INSTITUTE OF MEDICINE
OF THE NATIONAL ACADEMIES

Adviser to the Nation to Improve Health

THE NATIONAL ACADEMIES
Advisers to the Nation on Science, Engineering, and Medicine

The **National Academy of Sciences** is a private, nonprofit, self-perpetuating society of distinguished scholars engaged in scientific and engineering research, dedicated to the furtherance of science and technology and to their use for the general welfare. Upon the authority of the charter granted to it by the Congress in 1863, the Academy has a mandate that requires it to advise the federal government on scientific and technical matters. Dr. Bruce M. Alberts is president of the National Academy of Sciences.

The **National Academy of Engineering** was established in 1964, under the charter of the National Academy of Sciences, as a parallel organization of outstanding engineers. It is autonomous in its administration and in the selection of its members, sharing with the National Academy of Sciences the responsibility for advising the federal government. The National Academy of Engineering also sponsors engineering programs aimed at meeting national needs, encourages education and research, and recognizes the superior achievements of engineers. Dr. Wm. A. Wulf is president of the National Academy of Engineering.

The **Institute of Medicine** was established in 1970 by the National Academy of Sciences to secure the services of eminent members of appropriate professions in the examination of policy matters pertaining to the health of the public. The Institute acts under the responsibility given to the National Academy of Sciences by its congressional charter to be an adviser to the federal government and, upon its own initiative, to identify issues of medical care, research, and education. Dr. Harvey V. Fineberg is president of the Institute of Medicine.

The **National Research Council** was organized by the National Academy of Sciences in 1916 to associate the broad community of science and technology with the Academy's purposes of furthering knowledge and advising the federal government. Functioning in accordance with general policies determined by the Academy, the Council has become the principal operating agency of both the National Academy of Sciences and the National Academy of Engineering in providing services to the government, the public, and the scientific and engineering communities. The Council is administered jointly by both Academies and the Institute of Medicine. Dr. Bruce M. Alberts and Dr. Wm. A. Wulf are chair and vice chair, respectively, of the National Research Council.

www.national-academies.org

Staff

CATHARYN T. LIVERMAN, Study Director
LINDA D. MEYERS, Director, Food and Nutrition Board
ROSE MARIE MARTINEZ, Director, Board on Health Promotion and
Disease Prevention
VIVICA I. KRAAK, Senior Program Officer
JANICE RICE OKITA, Senior Program Officer
CARRIE SZLYK, Program Officer (through September 2003)
TAZIMA A. DAVIS, Research Associate
J. BERNADETTE MOORE, Science and Technology Policy Intern
(through June 2003)
ELISABETH RIMAUD, Financial Associate
SHANNON L. RUDDY, Senior Program Assistant

FOOD AND NUTRITION BOARD

vii

Reviewers

This report has been reviewed in draft form by individuals chosen for their diverse perspectives and technical expertise, in accordance with procedures approved by the National Research Council's Report Review Committee. The purpose of this independent review is to provide candid and critical comments that will assist the institution in making its published report as sound as possible and to ensure that the report meets institutional standards for objectivity, evidence, and responsiveness to the study charge. The review comments and draft manuscript remain confidential to protect the integrity of the deliberative process. We wish to thank the following individuals for their review of this report:

LINDA ADAIR, Carolina Population Center, University of North Carolina at Chapel Hill

TOM BARANOWSKI, Children's Nutrition Research Center, Baylor College of Medicine

EDWARD N. BRANDT, College of Public Health, University of Oklahoma

CUTBERTO GARZA, Division of Nutritional Sciences, Cornell University

MICHAEL S. JELLINEK, Newton Wellesley Hospital, Newton Lower Falls, MA

DAVID L. KATZ, Yale Prevention Research Center, Yale University

CARINE LENDERS, Department of Pediatrics, Boston Medical Center

AVIVA MUST, Department of Family Medicine and Community Health, Tufts University

VIVIAN PILANT, Office of School Food Services and Nutrition, South Carolina Department of Education

ALONZO PLOUGH, Department of Public Health-Seattle & King County, School of Public Health and Community Medicine, University of Washington

ROSSI RAY-TAYLOR, Minority Student Achievement Network, Ann Arbor, MI

JAMES F. SALLIS, San Diego State University, Active Living Research Program

MARILYN D. SCHORIN, Yum! Brands, Inc.

DONNA E. SHALALA, University of Miami

MICHAEL D. SLATER, Department of Journalism and Technical Communication, Colorado State University

SYLVIE STACHENKO, Centre for Chronic Disease Prevention and Control, Ottawa, Ontario

ROLAND STURM, RAND Corporation

BOYD SWINBURN, Centre for Physical Activity and Nutrition Research, Deakin University, Melbourne

MARGARITA S. TREUTH, Bloomberg School of Public Health, Johns Hopkins University

LINDA VAN HORN, Feinberg School of Medicine, Northwestern University

BARRY L. ZOUMAS, Department of Agricultural Economics and Rural Sociology, Pennsylvania State University

Although the reviewers listed above have provided many constructive comments and suggestions, they were not asked to endorse the conclusions or recommendations nor did they see the final draft of the report before its release. The review of this report was overseen by **ENRIQUETA C. BOND**, Burroughs Wellcome Fund, and **GORDON H. DEFRIESE**, Department of Social Medicine, University of North Carolina at Chapel Hill. Appointed by the National Research Council, they were responsible for making certain that an independent examination of this report was carried out in accordance with institutional procedures and that all review comments were carefully considered. Responsibility for the final content of this report rests entirely with the authoring committee and the institution.

Preface

In 2001, the U.S. Surgeon General issued the *Call to Action to Prevent and Decrease Overweight and Obesity* to stimulate the development of specific agendas and actions targeting this public health problem. In recognition of the need for greater attention directed to prevent childhood obesity, Congress, through the fiscal year 2002 Labor, Health and Human Services, Education Appropriations Act Conference Report, directed the Centers for Disease Control and Prevention (CDC) to request that the Institute of Medicine (IOM) develop an action plan targeted to the prevention of obesity in children and youth in the United States. In addition to CDC, this study was supported by the Department of Health and Human Services' Office of Disease Prevention and Health Promotion (ODPHP); National Institute of Diabetes and Digestive and Kidney Diseases (NIDDK); the National Heart, Lung, and Blood Institute (NHLBI); the National Institute of Child Health and Human Development (NICHD); the Division of Nutrition Research Coordination of the National Institutes of Health; and The Robert Wood Johnson Foundation (RWJF).

The charge to the IOM committee was to develop a prevention-focused action plan to decrease the prevalence of obesity in children and youth in the United States. The primary emphasis of the study's task was on examining the behavioral and cultural factors, social constructs, and other broad environmental factors involved in childhood obesity and identifying promising approaches for prevention efforts. To address this charge, the IOM appointed a 19-member multidisciplinary committee with expertise in child health and development, obesity, nutrition, physical activity, economics, education, public policy, and public health. Six meetings were held during the 24-month study and a variety of sources informed the committee's work. The committee obtained information through a literature review (Appendix C) and a commissioned paper discussing insights, strategies, and lessons learned from other public health issues and social change campaigns that might be relevant to the prevention of obesity in children and youth (Appendix D). The meetings included two workshops that were key elements of the committee's information-gathering process (Appendix E). Held in June 2003, the first workshop focused on strategies for developing school-based policies to promote nutrition and physical activity in children and youth. The second workshop was organized in December 2003 and addressed marketing and media influences on preventing childhood obesity and issues related to family dynamics. Each workshop included public forum sessions, and the committee benefited from the breadth of issues raised by nonprofit organizations, professional associations, and individuals.

Since the inception of this study, the committee recognized that it faced a broad task and a complex problem that has become an epidemic not only in the United States but also internationally. The committee appreciated the opportunity to develop an action plan on the prevention of obesity in children and youth and developed its recommendations to encompass the roles and responsibilities of numerous stakeholders and many sectors of society.

Children are highly cherished in our society. The value we attach to our children is fundamentally connected to society's responsibility to provide for their growth, development, and well-being. Extensive discussions will need to continue beyond this report so that shared understandings are reached and support is garnered for sustained societal and lifestyle changes that will reverse the obesity trends among our children and youth.

Jeffrey P. Koplan, *Chair*
Committee on Prevention of Obesity in
Children and Youth

Acknowledgments

It was a privilege to chair this Institute of Medicine (IOM) committee whose members not only brought their breadth and depth of expertise to this important topic but were actively engaged in the committee's work. This report represents the result of six meetings, two open sessions, numerous emails and phone conferences, and the extensive analysis and thoughtful writing contributed by the committee members who volunteered their time to work on this study. I thank each of the committee members for their dedication and perseverance in working through the diversity of issues in a truly interdisciplinary collaboration.

The committee greatly benefited from the opportunity for discussion with the individuals who made presentations and attended the committee's workshops and meetings, including: Neal Baer, Kelly Brownell, Harold Goldstein, Paula Hudson Collins, Mary Engle, Susan McHale, Alex Molnar, Eric Rosenthal, Mark Vallianatos, Jennifer Wilkins, and Judith Young, as well as all those who spoke during the open forums (Appendix E).

This study was sponsored by the U.S. Department of Health and Human Services' Centers for Disease Control and Prevention; Office of Disease Prevention and Health Promotion; National Heart, Lung, and Blood Institute; National Institute of Diabetes and Digestive and Kidney Diseases; National Institute of Child Health and Human Development; the Division of Nutrition Research Coordination of the National Institutes of Health; and The Robert Wood Johnson Foundation. The committee thanks Terry Bazzarre, William Dietz, Karen Donato, Gilman Grave, Van Hubbard,

Woodie Kessel, Kathryn McMurry, Pamela Starke-Reed, Susan Yanovski, and their colleagues for their support and guidance on the committee's task.

This study was conducted in collaboration with the IOM Board on Health Promotion and Disease Prevention (HPDP), and we wish to thank both Rose Martinez, director of the HPDP Board, for her thoughtful interactions and discussions with the committee, and Carrie Szlyk, who was of great assistance in the early phases of this study.

We appreciate the extensive analysis of lessons learned from other public health efforts and their relevance to preventing childhood obesity written by Michael Eriksen (Appendix D). Many thanks to Sally Ann Lederman and Lynn Parker for their technical review of sections of the report. Kathi Hanna's work as a consultant, financial oversight by Elisabeth Rimaud, and the editing work of Steven Marcus, Laura Penny, and Tom Burroughs are also greatly appreciated. The work of Rebecca Klima-Hudson and Stephanie Deutsch is also most appreciated. The report has been enhanced by the artwork of Becky Heavner, and we thank her for these creative efforts.

Last, but not least, I would like to thank the Food and Nutrition Board study staff, Linda Meyers, Cathy Liverman, Vivica Kraak, Janice Okita, Tazima Davis, and Shannon Ruddy, for their extraordinary competence, diligence, wisdom, and intellectual openness. Their in-depth knowledge of the subject matter, keen sense of policy and practice, and willingness to constantly work and revise to make this document as useful, thoughtful, and accurate as possible was invaluable in its creation.

Preventing Childhood Obesity: Health in the Balance presents a set of recommendations that, when implemented together, will catalyze synergistic actions among families, communities, schools, and the public and private sectors to effectively prevent the large majority of children and youth in the United States from becoming obese. Although the committee members have diverse backgrounds, over the course of this study we have gained a deeper appreciation for the difficulty and complexity of the steps necessary to prevent obesity in our nation's youth. We provide this guidance with the hope that it will benefit the health of our nation and future generations.

Jeffrey P. Koplan, *Chair*
Committee on Prevention of Obesity in
Children and Youth

Contents

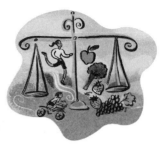

Executive Summary

Despite steady progress over most of the past century toward ensuring the health of our country's children, we begin the 21st century with a startling setback—an epidemic of childhood obesity. This epidemic is occurring in boys and girls in all 50 states, in younger children as well as adolescents, across all socioeconomic strata, and among all ethnic groups—though specific subgroups, including African Americans, Hispanics, and American Indians, are disproportionately affected. At a time when we have learned that excess weight has significant and troublesome health consequences, we nevertheless see our population, in general, and our children, in particular, gaining weight to a dangerous degree and at an alarming rate.

The increasing prevalence of childhood obesity[1] throughout the United States has led policy makers to rank it as a critical public health threat. Over the past three decades, its rate has more than doubled for preschool children aged 2 to 5 years and adolescents aged 12 to 19 years, and it has more than tripled for children aged 6 to 11 years. At present, approximately nine million children over 6 years of age are considered obese. These

---

[1]Reflecting classification based on the readily available measures of height and weight, this report uses the term "obesity" to refer to children and youth who have a body mass index (BMI) equal to or greater than the 95th percentile of the age- and gender-specific BMI charts of the Centers for Disease Control and Prevention (CDC). In most children, such BMI values are known to indicate elevated body fat and to reflect the presence or risk of related diseases.

trends mirror a similar profound increase over the same approximate period in U.S. adults as well as a concurrent rise internationally, in developed and developing countries alike.

Childhood obesity involves immediate and long-term risks to physical health. For children born in the United States in 2000, the lifetime risk of being diagnosed with diabetes at some point in their lives is estimated at 30 percent for boys and 40 percent for girls if obesity rates level off. Young people are also at risk of developing serious psychosocial burdens related to being obese in a society that stigmatizes this condition.

There are also considerable economic costs. The national health care expenditures related to obesity and overweight in adults alone have been estimated to range from approximately $98 billion to $129 billion after adjusting for inflation and converting estimates to 2004 dollars. Understanding the causes of childhood obesity, determining what to do about them, and taking appropriate action require attention to what influences eating behaviors and physical activity levels because obesity prevention involves a focus on energy balance (calories consumed versus calories expended). Although seemingly straightforward, these behaviors result from complex interactions across a number of relevant social, environmental, and policy contexts.

U.S. children live in a society that has changed dramatically in the three decades over which the obesity epidemic has developed. Many of these changes—such as both parents working outside the home, longer work hours by both parents, changes in the school food environment, and more meals eaten outside the home, together with changes in the physical design of communities often affect what children eat, where they eat, how much they eat, and the amount of energy they expend in school and leisure time activities. Other changes, such as the growing diversity of the population, influence cultural views and marketing patterns. Use of computers and video games, along with television viewing, often occupy a large percentage of children's leisure time and potentially influence levels of physical activity for children as well as for adults. Many of the social and cultural characteristics that the U.S. population has accepted as a normal way of life may collectively contribute to the growing levels of childhood obesity. An understanding of these contexts, particularly regarding their potential to be modified and how they may facilitate or impede development of a comprehensive obesity prevention strategy, is essential for reducing childhood obesity.

DEVELOPING AN ACTION PLAN FOR OBESITY PREVENTION

The Institute of Medicine Committee on Prevention of Obesity in Children and Youth was charged with developing a prevention-focused action plan to decrease the prevalence of obesity in children and youth in the United States. The primary emphasis of the committee's task was on examining the behavioral and cultural factors, social constructs, and other broad environmental factors involved in childhood obesity and identifying promising approaches for prevention efforts. The plan consists of explicit goals for preventing obesity in children and youth and a set of recommendations, all geared toward achieving those goals, for different segments of society (Box ES-1).

Obesity prevention requires an evidence-based public health approach to assure that recommended strategies and actions will have their intended effects. Such evidence is traditionally drawn from experimental (randomized) trials and high-quality observational studies. However, there is limited experimental evidence in this area, and for many environmental, policy, and societal variables, carefully designed evaluations of ongoing programs and policies are likely to answer many key questions. For this reason, the committee chose a process that incorporated all forms of available evidence—across different categories of information and types of study design—to enhance the biological, psychosocial, and environmental plausibility of its inferences and to ensure consistency and congruency of information.

Because the obesity epidemic is a serious public health problem calling for immediate reductions in obesity prevalence and in its health and social consequences, the committee believed strongly that actions should be based on the best *available* evidence—as opposed to waiting for the best *possible* evidence. However, there is an obligation to accumulate appropriate evidence not only to justify a course of action but to assess whether it has made a difference. Therefore, evaluation should be a critical component of any implemented intervention or change.

Childhood obesity prevention involves maintaining energy balance at a healthy weight while protecting overall health, growth and development, and nutritional status. The balance is between the energy an individual consumes as food and beverages and the energy expended to support normal growth and development, metabolism, thermogenesis, and physical activity. Although "energy intake = energy expenditure" looks like a fairly basic equation, in reality it is extraordinarily complex when considering the multitude of genetic, biological, psychological, sociocultural, and environmental factors that affect both sides of the equation and the interrelationships between these factors. For example, children are strongly influenced by the food- and physical activity-related decisions made by their families, schools, and communities. Furthermore, it is important to consider the kinds of foods and beverages that children are consuming over time, given that specific types and quantities of nutrients are required to support optimal growth and development.

BOX ES-1
Goals of Obesity Prevention in Children and Youth

The goal of obesity prevention in children and youth is to create—through directed social change—an environmental-behavioral synergy that promotes:

- **For the *population* of children and youth**
  - ◆ Reduction in the incidence of childhood and adolescent obesity
  - ◆ Reduction in the prevalence of childhood and adolescent obesity
  - ◆ Reduction of mean population BMI levels
  - ◆ Improvement in the proportion of children meeting Dietary Guidelines for Americans
  - ◆ Improvement in the proportion of children meeting physical activity guidelines
  - ◆ Achieving physical, psychological, and cognitive growth and developmental goals

- **For *individual* children and youth**
  - ◆ A healthy weight trajectory, as defined by the CDC BMI charts
  - ◆ A healthful diet (quality and quantity)
  - ◆ Appropriate amounts and types of physical activity
  - ◆ Achieving physical, psychosocial, and cognitive growth and developmental goals

Because it may take a number of years to achieve and sustain these goals, intermediate goals are needed to assess progress toward reduction of obesity through policy and system changes. Examples include:

- Increased number of children who safely walk and bike to school
- Improved access to and affordability of fruits and vegetables for low-income populations
- Increased availability and use of community recreational facilities
- Increased play and physical activity opportunities
- Increased number of new industry products and advertising messages that promote energy balance at a healthy weight
- Increased availability and affordability of healthful foods and beverages at supermarkets, grocery stores, and farmers markets located within walking distance of the communities they serve
- Changes in institutional and environmental policies that promote energy balance

---

Thus, changes at many levels and in numerous environments will require the involvement of multiple stakeholders from diverse segments of society. In the home environment, for example, incremental changes such as improving the nutritional quality of family dinners or increasing the time and frequency that children spend outside playing can make a difference.

Changes that lead to healthy communities, such as organizational and policy changes in local schools, school districts, neighborhoods, and cities, are equally important. At the state and national levels, large-scale modifications are needed in the ways in which society promotes healthful eating habits and physically active lifestyles. Accomplishing these changes will be difficult, but there is precedent for success in other public health endeavors of comparable or greater complexity and scope. This must be a national effort, with special attention to communities that experience health disparities and that have social and physical environments unsupportive of healthful nutrition and physical activity.

A NATIONAL PUBLIC HEALTH PRIORITY

Just as broad-based approaches have been used to address other public health concerns—including automobile safety and tobacco use—obesity prevention should be public health in action at its broadest and most inclusive level. **Prevention of obesity in children and youth should be a national public health priority.**

Across the country, obesity prevention efforts have already begun, and although the ultimate solutions are still far off, there is great potential at present for pursuing innovative approaches and creating linkages that permit the cross-fertilization of ideas. Current efforts range from new school board policies and state legislation regarding school physical education requirements and nutrition standards for beverages and foods sold in schools to community initiatives to expand bike paths and improve recreational facilities. Parallel and synergistic efforts to prevent adult obesity, which will contribute to improvements in health for the entire U.S. population, are also beginning. Grassroots efforts made by citizens and organizations will likely drive many of the obesity prevention efforts at the local level and can be instrumental in driving policies and legislation at the state and national levels.

The additional impetus that is needed is the political will to make childhood obesity prevention a national public health priority. Obesity prevention efforts nationwide will require federal, state, and local governments to commit adequate and sustained resources for surveillance, research, public health programs, evaluation, and dissemination. The federal government has had a longstanding commitment to programs that address nutritional deficiencies (beginning in the 1930s) and encourage physical fitness, but only recently has obesity been targeted. The federal government should demonstrate effective leadership by making a sustained commitment to support policies and programs that are commensurate to the scale of the problem. Furthermore, leadership in this endeavor will require coordination of federal efforts with state and community efforts, complemented by engagement of the private sector in developing constructive, socially responsible, and potentially profitable approaches to the promotion of a healthy weight.

State and local governments have especially important roles to play in obesity prevention, as they can focus on the specific needs of their state, cities, and neighborhoods. Many of the issues involved in preventing childhood obesity—including actions on street and neighborhood design, plans for parks and community recreational facilities, and locations of new schools and retail food facilities—require decisions by county, city, or town officials.

Rigorous evaluation of obesity prevention interventions is essential. Only through careful evaluation can prevention interventions be refined; those that are unsuccessful can be discontinued or refocused, and those that are successful can be identified, replicated, and disseminated.

Recommendation 1: *National Priority*
Government at all levels should provide coordinated leadership for the prevention of obesity in children and youth. The President should request that the Secretary of the Department of Health and Human Services (DHHS) convene a high-level task force to ensure coordinated budgets, policies, and program requirements and to establish effective interdepartmental collaboration and priorities for action. An increased level and sustained commitment of federal and state funds and resources are needed.

To implement this recommendation, the federal government should:

- Strengthen research and program efforts addressing obesity prevention, with a focus on experimental behavioral research and community-based intervention research and on the rigorous evaluation of the effectiveness, cost-effectiveness, sustainability, and scaling up of effective prevention interventions
- Support extensive program and research efforts to prevent childhood obesity in high-risk populations with health disparities, with a focus both on behavioral and environmental approaches
- Support nutrition and physical activity grant programs, particularly in states with the highest prevalence of childhood obesity
- Strengthen support for relevant surveillance and monitoring efforts, particularly the National Health and Nutrition Examination Survey (NHANES)
- Undertake an independent assessment of federal nutrition assistance programs and agricultural policies to ensure that they pro-

mote healthful dietary intake and physical activity levels for all children and youth
 • Develop and evaluate pilot projects within the nutrition assistance programs that would promote healthful dietary intake and physical activity and scale up those found to be successful

To implement this recommendation, state and local governments should:

 • Provide coordinated leadership and support for childhood obesity prevention efforts, particularly those focused on high-risk populations, by increasing resources and strengthening policies that promote opportunities for physical activity and healthful eating in communities, neighborhoods, and schools
 • Support public health agencies and community coalitions in their collaborative efforts to promote and evaluate obesity prevention interventions

HEALTHY MARKETPLACE AND MEDIA ENVIRONMENTS

Children, youth, and their families are surrounded by a commercial environment that strongly influences their purchasing and consumption behaviors. Consumers may initially be unsure about what to eat for good health. They often make immediate trade-offs in taste, cost, and convenience for longer term health. The food, beverage, restaurant, entertainment, leisure, and recreation industries share in the responsibilities for childhood obesity prevention and can be instrumental in supporting this goal. Federal agencies can strengthen industry efforts through general support, technical assistance, research expertise, and regulatory guidance.

Some leaders in the food industry are already making changes to expand healthier options for young consumers, offer products with reduced energy content, and reduce portion sizes. These changes must be adopted on a much larger scale, however, and marketed in ways that make acceptance by consumers (who may now have acquired entrenched preferences for many less healthful products) more likely. Coordinated efforts among the private sector, government, and other groups are also needed to create, support, and sustain consumer demand for healthful food and beverage products, appropriately portioned restaurant and take-out meals, and accurate and consistent nutritional information through food labels, health claims, and other educational sources. Similarly, the leisure, entertainment, and recreation industries have opportunities to innovate in favor of stimulating physical activity—as opposed to sedentary or passive-leisure pursuits—and portraying active living as a desirable social norm for adults and children.

Children's health-related behaviors are influenced by exposure to media messages involving foods, beverages, and physical activity. Research has shown that television advertising can especially affect children's food knowledge, choices, and consumption of particular food products, as well as their food-purchase decisions made directly and indirectly (through parents). Because young children under 8 years of age are often unable to distinguish between information and the persuasive intent of advertising, the committee recommends the development of guidelines for advertising and marketing of foods, beverages, and sedentary entertainment to children.

Media messages can also be inherently positive. There is great potential for the media and entertainment industries to encourage a balanced diet, healthful eating habits, and regular physical activity, thereby influencing social norms about obesity in children and youth and helping to spur the actions needed to prevent it. Public education messages in multiple types of media are needed to generate support for policy changes and provide messages to the general public, parents, children, and adolescents.

Recommendation 2: *Industry*
Industry should make obesity prevention in children and youth a priority by developing and promoting products, opportunities, and information that will encourage healthful eating behaviors and regular physical activity.

To implement this recommendation:

- Food and beverage industries should develop product and packaging innovations that consider energy density, nutrient density, and standard serving sizes to help consumers make healthful choices.
- Leisure, entertainment, and recreation industries should develop products and opportunities that promote regular physical activity and reduce sedentary behaviors.
- Full-service and fast food restaurants should expand healthier food options and provide calorie content and general nutrition information at point of purchase.

Recommendation 3: *Nutrition Labeling*
Nutrition labeling should be clear and useful so that parents and youth can make informed product comparisons and decisions to achieve and maintain energy balance at a healthy weight.

To implement this recommendation:

- The Food and Drug Administration should revise the Nutrition Facts panel to prominently display the total calorie content for items typically consumed at one eating occasion in addition to the standardized calorie serving and the percent Daily Value.
- The Food and Drug Administration should examine ways to allow greater flexibility in the use of evidence-based nutrient and health claims regarding the link between the nutritional properties or biological effects of foods and a reduced risk of obesity and related chronic diseases.
- Consumer research should be conducted to maximize use of the nutrition label and other food-guidance systems.

Recommendation 4: *Advertising and Marketing*
Industry should develop and strictly adhere to marketing and advertising guidelines that minimize the risk of obesity in children and youth.

To implement this recommendation:

- The Secretary of the DHHS should convene a national conference to develop guidelines for the advertising and marketing of foods, beverages, and sedentary entertainment directed at children and youth with attention to product placement, promotion, and content.
- Industry should implement the advertising and marketing guidelines.
- The Federal Trade Commission should have the authority and resources to monitor compliance with the food and beverage and sedentary entertainment advertising practices.

Recommendation 5: *Multimedia and Public Relations Campaign*
The DHHS should develop and evaluate a long-term national multimedia and public relations campaign focused on obesity prevention in children and youth.

To implement this recommendation:

- The campaign should be developed in coordination with other federal departments and agencies and with input from independent experts to focus on building support for policy changes; providing information to parents; and providing information to children and youth. Rigorous evaluation should be a critical component.

- Reinforcing messages should be provided in diverse media and effectively coordinated with other events and dissemination activities.
- The media should incorporate obesity issues into its content, including the promotion of positive role models.

HEALTHY COMMUNITIES

Encouraging children and youth to be physically active involves providing them with places where they can safely walk, bike, run, skate, play games, or engage in other activities that expend energy. But practices that guide the development of streets and neighborhoods often place the needs of motorized vehicles over the needs of pedestrians and bicyclists. Local governments should find ways to increase opportunities for physical activity in their communities by examining zoning ordinances and priorities for capital investment.

Community actions need to engage child- and youth-centered organizations, social and civic organizations, faith-based groups, and many other community partners. Community coalitions can coordinate their efforts and leverage and network resources. Specific attention must be given to children and youth who are at high risk for becoming obese; this includes children in populations with higher obesity prevalence rates and longstanding health disparities such as African Americans, Hispanic Americans, and American Indians, or families of low socioeconomic status. Children with at least one obese parent are also at high risk.

Health-care professionals, including physicians, nurses, and other clinicians, have a vital role to play in preventing childhood obesity. As advisors both to children and their parents, they have the access and influence to discuss the child's weight status with the parents (and child as age appropriate) and make credible recommendations on dietary intake and physical activity throughout children's lives. They also have the authority to encourage action by advocating for prevention efforts.

Recommendation 6: *Community Programs*
Local governments, public health agencies, schools, and community organizations should collaboratively develop and promote programs that encourage healthful eating behaviors and regular physical activity, particularly for populations at high risk of childhood obesity. Community coalitions should be formed to facilitate and promote cross-cutting programs and community-wide efforts.

To implement this recommendation:

• Private and public efforts to eliminate health disparities should include obesity prevention as one of their primary areas of focus and should support community-based collaborative programs to address social, economic, and environmental barriers that contribute to the increased obesity prevalence among certain populations.
• Community child- and youth-centered organizations should promote healthful eating behaviors and regular physical activity through new and existing programs that will be sustained over the long term.
• Community evaluation tools should incorporate measures of the availability of opportunities for physical activity and healthful eating.
• Communities should improve access to supermarkets, farmers' markets, and community gardens to expand healthful food options, particularly in low-income and underserved areas.

Recommendation 7: *Built Environment*
Local governments, private developers, and community groups should expand opportunities for physical activity including recreational facilities, parks, playgrounds, sidewalks, bike paths, routes for walking or bicycling to school, and safe streets and neighborhoods, especially for populations at high risk of childhood obesity.

To implement this recommendation:

Local governments, working with private developers and community groups, should:
• Revise comprehensive plans, zoning and subdivision ordinances, and other planning practices to increase availability and accessibility of opportunities for physical activity in new developments
• Prioritize capital improvement projects to increase opportunities for physical activity in existing areas
• Improve the street, sidewalk, and street-crossing safety of routes to school, develop programs to encourage walking and bicycling to school, and build schools within walking and bicycling distance of the neighborhoods they serve

Community groups should:
• Work with local governments to change their planning and capital improvement practices to give higher priority to opportunities for physical activity

The DHHS and the Department of Transportation should:
• Fund community-based research to examine the impact of changes to the built environment on the levels of physical activity in the relevant communities and populations.

Recommendation 8: *Health Care*
Pediatricians, family physicians, nurses, and other clinicians should engage in the prevention of childhood obesity. Health-care professional organizations, insurers, and accrediting groups should support individual and population-based obesity prevention efforts.

To implement this recommendation:

• Health-care professionals should routinely track BMI, offer relevant evidence-based counseling and guidance, serve as role models, and provide leadership in their communities for obesity prevention efforts.
• Professional organizations should disseminate evidence-based clinical guidance and establish programs on obesity prevention.
• Training programs and certifying entities should require obesity prevention knowledge and skills in their curricula and examinations.
• Insurers and accrediting organizations should provide incentives for maintaining healthy body weight and include screening and obesity preventive services in routine clinical practice and quality assessment measures.

HEALTHY SCHOOL ENVIRONMENT

Schools are one of the primary locations for reaching the nation's children and youth. In 2000, 53.2 million students were enrolled in public and private elementary and secondary schools in the United States. In addition, schools often serve as the sites for preschool, child-care, and after-school programs. Both inside and outside of the classroom, schools present opportunities for the concepts of energy balance to be taught and put into practice as students learn about good nutrition, physical activity, and their relationships to health; engage in physical education; and make food and physical activity choices during school meal times and through school-related activities.

All foods and beverages sold or served to students in school should be healthful and meet an accepted nutritional content standard. However, many of the "competitive foods" now sold in school cafeterias, vending machines, school stores, and school fundraisers are high in calories and low in nutritional value. At present, federal standards for the sale of competitive foods in schools are only minimal.

In addition, many schools around the nation have reduced their commitment to provide students with regular and adequate physical activity, often as a result of budget cuts or pressures to increase academic course offerings, even though it is generally recommended that children accumulate a minimum of 60 minutes of moderate to vigorous physical activity each day. Given that children spend over half of their day in school, it is not unreasonable to expect that they participate in at least 30 minutes of moderate to vigorous physical activity during the school day.

Schools offer many other opportunities for learning and practicing healthful eating and physical activity behaviors. Coordinated changes in the curriculum, the in-school advertising environment, school health services, and after-school programs all offer the potential to advance obesity prevention. Furthermore, it is important for parents to be aware of their child's weight status. Schools can assist in providing BMI, weight, and height information to parents and to children (as age appropriate) while being sure to sensitively collect and report on that information.

Recommendation 9: *Schools*
Schools should provide a consistent environment that is conducive to healthful eating behaviors and regular physical activity.

To implement this recommendation:

The U.S. Department of Agriculture, state and local authorities, and schools should:

- Develop and implement nutritional standards for all competitive foods and beverages sold or served in schools
- Ensure that all school meals meet the Dietary Guidelines for Americans
- Develop, implement, and evaluate pilot programs to extend school meal funding in schools with a large percentage of children at high risk of obesity

State and local education authorities and schools should:

- Ensure that all children and youth participate in a minimum of 30 minutes of moderate to vigorous physical activity during the school day
- Expand opportunities for physical activity through physical education classes; intramural and interscholastic sports programs and other physical activity clubs, programs, and lessons; after-school use of school facilities; use of schools as community centers; and walking- and biking-to-school programs
- Enhance health curricula to devote adequate attention to nutrition, physical activity, reducing sedentary behaviors, and energy balance, and to include a behavioral skills focus
- Develop, implement, and enforce school policies to create schools that are advertising-free to the greatest possible extent
- Involve school health services in obesity prevention efforts
- Conduct annual assessments of each student's weight, height, and gender- and age-specific BMI percentile and make this information available to parents
- Perform periodic assessments of each school's policies and practices related to nutrition, physical activity, and obesity prevention

Federal and state departments of education and health and professional organizations should:

- Develop, implement, and evaluate pilot programs to explore innovative approaches to both staffing and teaching about wellness, healthful choices, nutrition, physical activity, and reducing sedentary behaviors. Innovative approaches to recruiting and training appropriate teachers are also needed

HEALTHY HOME ENVIRONMENT

Parents (defined broadly to include primary caregivers) have a profound influence on their children by fostering certain values and attitudes, by rewarding or reinforcing specific behaviors, and by serving as role models. A child's health and well-being are thus enhanced by a home environment with engaged and skillful parenting that models, values, and encourages healthful eating habits and a physically active lifestyle. Economic and time constraints, as well as the stresses and challenges of daily living, may make healthful eating and increased physical activity a difficult reality on a day-to-day basis for many families.

Parents play a fundamental role as household policy makers. They make daily decisions on recreational opportunities, food availability at home, and children's allowances; they determine the setting for foods eaten in the home; and they implement countless other rules and policies that influence the extent to which various members of the family engage in healthful eating and physical activity. Older children and youth, meanwhile, have responsibilities to be aware of their own eating habits and activity patterns and to engage in health-promoting behaviors.

Recommendation 10: *Home*
Parents should promote healthful eating behaviors and regular physical activity for their children.

To implement this recommendation parents can:

- Choose exclusive breastfeeding as the method for feeding infants for the first four to six months of life
- Provide healthful food and beverage choices for children by carefully considering nutrient quality and energy density
- Assist and educate children in making healthful decisions regarding types of foods and beverages to consume, how often, and in what portion size
- Encourage and support regular physical activity
- Limit children's television viewing and other recreational screen time to less than two hours per day
- Discuss weight status with their child's health-care provider and monitor age- and gender-specific BMI percentile
- Serve as positive role models for their children regarding eating and physical-activity behaviors

CONFRONTING THE CHILDHOOD OBESITY EPIDEMIC

The committee acknowledges, as have many other similar efforts, that obesity prevention is a complex issue, that a thorough understanding of the causes and determinants of the obesity epidemic is lacking, and that progress will require changes not only in individual and family behaviors but also in the marketplace and the social and built environments (Box ES-2). As the nation focuses on obesity as a health problem and begins to address the societal and cultural issues that contribute to excess weight, poor food choices, and inactivity, many different stakeholders will need to make difficult trade-offs and choices. However, as institutions, organizations, and individuals across the nation begin to make changes, societal norms are

---

BOX ES-2
Summary of Findings and Conclusions

- Childhood obesity is a serious nationwide health problem requiring urgent attention and a population-based prevention approach so that all children may grow up physically and emotionally healthy.
- Preventing obesity involves healthful eating behaviors and regular physical activity with the goal of achieving and maintaining energy balance at a healthy weight.
- Individual efforts and societal changes are needed. Multiple sectors and stakeholders must be involved.

---

likely to change as well; in the long term, we can become a nation where proper nutrition and physical activity that support energy balance at a healthy weight will become the standard.

Recognizing the multifactorial nature of the problem, the committee deliberated on how best to prioritize the next steps for the nation in preventing obesity in children and youth. The traditional method of prioritizing recommendations of this nature would be to base these decisions on the strength of the scientific evidence demonstrating that specific interventions have a direct impact on reducing obesity prevalence and to order the evidence-based approaches based on the balance between potential benefits and associated costs including potential risks. However, a robust evidence base is not yet available. Instead, we are in the midst of compiling that much-needed evidence at the same time that there is an urgent need to respond to this epidemic of childhood obesity. Therefore, the committee used the best scientific evidence available—including studies with obesity as the outcome measure and studies on improving dietary behaviors, increasing physical activity levels, and reducing sedentary behaviors, as well as years of experience and study on what has worked in addressing similar public health challenges—to develop the recommendations presented in this report.

As evidence was limited, yet the health concerns are immediate and warrant preventive action, it is an explicit part of the committee's recommendations that all the actions and initiatives include evaluation efforts to help build the evidence base that continues to be needed to more effectively fight this epidemic.

From the ten recommendations presented above, the committee has identified a set of immediate steps based on the short-term feasibility of the actions and the need to begin a well-rounded set of changes that recognize the diverse roles of multiple stakeholders (Table ES-1). In discussions and interactions that have already begun and will follow with this report, each community and stakeholder group will determine their own set of priorities and next steps. Furthermore, action is urged for all areas of the report's recommendations, as the list in Table ES-1 is only meant as a starting point.

The committee was also asked to set forth research priorities. There is still much to be learned about the causes, correlates, prevention, and treatment of obesity in children and youth. Because the focus of this study is on prevention, the committee concentrated its efforts throughout the report on identifying areas of research that are priorities for progress toward preventing childhood obesity. The three research priorities discussed throughout the report are:

- Evaluation of obesity prevention interventions—The committee encourages the evaluation of interventions that focus on preventing an increase in obesity prevalence, improving dietary behaviors, increasing physical activity levels, and reducing sedentary behaviors. Specific policy, environmental, social, clinical, and behavioral intervention approaches should be examined for their feasibility, efficacy, effectiveness, and sustainability. Evaluations may be in the form of randomized controlled trials and quasi-experimental trials. Cost effectiveness research should be an important component of evaluation efforts.
- Behavioral research—The committee encourages experimental research examining the fundamental factors involved in changing dietary behaviors, physical activity levels, and sedentary behaviors. This research should inform new intervention strategies that are implemented and tested at individual, family, school, community, and population levels. This would include studies that focus on factors promoting motivation to change behavior, strategies to reinforce and sustain improved behavior, identification and removal of barriers to change, and specific ethnic and cultural influences on behavioral change.
- Community-based population-level research—The committee encourages experimental and observational research examining the most important established and novel factors that drive changes in population health, how they are embedded in the socioeconomic and built environments, how they impact obesity prevention, and how they affect society at large with regard to improving nutritional health, increasing physical activity, decreasing sedentary behaviors, and reducing obesity prevalence.

The recommendations that constitute this report's action plan to prevent childhood obesity commence what is anticipated to be an energetic and sustained effort. Some of the recommendations can be implemented immediately and will cost little, while others will take a larger economic investment and require a longer time for implementation and to see the benefits of the investment. Some will prove useful, either quickly or over the longer term, while others will prove unsuccessful. Knowing that it is impossible to produce an optimal solution a priori, we more appropriately adopt surveillance, trial, measurement, error, success, alteration, and dissemination as our course, to be embarked on immediately. Given that the health of today's children and future generations is at stake, we must proceed with all due urgency and vigor.

TABLE ES-1 Immediate Steps

Federal government	• Establish an interdepartmental task force and coordinate federal actions • Develop nutrition standards for foods and beverages sold in schools • Fund state-based nutrition and physical-activity grants with strong evaluation components • Develop guidelines regarding advertising and marketing to children and youth by convening a national conference • Expand funding for prevention intervention research, experimental behavioral research, and community-based population research; strengthen support for surveillance, monitoring, and evaluation efforts
Industry and media	• Develop healthier food and beverage product and packaging innovations • Expand consumer nutrition information • Provide clear and consistent media messages
State and local governments	• Expand and promote opportunities for physical activity in the community through changes to ordinances, capital improvement programs, and other planning practices • Work with communities to support partnerships and networks that expand the availability of and access to healthful foods
Health-care professionals	• Routinely track BMI in children and youth and offer appropriate counseling and guidance to children and their families
Community and nonprofit organizations	• Provide opportunities for healthful eating and physical activity in existing and new community programs, particularly for high-risk populations
State and local education authorities and schools	• Improve the nutritional quality of foods and beverages served and sold in schools and as part of school-related activities • Increase opportunities for frequent, more intensive and engaging physical activity during and after school • Implement school-based interventions to reduce children's screen time • Develop, implement, and evaluate innovative pilot programs for both staffing and teaching about wellness, healthful eating, and physical activity
Parents and families	• Engage in and promote more healthful dietary intakes and active lifestyles (e.g., increased physical activity, reduced television and other screen time, more healthful dietary behaviors)

1

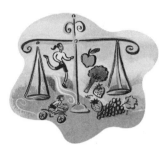

Introduction

AN EPIDEMIC OF CHILDHOOD OBESITY

Children's health in the United States has improved dramatically over the past century. Vaccines targeting previously common childhood infections—such as measles, polio, diphtheria, tetanus, rubella, and *Haemophilus influenza*—have nearly eliminated these scourges. Through the widespread availability of potable water, improved sanitation, and antibiotics, diarrheal diseases and infectious diseases such as tuberculosis and pneumonia have diminished in frequency and as primary causes of infant and child deaths in the United States (CDC, 1999). Pervasive food scarcity and essential vitamin and mineral deficiencies have largely disappeared in the U.S. population (IOM, 1991; Kessler, 1995). The net result is that infant mortality has been lowered by over 90 percent, contributing to the substantial increase in life expectancy—more than 30 years—since 1900 (CDC, 1999). Innovations such as seatbelts, child car seats, and bike helmets, meanwhile, have contributed to improved children's safety, and fluoridation of municipal drinking water has enhanced child and adolescent dentition (CDC, 1999).

Given this steady trajectory toward a healthier childhood and healthier children, we begin the 21st century with a startling setback—an epidemic[1]

---

[1]The term "epidemic" is used in reference to childhood obesity as there have been an unexpected and excess number of cases on a steady increase in recent decades.

of childhood obesity. This epidemic is occurring in boys and girls in all 50 states, in younger children as well as in adolescents, across all socioeconomic strata, and among all ethnic groups—though specific subgroups, including African Americans, Hispanics, and American Indians, are disproportionately affected (Ogden et al., 2002; Caballero et al., 2003). At a time when we have learned that excess weight has significant and troublesome health consequences, we nevertheless see our population, in general, and our children, in particular, gaining weight to a dangerous degree and at an alarming rate.

The increasing prevalence of childhood obesity throughout the United States has led policy makers to rank it as a critical public health threat for the 21st century (Koplan and Dietz, 1999; Mokdad et al., 1999, 2000; DHHS, 2001). Over the past three decades since the 1970s, the prevalence of childhood obesity (defined in this report as a gender- and age-specific body mass index [BMI] at or above the 95th percentile on the 2000 CDC BMI charts) has more than doubled for preschool children aged 2 to 5 years and adolescents aged 12 to 19 years, and it has more than tripled for children aged 6 to 11 years (see Chapter 2; Ogden et al., 2002). Approximately nine million American children over 6 years of age are already considered obese. These trends mirror a similar profound increase in U.S. adult obesity and co-morbidities over a comparable time frame, as well as a concurrent rise in the prevalence of childhood and adult obesity and related chronic diseases internationally, in developed and developing countries alike (WHO, 2002, 2003; Lobstein et al., 2004).

IMPLICATIONS FOR CHILDREN AND SOCIETY AT LARGE

Many of us consider our weight and height as personal statistics, primarily our own, and occasionally our physician's concern. Our weight is something we approximate on forms and applications requiring this information. Body size has been a cosmetic issue rather than a health issue throughout most of human history, but scientific study has changed this view. One's aesthetic preference for a lean versus a plump body type may be related to personal taste, cultural and social norms, and association of body type with wealth or well-being. However, the implications of a wholesale increase in BMIs are increasingly becoming a public health problem. Thus, we need to acknowledge the sensitive personal dimension of height and weight, while also viewing weight as a public health issue, especially as the weight levels of children, as a population, are proceeding on a harmful upward trajectory.

The as yet unabated epidemic of childhood obesity has significant ramifications for children's physical health, both in the immediate and long term, given that obesity is linked to several chronic disease risks. In a population-based sample, approximately 60 percent of obese children aged 5 to 10 years had at least one physiological cardiovascular disease (CVD) risk factor—such as elevated total cholesterol, triglycerides, insulin, or blood pressure—and 25 percent had two or more CVD risk factors (Freedman et al., 1999).

The increasing incidence of type 2 diabetes in young children (previously known as adult onset diabetes) is particularly startling. For individuals born in the United States in 2000, the lifetime risk of being diagnosed with diabetes at some point in their lives is estimated at 30 percent for boys and 40 percent for girls if obesity rates level off (Narayan et al., 2003).[2] The estimated lifetime risk for developing diabetes is even higher among ethnic minority groups at birth and at all ages (Narayan et al., 2003). Type 2 diabetes is rapidly becoming a disease of children and adolescents. In case reports limited to the 1990s, type 2 diabetes accounted for 8 to 45 percent of all new childhood cases of diabetes—in contrast with fewer than 4 percent before the 1990s (Fagot-Campagna et al., 2000). Young people are also at risk of developing serious psychosocial burdens related to being obese in a society that stigmatizes this condition, often fostering shame, self-blame, and low self-esteem that may impair academic and social func tioning and carry into adulthood (Schwartz and Puhl, 2003).

The growing obesity epidemic in children, and in adults, affects not only the individual's physical and mental health but carries substantial direct and indirect costs for the nation's economy as discrimination, economic disenfranchisement, lost productivity, disability, morbidity, and premature death take their tolls (Seidell, 1998). States and communities are obliged to divert resources to prevention and treatment, and the national health-care system is burdened with the co-morbidities of obesity such as type 2 diabetes, hypertension, CVD, osteoarthritis, and cancer (Ebbeling et al., 2002).

The obesity epidemic may reduce overall adult life expectancy (Fontaine et al., 2003) because it increases lifetime risk for type 2 diabetes and other serious chronic disease conditions (Narayan et al., 2003), thereby potentially reversing the positive trend achieved with the reduction of infectious diseases over the past century. The great advances of genetics and other biomedical discoveries could be more than offset by the burden of illness, disability, and death caused by too many people eating too much and moving too little over their lifetimes.

---

[2]These projections are based on data on the lifetime risk of diagnosed diabetes and do not account for undiagnosed cases. The data do not allow for differentiation between type 1 and type 2 diabetes. However, the major form of diabetes in the U.S. population is type 2, which accounts for an estimated 95 percent of diabetes cases (Narayan et al., 2003).

Aside from the statistics, we can see the evidence of childhood obesity in our community schoolyards, in shopping malls, and in doctors' offices. There are confirmatory journalistic reports of the epidemiologic trends in weight—from resizing of clothing to larger coffins to more spacious easy chairs to the increased need for seatbelt extenders. These would be of passing interest and minimal importance were it not for the considerable health implications of this weight gain for both adults and children. For example, compared with adults of normal weight, adults with a BMI of 40 or more have a seven-fold increased risk for diagnosed diabetes (Mokdad et al., 2003). Indeed, the obesity epidemic places at risk the long-term welfare and readiness of the U.S. military services by reducing the pool of individuals eligible for recruitment and decreasing the retention of new recruits. Nearly 80 percent of recruits who exceed the military accession weight-for-height standards at entry leave the military before they complete their first term of enlistment (IOM, 2003).

What might our population look like in the year 2025 if we continue on this course? In a land of excess calories ingested and insufficient energy expended, the inevitable scenario is a continued increase in average body size and an altered concept of what is "normal." Americans with a BMI below 30 will be considered small and obesity will no longer be newsworthy but accepted as the social norm.

While the existence and importance of the increase in the population-wide obesity problem are no longer debated, we are still mustering the determination to forge effective solutions. We must remind ourselves that social changes to transform public perceptions and behaviors regarding seatbelt use, smoking cessation, breastfeeding, and recycling would have sounded unreasonable just a few decades ago (Economos et al., 2001), yet we have acted vigorously and with impressive results. How to proceed similarly in meeting the formidable childhood obesity challenge is the focus of this Institute of Medicine (IOM) report.

The 19-member IOM committee was charged with developing a prevention-focused action plan to decrease the prevalence of obesity in children and youth in the United States. The primary emphasis of the committee's task was on examining the behavioral and cultural factors, social constructs, and other broad environmental factors involved in childhood obesity and identifying promising approaches for prevention efforts. This report presents the committee's recommendations for many different segments of society from federal, state, and local governments (Chapter 4), to industry and media (Chapter 5), local communities (Chapter 6), schools (Chapter 7), and parents and families (Chapter 8).

CONTEXTS FOR ACTION

Investigating the causes of childhood obesity, determining what to do about them, and taking appropriate action must address the variables that influence both eating and physical activity. Seemingly straightforward, these variables result from complex interactions across a number of relevant social, economic, cultural, environmental, and policy contexts.

U.S. children live in a society that has changed dramatically in the three decades over which the obesity epidemic has developed. Many of these changes, such as both parents working outside the home, often affect decisions about what children eat, where they eat, how much they eat, and the amount of energy they expend in school and leisure time activities (Ebbeling et al., 2002; Hill et al., 2003).

Other changes, such as the increasing diversity of the population, influence cultural views and marketing patterns. Lifestyle modifications, in part the result of media usage and content together with changes in the physical design of communities, affect adults' and children's levels of physical activity. Many of the social and cultural characteristics that the U.S. population has accepted as a normal way of life may collectively contribute to the growing levels of childhood obesity. The broad societal trends that impact weight outcomes are complex and clearly multifactorial. With such societal changes, it is difficult to tease out the quantitative and qualitative role of individual contributing factors. While distinct causal relationships may be difficult to prove, the dramatic rise in childhood obesity prevalence must be viewed within the context of these broad societal changes.

An understanding of these contexts, particularly regarding their potential to be modified and how they may facilitate or impede development of a comprehensive obesity prevention strategy, is therefore essential. This next section provides a useful background to understand the multidimensional nature of the childhood obesity epidemic.

Lifestyle and Demographic Trends

The interrelated areas of family life, ethnic diversity, eating patterns, physical activity, and media use—discussed below—are all aspects of societal change that must be considered. Singly and in concert, the trends in these areas will strongly influence prospects for preventive and corrective measures.

Family Life

The changing context of American families includes several distinct trends such as the shifting role of women in society, delayed marriage, childbearing outside of marriage, higher divorce rates, single parenthood, and work patterns of parents (NRC, 2003). Among the many important transformations that have occurred are expanded job opportunities for women, which have led to more women entering the workforce. Economic necessities have also prompted this trend. Moreover, married mothers are increasingly more likely than they were in the past to remain in the labor force throughout their childbearing years.

Women's participation in the labor force increased from 36 percent in 1960 to 58 percent in 2000 (Luckett Clark and Weismantle, 2003). Since 1975, the labor force participation rate of mothers with children under age 18 has grown from 47 to 72 percent, with the largest increase among mothers with children under 3 years of age (U.S. Department of Labor, 2004). Over the same period, men's labor force participation rates declined slightly from 78 percent to 74 percent (Population Reference Bureau, 2004b). In 2002, only 7 percent of all U.S. households consisted of married couples with children in which only the husband worked.

These trends, together with lower fertility rates, a decrease in average household size, and the shift in household demographics from primarily married couples with children to single person households and households without children, have caused the number of meal preparers in U.S. households who cook for three or more people to decline (Population Reference Bureau, 2003; Sloan, 2003).

It has been suggested that smaller households experience fewer economies of scale in home preparation of meals than do larger families. Preparing food at home involves a set amount of time for every meal that changes minimally with the number of persons served. Eating meals out involves the same marginal costs per person. Moreover, changes in salary and the lower prices of prepared foods may have reduced the value of time previously used to prepare at-home meals. Thus, incentives have been shifted away from home production toward eating more meals away from home (Sturm, 2004). Time-use trends for meal preparation at home reveal a gradual decline from 1965 to 1985 (44 minutes per day versus 39 minutes per day) and a steeper decline from 1985 to 1999 (39 minutes per day versus 32 minutes per day) (Robinson and Godbey, 1999; Sturm, 2004).

Ethnic Diversity

The racial and ethnic composition of children in the United States is becoming more diverse. In 2000, 64 percent of U.S. children were white non-Hispanic, 15 percent were black non-Hispanic, 4 percent were Asian/ Pacific Islander, and 1 percent were American Indian/Alaska Native. The proportion of children of Hispanic origin has increased more rapidly than the other racial and ethnic groups from 9 percent of the child population in

1980 to 16 percent in 2000 (Federal Interagency Forum on Child and Family Statistics, 2003).

Differences among ethnic groups (e.g., African American, American Indian, Hispanic, and Asian/Pacific Islanders) include variations in household composition and size—particularly larger household size in Hispanic and Asian populations (Frey, 2003)—and in other aspects of family life such as media use and exposure, consumer behavior, eating, and physical activity patterns (Tharp, 2001; Nesbitt et al., 2004).

Ethnic minorities are projected to comprise 40.2 percent of the U.S. population by 2020 (U.S. Census Bureau, 2001), and the food preferences of ethnic families are expected to have a significant impact on consumers' food preferences and eating patterns (Sloan, 2003). The higher-than-average prevalence of obesity in several ethnic minority populations may indicate differences in susceptibility to unfavorable lifestyle trends and the consequent need for specially designed preventive and corrective strategies (Kumanyika, 2002; Nesbitt et al., 2004).

Eating Patterns

As economic demands and the rapid pace of daily life increasingly constrain people's time, food trends have been marked by convenience, shelf stability, portability, and greater accessibility of foods throughout the entire day (Food Marketing Institute, 1996, 2003; French et al., 2001; Sloan, 2003). Food has become more available wherever people spend time. Because of technological advances, it is often possible to acquire a variety of highly palatable foods, in larger portion sizes, and at relatively low cost. Research has revealed a progressive increase, from 1977 to 1998, in the portion sizes of many types of foods and beverages available to Americans (Nielsen and Popkin, 2003; Smiciklas-Wright et al., 2003); and the concurrent rise in obesity prevalence has been noted (Nestle, 2003; Rolls, 2003).

Foods eaten outside the home are becoming more important in determining the nutritional quality of Americans' diets, especially for children (Lin et al., 1999b; French et al., 2001). Consumption of away-from-home foods comprised 20 percent of children's total calorie intake in 1977-1978 and rose to 32 percent in 1994-1996 (Lin et al., 1999b). In 1970, household income spent on away-from-home foods accounted for 25 percent of total food spending; by 1999, it had reached nearly one-half (47 percent) of total food expenditures (Clauson, 1999; Kennedy et al., 1999).

The trend toward eating more meals in restaurants and fast food establishments may be influenced not only by simple convenience but also in response to needs such as stress management, relief of fatigue, lack of time, and entertainment. According to a 1998 survey conducted by the National Restaurant Association, two-thirds of Americans indicated that patronizing a restaurant with family or friends allowed them to socialize and was a better use of their leisure time than cooking at home and cleaning up afterward (Panitz, 1999).

For food consumed at home, never has so much been so readily available to so many—that is, to virtually everyone in the household—at low cost and in ready-to-eat or ready-to-heat form (French et al., 2001; Sloan, 2003). Increased time demands on parents, especially working mothers, have shifted priorities from parental meal preparation toward greater convenience (French et al., 2001), and the effects of time pressures are seen in working mothers' reduced participation in meal planning, shopping, and food preparation (Crepinsek and Burstein, 2004). Industry has endeavored to meet this demand through such innovations as improved packaging and longer shelf stability, along with complementary technologies, such as microwaves, that have shortened meal preparation times.

Another aspect of this trend toward convenience is an increased prevalence, across all age groups of children and youth, of frequent snacking and of deriving a large proportion of one's total daily calories from energy-dense snacks (Jahns et al., 2001). At the same time, there has been a documented decline in breakfast consumption among both boys and girls, generally among adolescents (Siega-Riz et al., 1998) and in urban elementary school-age children as compared to their rural and suburban counterparts (Gross et al., 2004); further, children of working mothers are more likely to skip meals (Crepinsek and Burstein, 2004).

There are also indications that children and adolescents are not meeting the minimum recommended servings of five fruits and vegetables daily recommended by the Food Guide Pyramid (Cavadini et al., 2000; American Dietetic Association, 2004). This trend is partially explained by the limited variety of fruits and vegetables consumed by Americans. In 2000, five vegetables—iceberg lettuce, frozen potatoes, fresh potatoes, potato chips, and canned tomatoes—accounted for 48 percent of total vegetable servings and six fruits (out of more than 60 fruit products)—orange juice, bananas, apple juice, apples, fresh grapes, and watermelon—accounted for 50 percent of all fruit servings (Putnam et al., 2002).

These trends have contributed to an increased availability and consumption of energy-dense foods and beverages. As summarized in Table 1-1 and Figures 1-1 through 1-3, trends in the dietary intake of the general U.S. population parallel trends in the dietary intake of children and youth. A more in-depth discussion of caloric intake, energy balance, energy density, Dietary Guidelines for Americans, and the Food Guide Pyramid is included in Chapters 3, 5, and 7.

Physical Activity

Physical activity is often classified into different types including recreational or leisure time, utilitarian, household, and occupational. The direct surveillance of physical activity trends in U.S. adults began only in the 1980s and was limited to characterizing leisure-time physical activity. In 2001, CDC began collecting data on the overall frequency and duration of time spent in household, transportation, and leisure-time activity of both moderate and vigorous intensity in a usual week through the state-based Behavioral Risk Factor Surveillance System (BRFSS) (CDC, 2003c).

National surveys conducted over the past several decades suggest an increase in population-wide physical activity levels among American men, women, and older adolescents; however, a large proportion of these populations still do not meet the federal guidelines for recommended levels of total daily physical activity.[3] The data for children's and youth's leisure time and physical activity levels reveal a different picture than the adult physical activity trend data that are summarized in Table 1-2.

Trend data collected by the Americans' Use of Time Study, through time-use diaries, indicated that adults' free time increased by 14 percent between 1965 and 1985 from 35 hours to an average total of nearly 40 hours per week (Robinson and Godbey, 1999). Data from other population-based surveys, including the National Health Interview Survey, National Health and Nutrition Examination Survey (NHANES), BRFSS, and the Family Interaction, Social Capital and Trends in Time Use Data (1998-1999), together with trend data on sports and recreational participation, suggest minor to significant increases in reported leisure-time physical activity among adults (Pratt et al., 1999; French et al., 2001; Sturm, 2004).

Data from the 1990-1998 BRFSS[4] revealed only a slight increase in self-reported physical activity levels among adults (from 24.3 percent in 1990 to 25.4 percent in 1998), and a decrease in respondents reporting no physical activity at all (from 30.7 percent in 1990 to 28.7 percent in 1998) (CDC, 2001).

Women, older adults, and ethnic minority populations have been identified as having the greatest prevalence of leisure-time physical inactivity (CDC, 2004b). In general, the prevalence of self-reported, no leisure-time physical activity was highest in 1989, and declined to its lowest level in 15 years among all groups in 35 states and the District of Columbia based on

---

[3]The Surgeon General's report on physical activity and health suggests that significant health benefits can be obtained by Americans who include a moderate amount of physical activity (e.g., 30 minutes of brisk walking) on most if not all days of the week (DHHS, 1996).

[4]The BRFSS is a population-based, randomly selected, self-reported telephone survey conducted among the noninstitutionalized U.S. adult population aged 18 years and older throughout the 50 states (CDC, 2003c).

TABLE 1-1 Trends in Food Availability and Dietary Intake of the U.S. Population and of U.S. Children and Youth[a]

Dietary Intake Trend	U.S. Population	U.S. Children and Youth
Portion sizes of foods	Portion sizes of most foods consumed by adults both at home and away from home (except pizza) increased between 1977 and 1996 (Nielsen and Popkin, 2003).	Portion sizes for children aged 2 years and older increased for most foods consumed both at home and away from home between 1977 and 1996 (Nielsen and Popkin, 2003).
Total energy intake derived from away-from-home sources	Total energy intake increased from 18% to 34% for adults between 1977-1978 and 1995 (Lin et al., 1999a).	Total energy intake increased from 20% to 32% for children between 1977-1978 and 1994-1996 (Lin et al., 1999b).
Total energy intake	Between 1971 and 2000, average energy intake increased from 2,450 to 2,618 calories for men and 1,542 to 1,877 kcal for women (CDC, 2004a).	No significant increased trends in energy intake were observed in children aged 6-11 years between 1977-1978 and 1994-1996, 1998 (Enns et al., 2002).
	Between 1989 and1991 and 1994-1996, total energy increased 8.6% and 9.5%, according to food supply and CSFII data, respectively (Chanmugam et al., 2003).	Total calories consumed by adolescent boys aged 12 to 19 years increased by 243 between 1977-1978 and 1994-1996 from 2,523 to 2,766 calories (Enns et al., 2003). Total calories consumed by adolescent girls aged 12 to 19 years increased by 123 between 1977-1978 and 1994-1996 from 1,787 to 1,910 calories (Enns et al., 2003).
	Between 1983 and 2000, calories per capita increased by 20% (USDA, 2003) (Figure 1-1).	
Total fat consumption	Between 1971 and 2000, the percentage of calories from total fat decreased for men (from 36.9%to 32.8%) and women (from 36.1% to 32.8%) (CDC, 2004a). However, the intake of grams of total fat increased among women and decreased among men (CDC, 2004a) (Figure 1-2).	Between 1965 and 1996, the proportion of energy from total fat consumed by children decreased from 39% to 32%, and saturated fat from 15% to 12% (Cavadini et al., 2000). Children aged 6 to 11 years in 1994-1996, 1998 consumed 25% of calories from discretionary fat (USDA, 2000; Enns et al., 2002).

	For adolescents aged 12 to 19 years, girls consumed 25% and boys consumed 26% of their calories from added fat (USDA, 2000; Enns et al., 2003).
Added dietary sweeteners	Between 1977 and 2000, an 83 calorie/day increase in caloric sweeteners was observed in the U.S. for all individuals 2 years and older, representing a 22% increase in the proportion of energy derived from caloric sweeteners (Popkin and Nielsen, 2003).
	Children aged 6 to 11 years in 1994 to 1996 and 1998 consumed 21-23 teaspoons of added sugars in a 1,800-2,000 calorie diet which exceeded the Food Guide Pyramid recommendation of 6-12 teaspoons for a 1,600-2,200 calorie diet (USDA, 1996; Enns et al., 2002).
	Between 1982 and 1997, per capita consumption of sweeteners increased 28% (34 pounds) (Putnam and Gerrior, 1999).
Dairy and milk consumption	Between 1970 and 1997, the consumption of milk per capita decreased from 31 gallons to 24 gallons, while cheese consumption increased 146% from 11 pounds/person in 1970 to 28 pounds/person in 1997 (French et al., 2001).
	Milk consumption decreased by 37% in adolescent boys and 30% in adolescent girls between 1977-1978 and 1994 (Cavadini et al., 2000).
	Americans consumed 2.5 times as much cheese and drank 23% less milk per capita in 1997 than in 1970 (Putnam and Gerrior, 1999).
	In 1977-1978, children aged 6 to 11 years consumed four times as much milk as any other beverage, and adolescents aged 12 to 19 years drank 1.5 times as much milk as any other beverage. In 1994-1996 and 1998, children aged 6 to 11 consumed 1.5 times as much milk as soft drinks, and by 1994-1996 adolescents consumed twice as much soft drinks as milk (French et al., 2001).

continued

TABLE 1-1 Continued

Dietary Intake Trend	U.S. Population	U.S. Children and Youth
		Adolescent intake of whole milk decreased while cheese increased. In 1994-1996, for adolescents aged 12 to 19 years, only 12% of girls and 30% of boys consumed the number of dairy servings recommended by the Food Guide Pyramid (USDA, 2000; Enns et al., 2002, 2003).
Fruit and vegetable consumption	In 1997, Americans consumed 24% more fruit and vegetables per capita than they did in 1970 (French et al., 2001).	In 1977-1978 children aged 6 to 11 years consumed more total vegetables than children in 1994-1996, 1998 (Enns et al., 2002). In 1994-1996, 1998, only 24% of girls and 23% of boys consumed the number of Food Guide Pyramid recommended fruit servings (USDA, 2000; Enns et al., 2002).
		In 1994-1996 adolescents aged 12 to 19 years, only 18% of girls and 14% of boys consumed the number of Food Guide Pyramid recommended fruit servings (USDA, 2000; Enns et al., 2003).
Meat, poultry, and fish consumption	Total meat consumption per capita increased by 19 lbs from 1970 to 2000. In 2000, individual Americans consumed 16 pounds less red meat than in 1970, 32 lbs more poultry, and 3 lbs more fish and shellfish (Putnam et al., 2002).	In 1994-1996 and 1998 the percentages of children aged 6 to 11 years and adolescents aged 12 to 19 years consuming meat, poultry, fish, and eggs were lower than in 1977-1978 (USDA, 2000; Enns et al., 2002, 2003).

Beverage consumption	Annual soft drink consumption increased from 34.7 to 44.4 gallons per capita between 1987-1991 and 1997 (French et al., 2001).	Soft drink consumption nearly tripled among adolescent boys from 7 to 22 ounces per day between 1977-1978 and 1994 (Guthrie and Morton, 2000; French et al., 2003).
	Portion sizes of soft drinks increased by 49 calories (from 13.1 to 19.9 fl oz) between 1977 and 1996 (Nielsen and Popkin, 2003).	By 14 years of age, 32% of adolescent girls and 52% of adolescent boys consume three or more 8-ounce servings of soda daily (Gleason and Suitor, 2001).
		Children as young as 7 months old are consuming soda (Fox et al., 2004).

NOTE: CSFII = Continuing Survey of Food Intakes by Individuals.

aFood availability (per capita intake) is based on food supply data; dietary intake trends are based on measured or self-reported food consumption data.

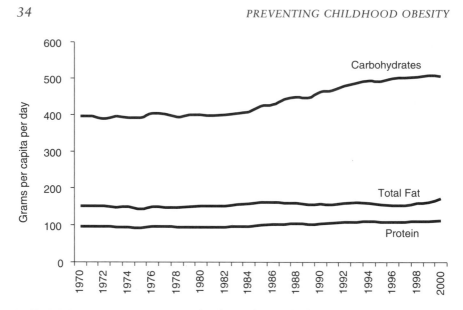

FIGURE 1-1 U.S. macronutrient food supply trends for carbohydrates, protein, and total fat, 1970-2000.
SOURCES: Putnam et al., 2002; USDA, 2003.

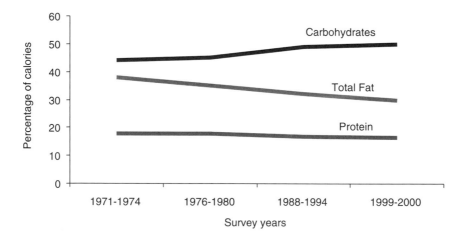

FIGURE 1-2 Percentage of calories from macronutrient intake for carbohydrates, protein, and total fat among adult men and women, 1970-2000.
SOURCE: CDC, 2004a.

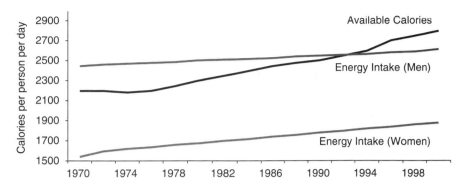

FIGURE 1-3 Available calories from the U.S. food supply, adjusted for losses,[a] and average energy intake for adult men and women,[b] 1970-2000.
SOURCES: Putnam et al., 2002; CDC, 2004a.

[a]Based on USDA food supply data, calories from the U.S. food supply adjusted for spoilage, cooking losses, plate waste, and other losses increased by 20 percent between 1983 and 2000 (Putnam et al., 2002; USDA, 2003).

[b]Dietary intake trends and percentage of calories from macronutrient intake are based on a CDC analysis of four NHANES, by survey year, for adult men and women aged 20 to 74 years from 1971 to 2000 for energy intake (kilocalories), protein, carbohydrates, total fat, and saturated fat (CDC, 2004a).

BRFSS data, although it is unclear why this occurred (CDC, 2004b). In 2001, BRFSS respondents were asked to report the overall frequency and duration of time spent in household, transportation, and leisure-time activity of both moderate and vigorous intensity (CDC, 2003c). Although 45.4 percent of adults reported having engaged in physical activities consistent with the recommendation of a minimum of 30 minutes of moderate intensity activity on most days of the week in 2001, more than one-half of U.S. adults (54.6 percent) were not sufficiently active to meet these recommendations (CDC, 2003c).

The physical activity trend data for children and youth are even more limited than for adults. Most available information is on the physical activity levels of high school youth, with limited data available on levels in younger children. Based on the Youth Risk Behavior Survey (YRBS), daily enrollment in physical education classes declined among high school students from 42 percent in 1991 to 25 percent in 1995 (DHHS, 1996) and increased slightly to 28.4 percent in 2003 (CDC, 2004c). Cross-sectional data collected through the YRBS for 15,214 high school students indicated that one-third (33.4 percent) of 9th to 12th graders nationwide are not engaging in recommended levels of moderate or vigorous physical activity

TABLE 1-2 Trends in Leisure Time and Physical Activity of U.S. Adults, Children, and Youth

Trend	Adults	Children and Youth
Available leisure time	Adults' free time increased by 14% between 1965 and 1985 to an average of nearly 40 hours per week based on Americans' Use of Time Study (Robinson and Godbey, 1999).	From 1981 to 1997, children aged 3 to 12 years experienced a decline in their free time by seven hours per week (Sturm, 2005a).
Leisure-time physical activity	There have been increases in reported leisure-time physical activity among U.S. adults based on NHES, NHANES, BRFSS, and trend data on sports and recreational participation (Pratt et al., 1999; French et al., 2001).

There was a slight increase in self-reported physical activity levels among adults, based on the 1990-1998 BRFSS, from 24.3% in 1990 to 25.4% in 1998 (CDC, 2001).

There was a slight decrease in adults reporting no physical activity at all (from 30.7% in 1990 to 28.7% in 1998) (CDC, 2001). | An estimated 61.5% of children aged 9 to 13 years do not participate in any organized physical activity during their nonschool hours and 22.6% do not engage in any free-time physical activity based on the 2002 YMCLS (CDC, 2003a).

From 1981 to 1997, children aged 3 to 12 years experienced an increase in time spent in organized sports and outdoor activities (Sturm, 2005a). |
| Moderate to vigorous physical activity | Based on the 2001 BRFSS, 45.4% of adults reported having engaged in physical activities consistent with the recommendation of a minimum of 30 minutes of moderate-intensity activity on most days of the week in 2001. However, 54.6% of U.S. adults were not sufficiently active to meet these recommendations (CDC, 2003c). | High school students in grades 9 to 12 are not engaging in recommended levels of moderate or vigorous physical activity based on the YRBS (CDC, 2003b, 2004c; see Chapter 7). |

TABLE 1-2 Continued

Trend	Adults	Children and Youth
Physical education classes	Not applicable	Daily enrollment in physical education classes declined among high school students from 42% in 1991 to 25% in 1995 (DHHS, 1996) and 28.4% in 2003 (CDC, 2004c).
Travel to and from school	Not applicable	From 1977 to 2001, there was a marked decline in children's walking to school as a percentage of total school trips made by children aged 5 to 15 years from 20.2% to 12.5% (Sturm, 2005b).

An estimated 25% of children aged 5 to 15 years who lived within a mile of school walked or bicycled at least once during the previous month based on the 1999 HealthStyles Survey (CDC, 2002). |

NOTE: BRFSS = Behavioral Risk Factor Surveillance System. NHES = National Health Examination Survey. NHANES = National Health and Nutrition Examination Surveys. YMCLS = Youth Media Campaign Longitudinal Survey. YRBS = Youth Risk Behavior Survey.

and an estimated 10 percent report that they are inactive (CDC, 2003b, 2004c; see Chapter 7).

In 2002, the CDC collected baseline data through the Youth Media Campaign Longitudinal Survey (YMCLS), a nationally representative survey of children aged 9 to 13 years and their parents, which revealed that 61.5 percent of youth in this age group do not participate in any organized physical activity during their nonschool hours and 22.6 percent do not engage in any free-time physical activity (CDC, 2003a).

Shifts in transportation patterns can affect energy balance. Many technological innovations have occurred over the past several decades such as the increased availability of labor-saving devices in the home, a decline in physically active occupations, and the dominance of automobiles for commuting to work and personal travel (Cutler et al., 2003). National data tracking trends on the physical activity levels and leisure or discretionary time of younger children and pre-adolescents are limited. However, an analysis of the available data for children aged 3 to 12 years from 1981 to 1997 (Hofferth and Sandberg, 2001) suggests a decline in their free time by six hours per week—attributed to an increase in time away from home in structured settings—and an increase in time spent in organized sports and outdoor activities over this time frame (Sturm, 2005a). However, it is not possible to determine the overall impact of these changes on children's physical activity levels.

One factor that has influenced overall transportation patterns in the United States is the change in the built environment. Through a number of mediating factors, the built environment can either promote or hinder physical activity, although the role and influence of the built environment on physical activity levels is a relatively new area of investigation. The ways in which land is developed and neighborhoods are designed may contribute to the level of physical activity residents achieve as a natural part of their daily lives (Frank, 2000).

There have been many changes in the built environment over the past century or more. For a variety of reasons, Americans moved away from central cities to lower density suburbs, many of the most recent of which necessitate driving for transportation.

In these areas, streets were often built without sidewalks, residential areas were segregated from other land uses, and shopping areas were designed for access by car. These characteristics discourage walking and biking as a means of transportation, historically an important source of physical activity.

Indeed, the amount of time that adults spend walking and biking for transportation has declined in the past two decades, largely because people are driving more (Sturm, 2004). In addition, the more time that Americans spend traveling, the less time they have available for other forms of physical activity. In 2000, Americans spent nearly 26 minutes commuting to their jobs, an increase from 22 minutes in 1990, and the average commuting time was 30 minutes or more in 25 of the 245 cities with at least 100,000 population (Population Reference Bureau, 2004a).

Children's motorized vehicle travel to and from school has increased, though this represents a small proportion of their overall travel. The 2001 National Household Travel Survey (NHTS) indicated that less than 15 percent of children aged 5 to 15 years walked to or from school and 1 percent bicycled (Bureau of Transportation Statistics, 2003). Even children living relatively close to school do not walk to this destination. The 1999 HealthStyles Survey found that among participating households, 25 percent of children aged 5 to 15 years who lived within a mile of school either walked or bicycled at least once during the previous month (CDC, 2002).

From 1977 to 2001, there was a marked decline in children's walking to school as a percentage of total school trips made by 5- to 15-year-olds from 20.2 percent to 12.5 percent (Sturm, 2005b). Based on data collected through the National Personal Transportation Surveys for 1977 and 1990, and the NHTS for 2001, there is little evidence of changes in walking trip length although distance traveled by bicycle has decreased (Sturm, 2005b). Although reduced physical activity has been identified as an unintended consequence of dependence on motorized travel, it is unclear how changes in children's transportation patterns have reduced their overall physical activity levels (Sturm, 2005b).

Media

The presence of electronic media in children's lives, and their time spent with such media, has grown considerably and has increased the time spent in sedentary pursuits, often with reduced outside play time. In 1999, the average American child lived in a home with three televisions, three radios, three tape players, two video cassette recorders (VCRs), one video game player, two compact disc players, and one computer (Roberts et al., 1999) (Figure 1-4). In 2003, nearly all children (99 percent) aged zero to six years lived in a home with a television set and the average number of VCRs or digital video discs (DVDs) in these young children's homes was 2.3 (Rideout et al., 2003). Television dominates the type of specific media used by children and youth and is the only form of electronic media for which trend data are available. In 1950, approximately 10 percent of U.S. households had a television (Putnam, 1995) in comparison with 98 percent in 1999 (Nielsen Media Research, 2000). The percent of American homes with more than one television set rose from 35 percent in 1970 (Lyle and Hoffman, 1972) to 88 percent in 1999 (Roberts et al., 1999). Moreover, there has been a ten-fold increase over the same period in the percent of American homes with three or more television sets (Rideout et al., 2003). In 2003, one-half (50 percent) of children aged zero to six years had three or more televisions, one-third (36 percent) had a television in their bedrooms, and nine out of ten children in this age range had watched television or DVDs (Rideout et al., 2003).

During a typical day, 36 percent of children watch television for one hour or less, 31 percent of children watch television for one to three hours, 16 percent watch television for three to five hours, and 17 percent watch television for more than 5 hours (Roberts et al., 1999) (Figure 1-5).

Two separate national data sources have tracked children's and adolescents' discretionary time spent watching television. Results indicate that the extent of television viewing differs by age, but also suggest an observed decline in television watching by children under 12 years by approximately four hours per week between 1981 and 1997 (Hofferth and Sandberg,

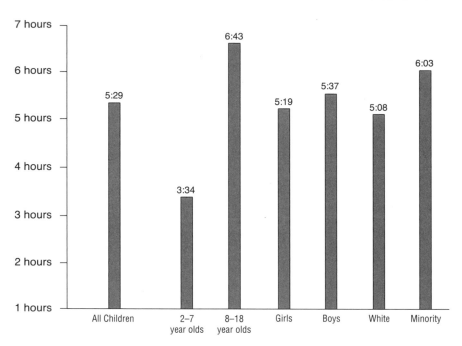

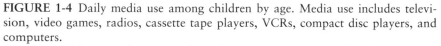

FIGURE 1-4 Daily media use among children by age. Media use includes television, video games, radios, cassette tape players, VCRs, compact disc players, and computers.
SOURCE: Rideout et al., 1999. This information was reprinted with permission from the Henry J. Kaiser Family Foundation.

2001). Based on the Monitoring the Future Survey from 1990 to 2001, there was a steady decrease in heavy television watching (three hours or more) among adolescents yet an observed increase in television viewing for one hour or less (Child Trends, 2002). Although children are using other types of electronic media including video games and computers (Roberts et al., 1999; Rideout et al., 2003), television viewing represents a significant amount of discretionary time among children and youth, which is a sedentary and modifiable activity (see Chapter 8).

Consumer Attitudes and Public Awareness

Trends in media coverage suggest a striking increase in public interest in obesity. The International Food Information Council (IFIC) has been following U.S. and international media coverage of the obesity issue since

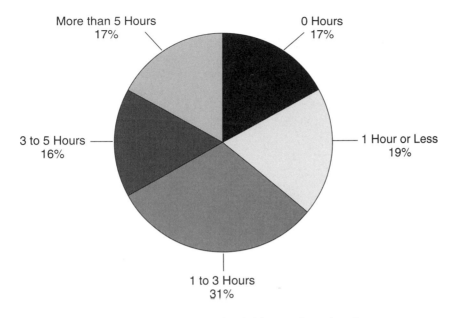

FIGURE 1-5 Daily television viewing by children and youth in hours.
SOURCE: Rideout et al., 1999. This information was reprinted with permission
from the Henry J. Kaiser Family Foundation.

1999 and has tracked a steady upward trend in the volume and breadth of issues covered (IFIC, 2004) (Figure 1-6).

This media focus, independent of the longstanding popularity of weight control as a consumer issue (Serdula et al., 1999), includes obesity-related topics ranging from popular diets and quick weight loss strategies to litigation against fast food restaurants to reports of new programs, policies, and research findings.

The media coverage on obesity is viewed by the public, parents, and other stakeholder groups in a variety of ways, depending on their personal beliefs regarding issues such as personal responsibility, the role of government and other institutions in promoting personal freedoms, media influences, free speech and the rights of advertisers, and the ways in which parents should raise their children, as well as on consequent responses to various population level approaches being proposed to address obesity.

While some people place a high value on the individual's right to choose what, when, where, and how to eat and be active, others are looking for advice, information, and enhanced opportunities, and may even favor government interventions that facilitate healthier choices (Kersh and Morone, 2002).

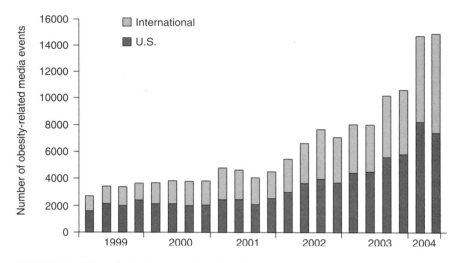

FIGURE 1-6 Trends in obesity-related media coverage, 1999-2004.
SOURCE: IFIC, 2004. Reprinted, with permission. Copyright 2004 by the International Food Information Council.

Recent opinion polls indicate that a large number of adults and parents are very concerned or somewhat concerned about childhood obesity (Field Research Corporation, 2003; Widmeyer Polling & Research, 2003). For example, a recent telephone survey of 1,068 randomly selected California residents suggested that for one out of three respondents, obesity-related behaviors, especially unhealthy eating habits or the lack of physical activity, represent the greatest risk to California children (Field Research Corporation, 2003). Although obesity is considered a health problem comparable to smoking, some research suggests that it remains low on the list of Americans' perceptions of serious health problems, which remain dominated by cancer, HIV/AIDS, and heart disease (Oliver and Lee, 2002; Lake Snell Perry & Associates, 2003; San Jose Mercury News/Kaiser Family Foundation, 2004). More recent national research shows that Americans are perceiving childhood obesity to be a serious problem, similar to tobacco use, underage drinking, and violence, but not as serious as drug abuse (Evans et al., 2004).

Families may vary in the value they place on different health outcomes related to obesity, and the merits they attribute to certain benefits or drawbacks of changing behaviors to address it (Whitaker, 2004). Research suggests that some parents do not perceive weight, per se, to be a health issue for their children (Baughcum et al., 2000; Jain et al., 2001; Borra et al., 2003), independent of their child's physical and social functioning. They think of their child as healthy if he or she has no serious medical conditions, and they embrace the hope that the overweight child will outgrow the problem. They may also hesitate to raise weight-related issues due to their concerns that this may lower the child's self-esteem and potentially encourage him or her to develop an eating disorder. School-age children, however, do not generally view obesity as a health problem as long as it does not significantly affect appearance and performance (Borra et al., 2003). Being obese, whether as a child or an adult, is highly stigmatized and viewed as a moral failing, among some educators (Price et al., 1987), health professionals (Teachman and Brownell, 2001), and even very young children (Cramer and Steinwert, 1998; Latner and Stunkard, 2003).

Further, individuals and consumers vary in the priority they place on healthy eating and an active lifestyle, and they hold a spectrum of views on health regarding weight management, weight control, and wellness (Buchanan, 2000; Strategy One, 2003). Consumer research reveals that Americans express not having enough time to fit everything into their day that they would like to, with the consequence that their health may be neglected (Strategy One, 2003).

In a recent national poll of 1,000 U.S. adult respondents, half of the respondents viewed obesity as a public health problem that society needs to solve while the other half considered it a personal responsibility or choice that should be dealt with privately (Lake Snell Perry & Associates, 2003).

However, Americans do appear more uniformly willing to support proactive actions to reduce obesity in children and youth, especially in the school setting (Lake Snell Perry & Associates, 2003; Robert Wood Johnson Foundation, 2003; Widmeyer Polling & Research, 2003). Childhood obesity presumably engenders more support for societal-level approaches because children, who are thought to have less latitude in food and activity choices than adults, are unlikely to be blamed by society for becoming obese. Understanding consumer perceptions and knowledge of public awareness about obesity will be essential in order to design an effective multimedia and public relations campaign supporting obesity prevention (see Chapter 5).

Emerging Programs and Policies

As it has done with many other child health concerns, from whooping cough, polio, and measles to use of toddlers' seats in automobiles, the United States is now addressing the growing problem of childhood obesity. State legislatures, federal agencies, school boards, teachers, youth programs, parents, and others are mobilizing to address the array of interrelated issues associated with the development, and potential prevention, of childhood obesity. Because adult overweight and obesity rates are even higher than those of children, many efforts focus on improving eating habits and encouraging physical activity for people of all ages.

The range of these efforts is quite broad, and many innovative approaches are under way. As discussed throughout the report, many of these efforts are occurring at the grassroots level—neighborhood-specific or community-wide programs and activities encouraging healthy eating and promoting regular physical activity. A number of U.S. school districts, for instance, have established new standards for the types of food and beverages that will be available in their school systems (Prevention Institute, 2003). Many communities are examining the local availability of opportunities for physical activity and are working to expand bike paths and improve the walkability of neighborhoods. Further, community child- and youth-centered organizations (such as the Girl Scouts and the Boys and Girls Clubs of America) are adding or expanding programs focused on increasing physical activity. A national cross-sector initiative, Shaping America's Youth, supported by the private sector (industry), nonprofit organizations, and the Department of Health and Human Services, is working to compile a registry of the relevant ongoing research and intervention programs across the country as well as funding sources. Evaluating these efforts and disseminating those that are most effective will be the challenge and goal for future endeavors.

In many other countries where childhood obesity is a growing problem, including the United Kingdom, Sweden, Germany, France, Canada, and Australia, a broad array of national and community-level efforts and policy options are being pursued. Among these are the banning of vending machines in schools, developing restrictions for television advertising to children, and using taxes derived from energy-dense foods to support physical activity programs.

PUBLIC HEALTH PRECEDENTS

Public health problems of comparably broad scope and complexity have been successfully addressed in the past (Economos et al., 2001), and this experience gives us not only the confidence that childhood obesity too can be moderated, even prevented, but supplies us with some of the needed tools. This solid public health history of achievements is exemplified in Box 1-1 (CDC, 1999; Appendix D).

Many of these problems were not apparent at first, and grew to become an accepted part of life before they were recognized and subsequently addressed. For example, in 1900, with only approximately 8,000 cars on the roads, it was surely inconceivable that motor vehicle deaths could reach a peak of 56,278 per year in 1972 (U.S. Department of Transportation, 1995; Waller, 2002). Multifocal interventions on vehicular safety and high-

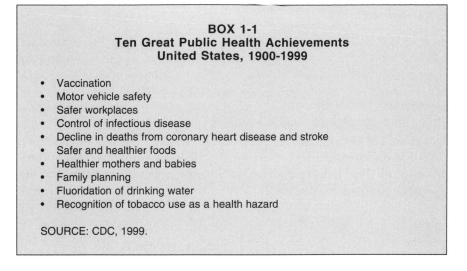

BOX 1-1
Ten Great Public Health Achievements
United States, 1900-1999

- Vaccination
- Motor vehicle safety
- Safer workplaces
- Control of infectious disease
- Decline in deaths from coronary heart disease and stroke
- Safer and healthier foods
- Healthier mothers and babies
- Family planning
- Fluoridation of drinking water
- Recognition of tobacco use as a health hazard

SOURCE: CDC, 1999.

way improvements have enabled us to make great progress in reducing motor vehicle deaths from this peak (Bolen et al., 1997; NSC, 1997). As the number of miles driven in the United States rose from 206 billion in 1930 to 2,467 billion in 1996, the death rate per 100 million miles declined dramatically from 15.97 in 1930 to 1.76 in 1996 (NSC, 1997; IOM, 1999). Even with this progress, however, we continue to record over 42,000 deaths a year from motor vehicle collisions (U.S. Department of Transportation, 2004).

Early in the 20th century, when cigarettes were hand-rolled, few would have predicted that cigarette smoking would become the major preventable cause of death in the United States a century later. Tobacco reform efforts can be traced back to the late 19th and early 20th century and were strengthened in the 1940s and 1950s as epidemiological studies began to convince the medical community and public about the health hazards of tobacco (Fee et al., 2002). In 1964, nearly 70 million people in the U.S. consumed tobacco on a regular basis; and according to the 1955 Current Population Survey, two-thirds of men (68 percent) and one-third of women (32.4 percent) 18 years and older were regular smokers of cigarettes. As revealed by these data, cigarette smoking was the social norm, its link with heart and lung diseases was not widely accepted, and the desire or ability to quit smoking in that era was very low (DHHS, 1964). The reduction in national prevalence of cigarette smoking from 41.9 percent in 1965 to 23 percent in 2001 (Kochanek and Smith, 2004) reflects changes in the social norms and the positive influence of public health and policy interventions (Public Health Service, 1994; Economos et al., 2001).

Recently, intensive effort has been devoted to reviewing the evidence of the effectiveness of community preventive services. The Guide to Community Preventive Services (Task Force on Community Preventive Services, 2004) has completed an analysis of the evidence in nine major areas (two health behaviors, six specific health conditions, and one addressing the social environment). Additional reports, including those central to preventing childhood obesity (e.g., school-based programs, community fruit and vegetable consumption, consumer literacy, and food and nutrition policy) are forthcoming. In the nine health areas examined to date, the Task Force found that certain categories of interventions appear to have strong evidence of effectiveness for multiple health behaviors and problems (Table 1-3). Further, based on the experience to date from the Guide

TABLE 1-3 Recommended Public Health Interventions Common to Multiple Health Behaviors and Conditions

Type of Intervention	Health Behavior or Condition
Community-wide campaigns	Physical activity** Motor vehicle occupant injuries* Oral health (water fluoridation)**
School-based interventions	Physical activity** Oral health (sealants)** Vaccine preventable diseases (requirement for school admission)* Skin cancer*
Mass media strategies	Tobacco initiation and cessation** Motor vehicle occupant injuries**
Laws and regulations	Reducing exposure to secondhand smoke** Motor vehicle occupant injuries**
Provider reminder systems	Vaccine preventable diseases** Tobacco cessation*
Reducing costs to patients	Tobacco cessation* Vaccine preventable diseases**
Home visits	Vaccine preventable diseases* Violence prevention**

* Sufficient Evidence.
** Strong Evidence.

SOURCE: Task Force on Community Preventive Services, 2004.

to Community Preventive Services, it appears that comprehensive programs that involve communities, schools, mass media, health providers, and laws and regulations are most likely to be effective for a number of health problems (see also Appendix D).

There is a general pattern to the interventions that have successfully addressed many of these public health problems (CDC, 1999). In nearly all cases, policy changes were followed by the emergence of new government leadership structures to effectively enforce the policies and oversee the development and implementation of pertinent programs. Such direction was aided by improved surveillance methods, control measures, technologies, and treatments, together with expanding systems of service delivery and provider education. By organizing the experiences, principles, and strategies underlying these multiple achievements into conceptual frameworks, we may likewise develop successful approaches to childhood obesity prevention.

SUMMARY

After working throughout the 20th century to improve children's physical health by reducing the incidence of disease and widening margins of safety, we now find ourselves bringing children into environments with some decidedly less-than-healthful features—fewer opportunities to be physically active and socially interactive, more opportunities to be sedentary and passively entertained, and frequent temptations to consume in the absence of hunger or need and to engage in other risky behaviors.

A complex of interacting cultural, social, economic, familial, and psychological issues have set the stage for these growing obesity risks for children. Although the need to take action to curb the epidemic is widely acknowledged, the debate about what to do and how to do it is just beginning in earnest. Important insights can potentially be obtained from an examination of past successes in overcoming, or at least alleviating, some other problems that also seemed insurmountable at first. Such insights are presented as part of the committee's charge to use theoretical and empirical findings to assess the potential utility of specific approaches within a comprehensive childhood obesity prevention strategy.

This report provides a broad-based examination of the problem of obesity in children and youth, and it presents an action plan—with recommendations on the roles and responsibilities of numerous stakeholders and many sectors of society—for addressing this problem. The committee hopes that the report will produce shared understandings and stimulate sustained societal and lifestyle changes so that the current obesity trends among our children and youth may be reversed.

REFERENCES

American Dietetic Association. 2004. Position of the American Dietetic Association: Dietary guidance for healthy children ages 2 to 11 years. *J Am Diet Assoc* 104(4):660-677.

Baughcum AE, Chamberlin LA, Deeks CM, Powers SW, Whitaker RC. 2000. Maternal perceptions of overweight preschool children. *Pediatrics* 106(6):1380-1386.

Bolen JR, Sleet DA, Chorba T, Brewer R, Dellinger A, Wallace LJD, Johnson VR. 1997. Overview of efforts to prevent motor-vehicle-related injury. In: *Prevention of Motor Vehicle-Related Injuries: A Compendium of Articles from the Morbidity and Mortality Weekly Report, 1985-1996*. Atlanta, GA: National Center for Injury Prevention and Control.

Borra ST, Kelly L, Shirreffs MB, Neville K, Geiger CJ. 2003. Developing health messages: Qualitative studies with children, parents, and teachers help identify communications opportunities for healthful lifestyles and the prevention of obesity. *J Am Diet Assoc* 103(6):721-728.

Buchanan DR. 2000. *An Ethic for Health Promotion*. New York: Oxford University Press.

Bureau of Transportation Statistics. 2003. *National Household Travel Survey*. [Online]. Available: http://www.bts.gov/programs/national_household_travel_survey/ [accessed July 27, 2004].

Caballero B, Himes JH, Lohman T, Davis SM, Stevens J, Evans M, Going S, Pablo J. 2003. Body composition and overweight prevalence in 1704 schoolchildren from 7 American Indian communities. *Am J Clin Nutr* 78:308-312.

Cavadini C, Siega-Riz AM, Popkin BM. 2000. US adolescent food intake trends from 1965 to 1996. *Arch Dis Child* 83(1):18-24.

CDC (Centers for Disease Control and Prevention). 1999. Ten great public health achievements—United States, 1990-1999. *MMWR* 48(12):241-243.

CDC. 2001. Physical activity trends—United States, 1990-1998. *MMWR* 50(9):166-169.

CDC. 2002. Barriers to children walking and bicycling to school—United States, 1999. *MMWR* 51(32):701-704.

CDC. 2003a. Physical activity levels among children aged 9-13 years—United States, 2002. *MMWR* 52(33):785-788.

CDC. National Center for Health Statistics. 2003b. *Health, United States, 2003 with Chartbook on Trends in the Health of Americans*. [Online]. Available: http://www.cdc.gov/nchs/data/hus/tables/2003/03hus059.pdf [accessed May 25, 2004].

CDC. 2003c. Prevalence of physical activity, including lifestyle activites among adults—United States, 2000-2001. *MMWR* 52(32):764-769.

CDC. 2004a. Trends in intake of energy and macronutrients—United States, 1971-2000. *MMWR* 53(4):80-82.

CDC. 2004b. Prevalence of no leisure-time physical activity—35 states and the District of Columbia, 1988-2002. *MMWR* 53(4):82-86.

CDC. 2004c. Youth Risk Behavior Surveillance—United States, 2003. *MMWR* 53(SS-2):21-24.

Chanmugam P, Guthrie J, Cecilio S, Morton J, Basiotis P, Anand R. 2003. Did fat intake in the United States really decline between 1989-1991 and 1994-1996? *J Am Diet Assoc* 103(7):867-872.

Child Trends. 2002. *Watching Television*. [Online]. Available: http://www.childtrendsdatabank.org/pdf/55_PDF.pdf [accessed September 3, 2004].

Clauson A. 1999. Share of food spending for eating out reaches 47 percent. *Food Rev* 22(3):15-17.

Cramer P, Steinwert T. 1998. Thin is good, fat is bad: How early does it begin? *J Appl Dev Psych* 19:429-451.

Crepinsek MK, Burstein NR. 2004. *Maternal Employment and Children's Nutrition. Volume II, Other Nutrition-Related Outcomes*. E-FAN-04-006-1. Washington, DC: Economic Research Service, USDA.

Cutler D, Glaeser E, Shapiro J. 2003. *Why Have Americans Become More Fat?* NBER Working Paper No. W9446. Cambridge, MA: National Bureau of Economic Research.

DHHS (U.S. Department of Health and Human Services). 1964. *Surgeon General Report: Smoking and Health*. Washington, DC: Report of the Advisory Committee to the Surgeon General of the Public Health Service.

DHHS. 1996. *Physical Activity and Health: A Report of the Surgeon General*. Atlanta, GA: USDHHS, CDC, NCCDPHP.

DHHS. 2001. *The Surgeon General's Call to Action to Prevent and Decrease Overweight and Obesity*. Rockville, MD: Public Health Service, Office of the Surgeon General.

Ebbeling CB, Pawlak DB, Ludwig DS. 2002. Childhood obesity: Public-health crisis, common sense cure. *Lancet* 360(9331):473-482.

Economos CD, Brownson RC, DeAngelis MA, Novelli P, Foerster SB, Foreman CT, Gregson J, Kumanyika SK, Pate RR. 2001. What lessons have been learned from other attempts to guide social change? *Nutr Rev* 59(3 Pt 2):S40-S56.

Enns CW, Mickle SJ, Goldman JD. 2002. Trends in food and nutrient intakes by children in the United States. *Fam Econ Nutr Rev* 14(2):56-68.

Enns CW, Mickle SJ, Goldman JD. 2003. Trends in food and nutrient intakes by adolescents in the United States. *Fam Econ Nutr Rev* 15(2):15-27.

Evans WD, Finkelstein EA, Kamerow DB, Renaud JM. June 2-4, 2004. *Public Perceptions of Childhood Obesity*. Presentation at the Time/ABC News Obesity Summit, Williamsburg, VA.

Fagot-Campagna A, Pettitt DJ, Engelgau MM, Burrows NR, Geiss LS, Valdez R, Beckles GL, Saaddine J, Gregg EW, Williamson DF, Narayan KM. 2000. Type 2 diabetes among North American children and adolescents: An epidemiologic review and a public health perspective. *J Pediatr* 136(5):664-672.

Federal Interagency Forum on Child and Family Statistics. 2003. *America's Children: Key National Indicators of Child Well-Being, 2003*. Washington, DC: U.S. Government Printing Office.

Fee E, Brown TM, Lazarus J, Theerman P. 2002. The smoke nuisance. *Am J Public Health* 92(6):931.

Field Research Corporation. 2003. *A Survey of Californians about the Problem of Childhood Obesity*. Conducted for the California Endowment. October-November 2003. [Online]. Available: http://www.calendow.org/obesityattitudes/index.htm [accessed April 9, 2004].

Fontaine KR, Redden DT, Wang C, Westfall AO, Allison DB. 2003. Years of life lost due to obesity. *J Am Med Assoc* 289(2):187-193.

Food Marketing Institute. 1996. *Trends in the United States: Consumer Attitudes & the Supermarket, 1996*. Washington, DC: Food Marketing Institute.

Food Marketing Institute. 2003. *Trends in the United States: Consumer Attitudes & the Supermarket 2003*. Washington, DC: Food Marketing Institute.

Fox MK, Pac S, Devaney B, Jankowski L. 2004. Feeding Infants and Toddlers Study: What foods are infants and toddlers eating? *J Am Diet Assoc* 104(1 Suppl 1):S22-S30.

Frank LD. 2000. Land use and transportation interaction: Implications on public health and quality of life. *J Plan Educ Res* 20:6-22.

Freedman DS, Dietz WH, Srinivasan SR, Berenson GS. 1999. The relation of overweight to cardiovascular risk factors among children and adolescents: The Bogalusa Heart Study. *Pediatrics* 103(6 Pt 1):1175-1182.

French SA, Story M, Jeffery RW. 2001. Environmental influences on eating and physical activity. *Annu Rev Public Health* 22:309-335.

French SA, Lin BH, Guthrie JF. 2003. National trends in soft drink consumption among children and adolescents age 6 to 17 years: Prevalence, amounts, and sources, 1977/ 1978 to 1994/1998. *J Am Diet Assoc* 103(10):1326-1331.

Frey WH. 2003. Married with children. *Am Demogr* 25(2):17-19.

Gleason P, Suitor C. 2001. *Children's Diets in the Mid-1990's: Dietary Intake and Its Relationship with School Meal Participation.* Alexandria, VA: U.S. Department of Agriculture. Report No. CN-01-CD1.

Gross SM, Bronner Y, Welch C, Dewberry-Moore N, Paige DM. 2004. Breakfast and lunch meal skipping patterns among fourth-grade children from selected public schools in urban, suburban, and rural Maryland. *J Am Diet Assoc* 104(3):420-423.

Guthrie JF, Morton JF. 2000. Food sources of added sweeteners in the diets of Americans. *J Am Diet Assoc* 100(1):43-51.

Hill JO, Wyatt HR, Reed GW, Peters JC. 2003. Obesity and the environment: Where do we go from here? *Science* 299(5608):853-855.

Hofferth SL, Sandberg JF. 2001. Changes in American children's time, 1981-1997. In: Owens T, Hofferth S, eds. *Children at the Millennium: Where Have We Come From, Where Are We Going?* Advances in Life Course Research. New York: Elsevier Science.

IFIC (International Food Information Council). 2004. *Trends in Obesity-Related Media Coverage.* Washington, DC. [Online]. Available: http://www.ific.org/research/obesitytrends. cfm [accessed July 26, 2004].

IOM (Institute of Medicine). 1991. *Improving America's Diet and Health.* Washington, DC: National Academy Press.

IOM. 1999. *Reducing the Burden of Injury: Advancing Prevention and Treatment.* Washington, DC: National Academy Press.

IOM. 2003. *Weight Management: State of the Science and Opportunities for Military Programs.* Washington, DC: The National Academies Press.

Jahns L, Siega-Riz AM, Popkin BM. 2001. The increasing prevalence of snacking among US children from 1977 to 1996. *J Pediatr* 138(4):493-498.

Jain A, Sherman SN, Chamberlin DL, Carter Y, Powers SW, Whitaker RC. 2001. Why don't low-income mothers worry about their preschoolers being overweight? *Pediatrics* 107(5): 1138-1146.

Kennedy E, Blaylock J, Kuhn B. 1999. Introduction. On the road to better nutrition. In: Frazao E, ed. *America's Eating Habits: Changes and Consequences.* Washington, DC: USDA.

Kersh R, Morone J. 2002. How the personal becomes political: Prohibitions, public health, and obesity. *Stud Am Polit Dev* 16:162-175.

Kessler DA. 1995. The evolution of national nutrition policy. *Annu Rev Nutr* 15:xiii-xxvi.

Kochanek KD, Smith BL. 2004. Deaths: Preliminary data for 2002. *Natl Vital Stat Rep* 52(13):1-47.

Koplan JP, Dietz WH. 1999. Caloric imbalance and public health policy. *J Am Med Assoc* 282(16):1579-1581.

Kumanyika S. 2002. The minority factor in the obesity epidemic. *Ethn Dis* 12(3):316-319.

Lake Snell Perry & Associates. 2003. *Obesity as a Public Health Issue: A Look at Solutions.* [Online]. Available: http://www.phsi.harvard.edu/health_reform/harvard_forum_release. pdf [accessed January 28, 2004].

Latner JD, Stunkard AJ. 2003. Getting worse: The stigmatization of obese children. *Obes Res* 11(3):452-456.

Lin BH, Guthrie J, Frazao E. 1999a. Nutrient contribution of food away from home. In: Frazao E, ed. *America's Eating Habits: Changes and Consequences.* Washington, DC: USDA.

Lin BH, Guthrie J, Frazao E. 1999b. Quality of children's diets at and away from home: 1994-96. *Food Rev* 2-10.

Lobstein T, Baur L, Uauy R, IASO International Obesity TaskForce. 2004. Obesity in children and young people: A crisis in public health. *Obes Rev* 5(Suppl 1):4-85.

Luckett Clark S, Weismantle M. 2003. *Employment Status: 2000.* Census 2000 Brief. U.S. Department of Commerce. [Online]. Available: http://www.census.gov/prod/2003pubs/c2kbr-18.pdf [accessed July 23, 2004].

Lyle J, Hoffman HR. 1972. Children's use of television and other media. In: Rubenstein EA, Comstock GA, Murray JP, eds. *Television and Social Behavior.* Vol. 4. Washington, DC: U.S. Government Printing Office. Pp. 257-273.

Mokdad AH, Serdula MK, Dietz WH, Bowman BA, Marks JS, Koplan JP. 1999. The spread of the obesity epidemic in the United States, 1991-1998. *J Am Med Assoc* 282(16):1519-1522.

Mokdad AH, Serdula MK, Dietz WH, Bowman BA, Marks JS, Koplan JP. 2000. The continuing epidemic of obesity in the United States. *J Am Med Assoc* 284(13):1650-1651.

Mokdad AH, Ford ES, Bowman BA, Dietz WH, Vinicor F, Bales VS, Marks JS. 2003. Prevalence of obesity, diabetes, and obesity-related health risk factors, 2001. *J Am Med Assoc* 289(1):76-79.

Narayan KM, Boyle JP, Thompson TJ, Sorensen SW, Williamson DF. 2003. Lifetime risk for diabetes mellitus in the United States. *J Am Med Assoc* 290(14):1884-1890.

Nesbitt SD, Aahaye MO, Stettler N, Sorof JM, Goran MI, Parekh R, Falkner BE. 2004. Overweight as a risk factor in children: A focus on ethnicity. *Ethn Dis* 14(1):94-110.

Nestle M. 2003. Increasing portion sizes in American diets: More calories, more obesity. *J Am Diet Assoc* 103(1):39-40.

Nielsen Media Research. 2000. *2000 Report on Television: The First 50 Years.* New York: AC Nielsen Company.

Nielsen SJ, Popkin BM. 2003. Patterns and trends in food portion sizes, 1977-1998. *J Am Med Assoc* 289(4):450-453.

NRC (National Research Council), IOM. 2003. *Working Families and Growing Kids: Caring for Children and Adolescents.* Washington, DC: The National Academies Press.

NSC (National Safety Council). 1997. *Accident Facts.* Ithaca, IL: NSC.

Ogden CL, Flegal KM, Carroll MD, Johnson CL. 2002. Prevalence and trends in overweight among US children and adolescents, 1999 2000. *J Am Med Assoc* 288(14):1728-1732.

Oliver JE, Lee T. 2002. *Public Opinion and the Politics of America's Obesity Epidemic.* KSG Working Paper No. RWP02-017. [Online]. Available: http://ksgnotes1.harvard.edu/Research/wpaper.nsf/rwp/RWP02-017?OpenDocument [accessed August 9, 2004].

Panitz B. 1999. Year of the restaurant: Unwrapping what the industry has to offer. *Restaurants USA*, February, Pp. 26-30. [Online]. Available: http://www.restaurant.org/rusa/magArticle.cfm?ArticleID=338 [accessed December 16, 2003].

Popkin BM, Nielsen SJ. 2003. The sweetening of the world's diet. *Obes Res* 11(11):1325-1332.

Population Reference Bureau. 2003. *Traditional Families Account for 7 Percent of U.S. Households.* [Online]. Available: http://www.ameristat.org/pdf/TraditionalFamiliesAccountfor7Percent.pdf [accessed April 15, 2004].

Population Reference Bureau. 2004a. *Going to Work: America's Commuting Patterns in 2000.* [Online]. Available: http://www.prb.org/AmeristatTemplate.cfm?Section=2000Census1 [accessed April 15, 2004].

Population Reference Bureau. 2004b. *Record Number of Women in the U.S. Labor Force.* [Online]. Available: http://www.prb.org/AmeristatTemplate.cfm?Section=Labor__Employment &template=/ContentManagement/ContentDisplay.cfm&ContentID=7880 [accessed April 15, 2004].

Pratt M, Macera CA, Blanton C. 1999. Levels of physical activity and inactivity in children and adults in the United States: Current evidence and research issues. *Med Sci Sports Exerc* 31(11 Suppl):S526-S533.

Prevention Institute. 2003. *Environmental and Policy Approaches to Promoting Healthy Eating and Activity Behaviors.* Oakland, CA: Prevention Institute.

Price JH, Desmond SM, Stelzer CM. 1987. Elementary school principals' perceptions of childhood obesity. *J Sch Health* 57(9):367-370.

Public Health Service. 1994. *For a Healthy Nation: Returns on Investment in Public Health.* Atlanta, GA: DHHS.

Putnam J, Gerrior S. 1999. Trends in the U.S. food supply. In: Frazao E, ed. *America's Eating Habits: Changes and Consequences.* Washington, DC: USDA. Pp. 133-160.

Putnam J, Allshouse J, Kantor LS. 2002. U.S. per capita food supply trends: More calories, refined carbohydrates, and fats. *Food Rev* 25(3):2-15.

Putnam RD. 1995. Tuning in, tuning out: The strange disappearance of social capital in America. *Political Science* 28:664-683.

Rideout VJ, Foehr UG, Roberts DF, Brodie M. 1999. *Kids & Media @ the New Millennium: Executive Summary.* Menlo Park, CA: Henry J. Kaiser Family Foundation. [Online] Available: http://www.kff.org/content/1999/1535/KidsExecSum%20FINAL.pdf [accessed November 20, 2003].

Rideout VJ, Vandewater EA, Wartella EA. 2003. *Zero to Six: Electronic Media in the Lives of Infants, Toddlers and Preschoolers.* Menlo Park, CA: Henry J. Kaiser Family Foundation.

Robert Wood Johnson Foundation. 2003. *Healthy Schools for Healthy Kids.* Princeton, NJ: Robert Wood Johnson Foundation.

Roberts D, Foehr U, Rideout V, Brodie M. 1999. *Kids and Media @ the New Millennium.* Menlo Park, CA: Henry J. Kaiser Family Foundation.

Robinson JP, Godbey G. 1999. *Time for Life. The Surprising Ways That Americans Use Their Time.* 2nd edition. University Park, PA: The Pennsylvania State University Press.

Rolls BJ. 2003. The supersizing of America. Portion size and the obesity epidemic. *Nutr Today* 38(2):42-53.

San Jose Mercury News/Kaiser Family Foundation. 2004. *Survey on Childhood Obesity.* Menlo Park, CA: Henry J. Kaiser Family Foundation.

Schwartz MB, Puhl R. 2003. Childhood obesity: A societal problem to solve. *Obes Rev* 4(1):57-71.

Seidell JC. 1998. Societal and personal costs of obesity. *Exp Clin Endocrinol Diabetes* 106(Suppl 2):7-9.

Serdula MK, Mokdad AH, Williamson DF, Galuska DA, Mendlein JM, Heath GW. 1999. Prevalence of attempting weight loss and strategies for controlling weight. *J Am Med Assoc* 282(14):1353-1358.

Siega-Riz AM, Popkin BM, Carson T. 1998. Trends in breakfast consumption for children in the United States from 1965-1991. *Am J Clin Nutr* 67(4):748S-756S.

Sloan EA. 2003. What, when, and where Americans eat. *Food Techn* 57(8):48-66.

Smiciklas-Wright H, Mitchell D, Mickle S, Goldman J, Cook A. 2003. Foods commonly eaten in the United States, 1989-1991 and 1994-1996: Are portion sizes changing? *J Am Diet Assoc* 103(1):41-47.

Strategy One. 2003. *Addressing the Obesity Debate: A Consumer Point of View.* Washington, DC: International Food Information Council.

Sturm R. 2004. The economics of physical activity: Societal trends and rationales for interventions. *Am J Prev Med* 27(3S):126-135.

Sturm R. 2005a. Childhood obesity—What can we learn from existing data on societal trends. Part 1. *Preventing Chronic Disease* [Online]. Available: http://www.cdc. gov/pcd/issues/2005/jan/04_0038.htm.

Sturm R. 2005b (in press). Childhood obesity—What can we learn from existing data on societal trends. Part 2. *Preventing Chronic Disease* [Online]. Available: http://www.cdc. gov/pcd/issues/2005/apr/04_0039.htm.

Task Force on Community Preventive Services. 2004. *Guide to Community Preventive Services. Task Force Recommendations.* [Online] Available: http://www.thecommunity guide.org/overview/recs-to-date.pdf [accessed May 25, 2004].

Teachman BA, Brownell KD. 2001. Implicit anti-fat bias among health professionals: Is anyone immune? *Int J Obes Relat Metab Disord* 25(10):1525-1531.

Tharp MC. 2001. *Marketing and Consumer Identity in Multicultural America.* Thousand Oaks, CA: Sage Publications.

U.S. Census Bureau. 2001. *U.S. Interim Projections by Age, Sex, Race, and Hispanic Origin.* [Online]. Available: http://www.census.gov/ipc/www/usinterimproj/ [accessed June 11, 2004].

USDA (U.S. Department of Agriculture). Center for Nutrition Policy and Promotion. 1996. *The Food Guide Pyramid.* Washington, D.C.: U.S. Government Printing Office.

USDA. 2000. *Pyramid Servings Intakes by U.S. Children and Adults: 1994-96, 1998.* Agricultural Research Service, Community Nutrition Research Group. Table Set No. 1.

USDA. 2003. Profiling food consumption in America. In: *Agriculture Fact Book 2001-2002.* Washington, DC: USDA. U.S. Government Printing Office.

U.S. Department of Labor. 2004. *Women in the Labor Force: A Databook.* Bureau of Labor Statistics. Report 973. [Online]. Available: http://www.bls.gov/cps/wlf-databook.pdf [accessed April 15, 2004].

U.S. Department of Transportation. 1995. *Highway Statistics Summary to 1995.* Washington, DC: Federal Highway Administration. Office of Highway Information Management. [Online]. Available: http://www.fhwa.dot.gov/ohim/summary95/ [accessed June 18, 2004].

U.S. Department of Transportation. 2004. *Fatality Analysis Reporting System (FARS) Web-Based Encyclopedia.* Washington, DC: National Center for Statistics and Analysis. National Highway Traffic Safety Administration. [Online]. Available: http://www-fars.nhtsa.dot.gov/ [accessed September 28, 2004].

Waller PF. 2002. Challenges in motor vehicle safety. *Annu Rev Public Health* 23:93-113.

Whitaker RC. 2004. *Informational Report on Evidence-Based Literature for Development of a Childhood Obesity Interactive Tool.* Princeton, NJ: Mathematica Policy Research.

WHO (World Health Organization). 2002. *World Health Report: Reducing Risks, Promoting Healthy Life.* Geneva: WHO.

WHO. 2003. *Diet, Nutrition and the Prevention of Chronic Diseases.* Technical Report Series No. 916. Geneva: WHO.

Widmeyer Polling & Research. 2003. *Summary of Study Findings: Americans' Attitudes on Fighting Obesity.* American Public Health Association Obesity Poll. Washington, DC.

2

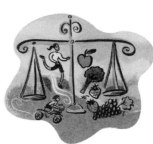

Extent and Consequences of Childhood Obesity

Overall trend data clearly indicate that obesity prevalence in U.S. children and youth has risen to distressing proportions, but many questions remain about the nature, extent, and consequences of this problem. How much do we really know about how this epidemic is unfolding? Which population groups are most affected? What does the available evidence tell us about how to address this problem? Finally, what are the potential consequences of inaction with respect to social, developmental, and health outcomes and the associated health-care system costs? This chapter's discussion of these questions informs the recommendations throughout the remainder of this report.

PREVALENCE AND TIME TRENDS

Because direct measures of body fat are neither feasible nor available for nationwide assessments of the prevalence of obesity, the National Health and Nutrition Examination Surveys (NHANES),[1] conducted by the National Center for Health Statistics, have been using body mass index (BMI) as a surrogate measure for body fatness. The prevalence of childhood and

---

[1]NHANES is a series of cross-sectional, nationally representative examination surveys that became a continuous survey in 1999. Previous surveys include NHANES III (conducted from 1988 to 1994), NHANES II (conducted from 1976 to 1980), NHANES I (conducted from 1971 to 1974), the National Health Examination Survey (NHES) cycle 3 (conducted from 1966 to 1970), and the NHES cycle 2 (conducted from 1963 to 1965).

adolescent obesity is equated to the proportion of those who are in the upper end of the BMI distribution—specifically, at or above the age- and gender-specific 95th percentile of the Centers for Disease Control and Prevention's (CDC's) BMI charts for children and youth aged 2 through 19 years[2] (Kuczmarski et al., 2000) (see Chapter 3 for a more extensive discussion about the use of terms for childhood overweight and childhood obesity).

If BMI is normally distributed and survey-specific percentile distributions are presented, then by definition, 5 percent of children in each survey will be above the 95th percentile BMI of the survey sample. Thus, reports based on the survey-specific BMI percentiles would always designate 5 percent of children as obese and would fail to detect any true increasing prevalence of obesity across surveys. The CDC therefore developed a revised growth reference in 2000 that established the age- and gender-specific 95th percentile of BMI. The growth reference data were based on BMI distributions from national surveys between 1963 and 1980 for children aged 6 to 19 years, and between 1971 and 1994 for children aged 2 through 5 years (Kuczmarski et al., 2002; Ogden et al., 2002b). There are no BMI-for-age references or accepted definitions for children younger than 2 years of age. However, the Special Supplemental Nutrition Program for Women, Infants and Children (WIC) has defined the term overweight for children under 2 years who are at or above the 95th percentile of weight-for-length and uses this standard for determining WIC program eligibility (Ogden et al., 2002a).

Overall Burden

The term "epidemic" suggests a condition that is occurring more frequently and extensively among individuals in a community or population than is expected. This characterization clearly appears to apply to childhood obesity. In 2000, obesity was two to three times more common in children and youth than in a reference period in the early 1970s. **The increase in obesity prevalence has been particularly striking since the late 1970s. The obesity epidemic affects both boys and girls and has occurred in all age, race, and ethnic groups throughout the United States (Ogden et al., 2002a).**

The 1999-2000 NHANES found that approximately 10 percent of 2- to 5-year-old children were at or above the 95th percentile of BMI, repre-

---

[2]The NHANES series use the term "overweight" rather than "obese" to describe all children who are at or above the age- and gender-specific 95th percentile of BMI. However, this report uses the term "obese" to refer to those children (see Chapter 3).

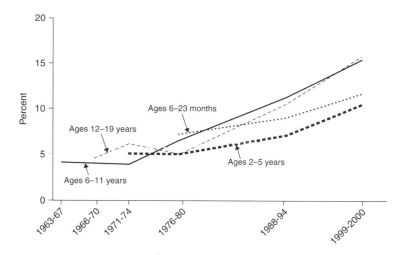

FIGURE 2-1 Age-specific trends in child and adolescent obesity.
NOTE: Obesity is defined as a BMI at or above the age- and gender-specific 95th
percentile cutoff points from the 2000 CDC BMI charts. Weight-for-length is used
to track children aged 6 to 23 months (under 2 years of age).
SOURCES: Ogden et al., 2002a; CDC, 2003.

senting twice the expected percentage; and that more than 15 percent of 6-
to 19-year-olds met this criterion, representing about three times the expected percentage (Ogden et al., 2002a). No significant increases in obesity
prevalence were reported between the 1999-2000 and the 2001-2002
NHANES (Hedley et al., 2004).

A significant, unabated increase in the prevalence of childhood obesity
across all age groups is clearly seen in an analysis of serial national surveys
from the early 1970s through the year 2000 (Figure 2-1). In the nearly 30
years between the 1971-1974 NHANES and the 1999-2000 NHANES, the
prevalence of childhood obesity more than doubled for youth aged 12 to 19
years (from 6.1 percent to 15.5 percent) and more than tripled for children
aged 6 to 11 years (4 percent to 15.3 percent). Even for preschool children,
aged 2 to 5 years, the prevalence also more than doubled (5 percent to 10.4
percent) between these two national surveys (Ogden et al., 2002a). Data for
children younger than 2 years of age, based on weight-for-length data
available from NHANES II (6-23 months) onward also suggest an upward
trend (Ogden et al., 2002a).

The same trends, stratified by gender, are shown in Figure 2-2 for
infants and preschool children and in Figure 2-3 for school-aged children
and adolescents. Among children older than 2 years of age, the increased
prevalence of obesity over time has occurred to a similar degree in both

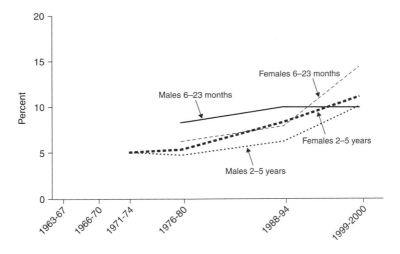

FIGURE 2-2 Trends in infant and child obesity, boys and girls aged 6 months through 5 years.
NOTE: Obesity is defined as a BMI at or above the age- and gender-specific 95th percentile cutoff points from the 2000 CDC BMI charts. Weight-for-length is used to track children aged 6 to 23 months (under 2 years of age).
SOURCE: Ogden et al., 2002a.

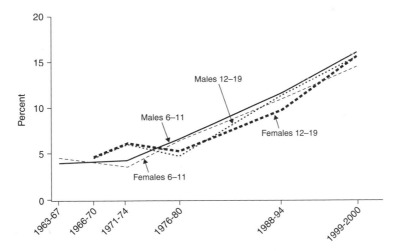

FIGURE 2-3 Trends in child and adolescent obesity, girls and boys aged 6 through 19 years.
NOTE: Obesity is defined as a BMI at or above the age- and gender-specific 95th percentile cutoff points from the 2000 CDC BMI charts.
SOURCES: Ogden et al., 2002a; CDC, 2003.

boys and girls. However, in those children under 2 years of age,[3] the increased prevalence is more marked in girls than in boys.

High-Risk Population Subgroups

Although no demographic group in the United States has been untouched by the childhood obesity epidemic, there is evidence that some subgroups of the U.S. population have been affected more than others. As discussed below, certain ethnic minority populations, children in low-socio-economic-status families, and children in the country's southern region tend to have higher rates of obesity than the rest of the population. Either the factors driving the obesity epidemic are more pronounced in these high-risk populations and communities, or their children and adolescents may be more sensitive to, or less able to avoid, the causal factors when present. Additional efforts will be needed to identify the nature of the risk for obesity in these high-risk population subgroups.

High-Risk Ethnic Groups

Cross-sectional population-based estimates of obesity prevalence at 6 to 19 years of age are available for U.S. children and adolescents overall, and specifically for non-Hispanic blacks, non-Hispanic whites, and Mexican Americans (Figure 2-4).[4]

Although obesity is prevalent among children and youth throughout the entire population, Hispanic, non-Hispanic black, and Native-American children and adolescents are disproportionately affected when compared to the general population (Ogden et al., 2002a). With both sexes combined, up to 24 percent of non-Hispanic black and Mexican-American adolescents are above the 95th percentile. Among boys, the highest prevalence of obesity is observed in Mexican Americans and among girls, the highest prevalence is observed in non-Hispanic blacks (Ogden et al., 2002a). American-

---

[3]There are no BMI-for-age references or accepted definitions for children younger than 2 years of age. Weight-for-length greater than the 95th percentile is used by the CDC and the WIC program to define overweight in children under 2 years of age (see Chapter 3).

[4]Standard terms used in the NHANES series include non-Hispanic whites, non-Hispanic blacks, and Mexican Americans. The ethnic and racial categories discussed throughout this chapter use those that specific researchers used for different data sets. This report generally uses the terms African Americans to refer to non-Hispanic blacks; Hispanics to refer to Mexican Americans and populations from other Latin-American countries of Hispanic descent; American Indians to refer to Native Americans; and whites to refer to non-Hispanic whites. The report also uses the term Asian/Pacific Islanders (which includes Native Hawaiians).

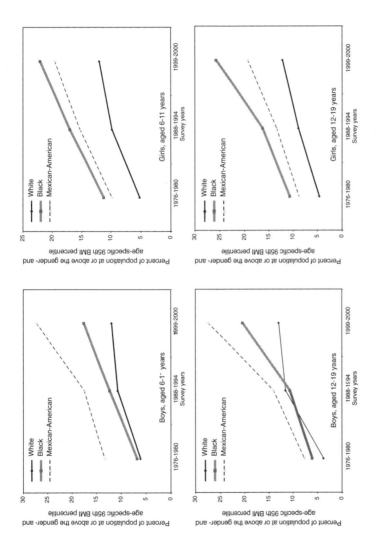

FIGURE 2-4 Trends in obesity prevalence for non-Hispanic white, non-Hispanic Black, and Mexican-American boys and girls.
NOTE: Obesity is defined as a BMI at or above the age- and gender-specific 95th percentile cutoff points from the 2000 CDC BMI charts. The following datapoints have a relative standard error of 20 to 30 percent: 1999-2000 boys, aged 6 to 11 years (white); 1999-2000 girls, aged 6 to 11 years (white); 1988-1994 girls, aged 12 to 19 years (Mexican American).

Indian children and youth, although not reported separately in the NHANES data, are also particularly affected by obesity (Caballero et al., 2003). For example, the prevalence of obesity in 7-year-old American-Indian children has been estimated recently at nearly 30 percent, representing twice the current estimated prevalence among all U.S. children of that age (Caballero et al., 2003).

Moreover, ethnicity-specific plots of the cross-sectional NHES and NHANES data for children aged 6 to 19 years suggest accelerated rates of increase in obesity prevalence for non-Hispanic black and Mexican-American children of both sexes (Figure 2-4), creating a disparity in obesity prevalence between non-Hispanic white and black children (particularly among girls) (CDC, 2003).

Additional evidence that some ethnic disparities for obesity are increasing over time is drawn from the National Longitudinal Survey of Youth (NLSY). Between 1986 and 1998, the prevalence of obesity increased 120 percent among African Americans and Hispanics while it increased 50 percent among non-Hispanic whites (Strauss and Pollack, 2001).

Socioeconomic Difference

Evidence also suggests significant variation in BMI as a function of both socioeconomic status and ethnicity based on NHANES III in girls aged 6 to 9 years (Winkelby et al., 1999). An increase in obesity prevalence among African Americans appears greatest for those at the lowest income (Strauss and Pollack, 2001). But uncertainties remain. These disparities are not the same across ethnic groups and they do not emerge at comparable times during childhood. Also, there is almost no consensus, despite many theories, about the mechanisms by which they occur. For instance, analysis of the data from the 1988-1994 NHANES shows that the prevalence of obesity in white adolescents is higher among those in low-income families but there is no clear relationship between family income and obesity in other age or ethnic subgroups (Troiano and Flegal, 1998; Ogden et al., 2003).

Nonetheless, two analyses of nationally representative longitudinal data—the NLSY (Strauss and Knight, 1999; Strauss and Pollack, 2001) and the National Longitudinal Study of Adolescent Health (Goodman, 1999; Goodman et al., 2003)—have suggested that family socioeconomic status is inversely related to obesity prevalence in children and that the effects of socioeconomic status and race or ethnicity were independent of other variables.

One explanation is insurance status, which is related to socioeconomic status; the uninsured may face barriers to accessing health care (Haas et al., 2003). Insurance coverage has been associated with the prevalence of obesity in youth. An analysis of the 1996 Medical Expenditure Panel Survey Household Component found that a combination of lacking health insurance and having public insurance (Medicaid, Medicare, or other public hospital coverage) were directly associated with obesity among adolescents (Haas et al., 2003).

Regional Differences

Regional differences in the prevalence of U.S. childhood obesity were already apparent in 1998 based on NLSY data (10.8 percent in western states and 17.1 percent in southern states) (Strauss and Pollack, 2001). However, most data available for regional differences are for adults. In 1998, adult obesity prevalence based on the CDC Behavioral Risk Factor Surveillance System (BRFSS) exceeded 20 percent in several states—Alabama (20.7 percent), Alaska (20.7 percent), Louisiana (21.3 percent), South Carolina (20.2 percent) and West Virginia (22.9 percent)—predominantly in the Southeast (Mokdad et al., 1999). By 2002, BRFSS data revealed that seven states had adult obesity prevalence rates greater than 25 percent: Alabama, Louisiana, Michigan, Mississippi, South Carolina, Texas, and West Virginia (CDC, 2002). Systematic data reflecting regional differences in obesity prevalence for children and youth are currently not available.

Shifts in the Population BMI Distribution

Researchers can monitor changes in the nature of the obesity epidemic by comparing the BMI distribution curves derived from population-based surveys and noting shifts in any particular distribution over time. A shift toward higher BMIs over the entire distribution would indicate that virtually everyone is becoming heavier, with lean individuals gradually moving into the overweight range, overweight individuals moving into the obese range, and the number of obese individuals becoming more severely obese. However, a graphical analysis comparing NHANES III (1988-1994) with earlier data found that the distributional patterns of BMIs differed among age groups (Flegal and Troiano, 2000).

For adults, there was a general shift upward in the BMI distribution, with the greatest shift occurring at the upper end of the distribution, reflected by the heaviest subgroups becoming heavier. For younger children aged 6 to 11 years, and to a lesser extent in adolescents, the distributions of BMI values were characterized by little or no difference in the lower part of the distribution, though there was also a greater shift at the upper end, as shown schematically in Figures 2.5a and 2.5b (Flegal and Troiano, 2000). The results of this study indicate that the heaviest children and youth were heavier in NHANES III than in earlier surveys; the authors caution, how-

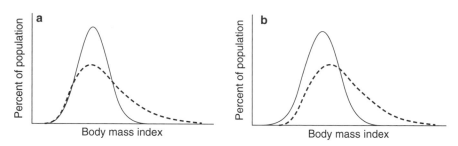

FIGURE 2-5 Schematic representations of BMI distribution models.
NOTE: **Figure 2-5a** shows a schematic representation of increased skewness (lack of symmetry) at the upper end of the BMI distribution with little change at the lower end, as has been observed in U.S. children and adolescents. **Figure 2-5b** shows a schematic representation of both a rightward shift in the distribution and increased skewness at the upper end of the distribution, as has been observed in U.S. adults.
SOURCE: Reprinted, with permission, from Flegal and Troiano, 2000. Copyright 2000 by the *International Journal of Obesity and Related Metabolic Disorders.*

ever, that the unweighted sample sizes for 6- to 17-year-olds, particularly for adolescents, are small (Flegal and Troiano, 2000). Strauss and Pollack (2001) came to a similar conclusion based on their analyses of NLSY data.

Changes in BMI distributions have impacts on the population's health. In adults, the major health-related co-morbidities that occur with obesity do not have a linear relationship with BMI. For example, although relationships between BMI and hypertension, diabetes, dyslipidemia, and even death occur across a wide range of BMIs, these relationships strengthen considerably at the highest levels of BMI (Solomon and Manson, 1997; Must et al., 1999).

Similarly, children at the highest levels of BMI are generally at the greatest risk of adverse health outcomes. Elevated blood pressure and insulin were both observed to be twice as common in children with BMIs above the 97th percentile as in children within the 95th to 97th percentile (Freedman et al., 1999). But the prevalence of these health outcomes is low between the 25th and 75th BMI percentiles, increasing modestly, if at all, across that span. Thus, with the childhood obesity epidemic characterized by a disproportionate number of children at the extreme ranges of BMI, there are likely to be higher obesity-related morbidity rates in children than if the epidemic mostly resulted from an upward shift in BMI across their entire population.

Relationship Between the Childhood and Adult Obesity Epidemics

The obesity epidemic that began in the early 1970s and escalated after 1980 for children and youth has progressed similarly in adults over the same time period. As depicted in Figures 2-6 and 2-7, between the 1971-1974 NHANES and the 1999-2000 NHANES the prevalence of obesity— defined as a BMI at or above 30 kg/m^2—more than doubled (from 14.5

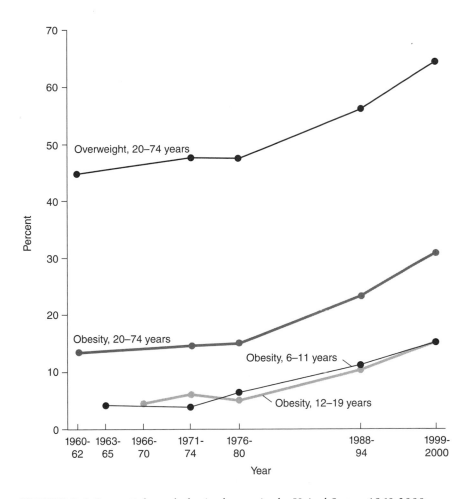

FIGURE 2-6 Overweight and obesity by age in the United States, 1960-2000. NOTE: Percents for adults are age-adjusted. Obesity for children is defined as a BMI at or above the age- and gender-specific 95th percentile BMI cutpoints from the 2000 CDC BMI charts. Obesity for adults is defined as a BMI greater than or equal to 30. Obesity is a subset of the percent of overweight. SOURCE: CDC, 2003.

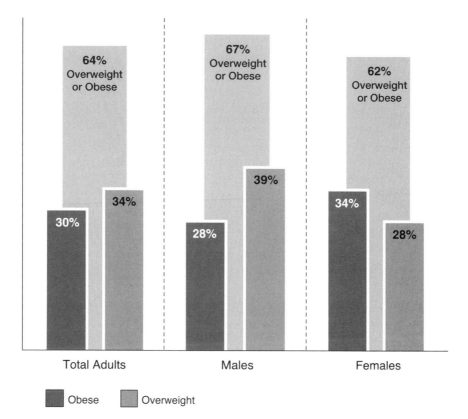

Total Adults   Males   Females

■ Obese   ▮ Overweight

FIGURE 2-7 Prevalence of overweight and obesity among adults 20 years of age and older, NHANES 1999-2000.
SOURCE: CDC, 2003. Reprinted with permission from Salinsky and Scott, 2003. Copyright by the National Health Policy Forum.

percent to 30.5 percent) among 60 million U.S. adults. Between 1999-2000 and 2001-2002 there were no significant changes in the prevalence of obesity in adults (30.5 percent versus 30.6 percent) (Hedley et al., 2004). These trends, underscored by similar findings at the state level (Mokdad et al., 2001), have paralleled childhood and youth obesity prevalence, suggesting that the epidemics may be linked.

The observation that children and adults are both experiencing epidemics of obesity over the same time frame has important implications for understanding causes and formulating prevention interventions. Many of the same sociocultural factors that have contributed to the adult obesity epidemic have likely contributed to the childhood obesity epidemic.

The average parents today are twice as likely to be obese as 30 years ago, even though their genetic susceptibility and that of their child has not changed over this period. Parental obesity more than doubles the risk of adult obesity among both obese and nonobese children under 10 years of age (Whitaker et al., 1997). For example, an obese preschool child with normal weight parents has approximately a 25 percent chance of being obese as an adult. However, this same preschool child with an obese parent has more than a 60 percent chance of being an obese adult (Whitaker et al., 1997). An additional implication of the adult and childhood obesity co-epidemics relates to intergenerational transmission. There are a number of potential mechanisms by which maternal obesity in pregnancy may promote offspring obesity (Whitaker and Dietz, 1998; Levin, 2000; Oken and Gillman, 2003), and further research is needed to examine these mechanisms.

Children can inherit obesity susceptibility genes from an obese parent or parents, or can be exposed, after birth, to diet and activity patterns that promote obesity. Moreover, recent research suggests that an altered intrauterine environment may be a third mechanism (see Chapter 8). For example, obese mothers are more likely to experience diabetes in pregnancy, and some evidence suggests that the offspring of mothers who have diabetes in pregnancy may have an increased risk of developing obesity later in life (Silverman et al., 1998).

In a study of low-income families enrolled in the WIC program, children born to mothers who were obese at the time of conception were twice as likely to be obese at 4 years of age (Whitaker, 2004b). Although much remains to be learned about the mechanisms of intergenerational obesity, these data suggest that it may be important to consider the promotion of healthy body weights among pregnant mothers as part of childhood obesity prevention efforts, and obesity research efforts should examine prevention interventions for pregnant mothers who are obese as well as for their children.

CONSIDERING THE COSTS FOR CHILDREN AND FOR SOCIETY

The primary concern about childhood obesity is its potential impact on well-being, not only in childhood but into adulthood, with the term "well-being" reflecting the committee's view that social and emotional health is as important as physical health. As discussed in Chapter 1, families may differ in the value they place on the different health outcomes of obesity, and the merits they attribute to certain benefits or drawbacks of changing behaviors to address it (Whitaker, 2004a). Research suggests that some parents do not perceive weight to be a health issue for their children (Baughcum et al., 2000; Jain et al., 2001; Borra et al., 2003), independent of their child's physical and social functioning. Thus, individuals may differ in the value they place on various aspects of their well-being (Buchanan, 2000). Depending on these values, childhood obesity may represent a greater concern to some than to others. Failing to reverse the trend in childhood obesity means that many obese children, over their lifetimes, could experience significant impairments in multiple domains of functioning. They are more likely to be chronically ill, to have a negative impact on their earning potential, and to even die prematurely.

Social and Emotional Health

While childhood obesity may not result in recognized clinical symptoms until later in life, the social and emotional correlates often have immediate effects on children's lives. Research on the short- and long-term impacts of obesity on children's emotional and social functioning has been extensively reviewed (French et al., 1995; Dietz, 1998b; Must and Strauss, 1999; Puhl and Brownell, 2001; Styne, 2001; Must and Anderson, 2003; Schwartz and Puhl, 2003), and the collective body of research clearly indicates that obese children and youth are stigmatized, and subject to negative stereotyping and discrimination by their peers (Schwartz and Puhl, 2003; Strauss and Pollack, 2003).

This sort of treatment, which is hypothesized to produce adverse emotional consequences such as low self-esteem, negative body image, and depressive symptoms for obese children, is not limited to peers; it may also come from adults, including parents, teachers, and health-care providers (Strauss et al., 1985). Even though obesity in children has become more common, such negative treatment has not diminished (Latner and Stunkard, 2003), as revealed by obese children who continue to be socially marginalized by their peers (Strauss and Pollack, 2003).

The results of studies on the emotional well-being of obese children are difficult to succinctly summarize, given the differences between studies. Variations include the outcome measures used, the characteristics of the study subjects (particularly age, gender, racial/ethnic status, and degree of obesity), and whether the samples were clinical or community-based. Furthermore, because many of the study designs are cross-sectional, it is often impossible to distinguish between time course, and impossible to determine whether the associations are causal. Nonetheless, a few general statements can be made.

In one longitudinal study, associations between obesity and low self-esteem appear to emerge by early adolescence and were strongest in Hispanic and white adolescent girls but not in African-American girls (Strauss, 2000). The emotional consequences are somewhat stronger in girls than in boys, increase with age, and may be greater in those obese children who seek treatment (Schwartz and Puhl, 2003). Having concerns about being obese, regardless of actual body weight, appears to be a primary factor associated with depressive symptoms among preadolescent girls (Erickson et al., 2000).

The social and emotional impacts of obesity can also be long term. In a longitudinal U.S. cohort with a seven-year follow-up, women 16 to 24 years of age at baseline who had been overweight completed fewer years of school, earned less money, and were less likely to be married (Gortmaker et al., 1993). The impact of adolescent obesity on the subsequent lower earnings of women was also demonstrated in a British cohort study (Sargent and Blanchflower, 1994).

Physical Health

Several thorough reviews (Dietz, 1998a,b; Must and Strauss, 1999; Deckelbaum and Williams, 2001; Styne, 2001; Must and Anderson, 2003) have found childhood obesity to be associated with a wide array of disorders that affect multiple organ systems. These disorders include hypertension, dyslipidemia, glucose intolerance/insulin resistance, hepatic steatosis, cholelithiasis, sleep apnea, menstrual abnormalities, impaired balance, and orthopedic problems. Some of these conditions produce clinical symptoms in obese children, while others do not; however, the metabolic and physiologic changes associated with childhood obesity, along with the obesity itself, tend to track into adult life and eventually enhance the risks of disease, disability, and death.

In 2000, it was estimated that 400,000 deaths were attributed to poor diet and physical inactivity in the United States (Mokdad et al., 2004), an increase of one-third from 300,000 annual deaths attributed to diet and sedentary activities in 1990 (McGinnis and Foege, 1993). Although these risk factors represent the second leading cause of deaths among Americans, diet and physical inactivity are predicted to exceed tobacco as the leading cause of deaths in the future (Mokdad et al., 2004).

Of the multiple health correlates of the childhood obesity epidemic, perhaps the one that has received greatest attention is the increased prevalence of type 2 diabetes in children.[5] By one population-based estimate from southwestern Ohio, a ten-fold increase in the prevalence of type 2 diabetes in children between 1982 and 1994 accounted for one-third of all new cases of diabetes (including type 1 and type 2) in children by 1994 (Pinhas-Hamiel et al., 1996). For individuals born in the United States in 2000, the lifetime risk of being diagnosed with diabetes at some point in their lives is estimated at 30 percent for boys and 40 percent for girls if

---

[5]Type 2 diabetes was previously referred to as adult-onset diabetes and type 1 diabetes was previously called juvenile-onset diabetes.

obesity rates level off (Narayan et al., 2003). Nearly all children with type 2 diabetes are obese, and a disproportionate number are Native American, African American, Hispanic, or Asian/Pacific Islander (Fagot-Campagna et al., 2000; Goran et al., 2003; Davis et al., 2004).

Several risk factors—including increased body fat (especially abdominal fat), insulin resistance, ethnicity, and the onset of puberty—have been identified as contributors to the development of type 2 diabetes, and they appear to have an additive influence (Goran et al., 2003). Accurate estimates of the prevalence of diabetes in U.S. children are difficult to determine. It has been estimated that the prevalence of diabetes is 0.41 percent in U.S. youth aged 12-19 years (approximately 100,000 U.S. adolescents) and the prevalence of impaired fasting glucose is 1.76 percent (approximately 500,000 U.S. adolescents) (Fagot-Campagna et al., 2001). Better estimates for children are not possible because the prevalence of type 2 diabetes in this population is still relatively low. NHANES is the only current national data collection effort that could potentially make such an estimate. However, the sample sizes from NHANES are not large enough to make a stable point estimate of the prevalence.

The childhood obesity epidemic may result in increased risk of type 2 diabetes. One study found that for each adolescent diagnosed with type 2 diabetes, there are 5 others with impaired fasting glucose, an indicator of insulin resistance below the diagnostic threshold for type 2 diabetes (Fagot-Campagna et al., 2001). Furthermore, the degree of insulin resistance in children increases with the severity of body fatness, as it does in adults (ADA, 2000). Thus, the combination of more obese children and the increased severity of obesity suggests that larger numbers of children will reach the diagnostic threshold for type 2 diabetes. Finally, it is estimated that approximately three-fourths of obese adolescents will be overweight as young adults (Guo et al., 2002) and will likely face the persistent risk of developing type 2 diabetes.

The increased prevalence of obesity among adults of all ages also has been associated with a similar increase in the prevalence of diabetes (Mokdad et al., 2001). In fact, the increase in diabetes prevalence has been greatest in young adults aged 30 to 39 years, with prevalence almost doubling between 1990 and 2001 (Mokdad et al., 2000, 2003). Moreover, the development of all of the major complications of diabetes, including retinopathy, nephropathy, and neuropathy, are related to duration of disease. Those who develop diabetes earlier in life generally will develop costly complications earlier with the potential for premature mortality. For example, among 79 individuals in a Canadian referral clinic who were diagnosed with type 2 diabetes before the age of 17 and who were followed up from ages 18 to 33 years, two had died suddenly while on dialysis and three more were currently receiving dialysis (Dean and Flett, 2002).

A potentially even more important complication of childhood obesity may be the metabolic syndrome, diagnosed when a person has at least three of five metabolic abnormalities: glucose intolerance, abdominal obesity, hypertriglyceridemia, low high-density lipoprotein (HDL) cholesterol, and high blood pressure (NHLBI, 2002). The metabolic syndrome is now present in approximately one-quarter of all U.S. adults (Ford et al., 2002; Park et al., 2003) and in nearly 30 percent of U.S. children and youth who are obese (Cook et al., 2003).

Among adults, the metabolic syndrome is associated not only with type 2 diabetes (Haffner et al., 1992; Cook et al., 2003) but also with cardiovascular disease (Isomaa et al., 2001; Cook et al., 2003) and a higher mortality rate (Lakka et al., 2002; Cook et al., 2003). Even among those obese youth who do not yet have clinical diabetes, components of the metabolic syndrome appear to contribute to the development of atherosclerosis (Mahoney et al., 1996; Berenson et al., 1998; McGill et al., 2002). Ultimately, it may be the association of childhood obesity with the metabolic syndrome, rather than exclusively with diabetes, that may comprise the greatest physical health threat of childhood obesity.

It is possible that if the childhood obesity epidemic continues at its current rate, conditions related to type 2 diabetes—such as blindness, amputation, coronary artery disease, stroke, and kidney failure—will become ordinary in middle-aged people. Additionally, risk factors for cancer in obese adults, such as hormone alterations, may be present in obese children and contribute to a higher incidence of certain types of cancer later in life (Gascon et al., 2004). Thus, these conditions may affect a greater proportion of the population than current morbidity. This is a serious prospect given that obesity accounts for a level of morbidity comparable to that of smoking and poverty (Sturm and Wells, 2001).

Integrated View of the Consequences of Childhood Obesity

In reviews of the correlates of childhood obesity, discussions of the physical impacts and of the social and emotional impacts are often separate. But this distinction may be artificial. First, although the brain plays a central role in the regulation of energy balance and obesity (Schwartz et al., 2000), it is also the central organ for integrating social stimuli, regulating emotion, and executing social interaction. Not surprisingly, cues that affect both eating and activity behaviors are often social in nature, ranging from sadness to anxiety to boredom.

Social and emotional factors must therefore be recognized not only as potential consequences of obesity but also as potential causes. For example, depressed mood in children and adolescents may precede the development of obesity and not just follow it (Pine et al., 2001; Goodman and Whitaker,

2002; Richardson et al., 2003). In a nationally representative sample of 8- to 11-year-olds, clinically meaningful behavioral problems have been shown to be associated with the development of obesity over a 2-year period among children not obese at baseline (Lumeng et al., 2003). Affective factors, such as depressive symptoms, are also the likely mediators of the observed association between adult obesity and traumatic childhood experiences (e.g., physical abuse, sexual abuse) (Williamson et al., 2002).

There is accruing evidence that even the metabolic syndrome itself may be a consequence of how the brain processes environmental stimuli that are social in nature. For instance, the brain's response to stress may alter the hypothalamic-pituitary-adrenal (or gonadal) axis in a way that promotes central fat deposition and insulin resistance in adults (Bjorntorp, 2001). Because children also experience stress, the part of the brain that regulates emotion may not only influence whether a child overeats, but also the metabolic consequences of that excess energy.

The fact that the physiologic response to stress is conditioned in childhood (Gunnar and Donzella, 2002) emphasizes the potential importance of optimizing the social and emotional health of children as a strategy for preventing obesity over a lifetime. Failure to recognize this connection between social or emotional health and physical health could result in prevention strategies that are poorly conceptualized, and underscores the need to consider the broadest possible definition of health to include the physical, mental, and emotional aspects (Table 2-1), because the foundations of all three develop during childhood and are interconnected.

Health-Care Costs

A RAND study has calculated that the costs imposed on society by people with sedentary lifestyles (i.e., the "external" costs generated) may be greater than those imposed by smokers (Keeler et al., 1989). More recent computations of national health-care expenditures related to obesity and overweight in adults showed large lifetime external costs related to these conditions. After adjusting for inflation and converting estimates to 2004 dollars, the national direct and indirect health-care costs related to overweight and obesity range from $98 billion (Finkelstein et al., 2003) to $129 billion (DHHS, 2001a).[6] It has been suggested that overweight and obesity may account for nearly one-third (27 to 31 percent) of total direct costs related to 15 co-morbid diseases (Lewin Group, 2000) and account for 9

---

[6]The $98 billion is based on an estimate of $93 billion in year 2002 dollars (Finkelstein et al., 2003) and the $129 billion is based on an estimate of $117 billion in year 2000 dollars (DHHS, 2001a) calculated from the 2004 Consumer Price Index (U.S. Bureau of Labor Statistics, 2004).

TABLE 2-1 Physical, Social, and Emotional Health Consequences of Obesity in Children and Youth

Physical Health
- Glucose intolerance and insulin resistance
- Type 2 diabetes
- Hypertension
- Dyslipidemia
- Hepatic steatosis
- Cholelithiasis
- Sleep apnea
- Menstrual abnormalities
- Impaired balance
- Orthopedic problems

Emotional Health
- Low self-esteem
- Negative body image
- Depression

Social Health
- Stigma
- Negative stereotyping
- Discrimination
- Teasing and bullying
- Social marginalization

percent of total U.S. medical spending (Finkelstein et al., 2003). Less than a decade ago, by contrast, the estimated direct health-care costs attributable to obesity ranged from 1 to 6 percent of total health-care expenditures, depending on the definition of obesity and the methods of calculation used (Seidell, 1995; Wolf and Colditz, 1998). Annual medical expenditures in the United States related to obesity are estimated at $75 billion (in 2003 dollars) with approximately half of the expenditures financed by Medicaid and Medicare (Finkelstein et al., 2004). California, the most populous state, spent the most in public funds on health care for obese people in that year, a total of $7.7 billion (Finkelstein et al., 2004).

The direct health-care costs of physical inactivity, which contribute to the obesity epidemic, have been estimated to exceed $77 billion annually (Pratt et al., 2000). In addition, there are indirect costs of physical inactivity, such as those associated with dependence on motorized travel. For example, the national cost of traffic congestion in 2002 was estimated at 3.5 billion hours of delay, costing the nation $69.5 billion—an increase of $4.5 billion from the previous year (Schrank and Lomax, 2003).

Additionally, the estimated national health-care expenditures for Americans with diabetes exceeded $132 billion in 2002, and it has been suggested that people with diabetes have health-care costs that are on average 2.4 times higher than those of people without diabetes (ADA, 2003). Obesity-linked type 2 diabetes, by far the most common form of the disease, is largely preventable. The cost of obesity has recently been compared to other health-care costs, and research suggests that it outranks both smoking and drinking in adverse health effects and health-care costs, adding an average of $395 per patient per year to health-care costs (Sturm, 2002).

The direct economic burden of obesity in youth aged 6 to 17 years has been estimated, based on the 1979-1999 National Hospital Discharge Survey (Wang and Dietz, 2002). Obesity-associated hospital costs were determined from hospital discharges that listed obesity as either the primary or secondary diagnosis. Results indicate that the percentage of discharges with obesity-related diseases increased dramatically from 1979-1981 to 1997-1999. Discharges for diabetes doubled, gallbladder disease tripled, and sleep apnea increased five-fold during this time frame. In 2001 dollars, obesity-associated annual hospital costs for children and youth were estimated to have more than tripled from $35 million (1979-1981) to $127 million (1997-1999) (Wang and Dietz, 2002).

In 2000, the United States spent approximately 14 percent of its gross national product on health care—representing the largest share for any developed country over the past decade—and its per capita health-care expenditures were greater than those of any other nation (OECD Health Data, 2003). But although it is estimated that preventive measures could impact 70 percent of the causes of early deaths in the United States (McGinnis et al., 2002), most of the $1.4 trillion that the United States spends per year on health is used for direct medical care service. The national investment in preventing disease and promoting health is estimated to be only 5 percent of the total annual health-care costs (DHHS, 2001b; Kelley et al., 2004). This imbalance underscores the need for the health-care systems in the United States to establish a greater preventive orientation (Mokdad et al., 2004), particularly for childhood obesity, a largely preventable condition that has been shown to be a major determinant of health-care costs.

SUMMARY

Representative population surveys have found significant increases in the prevalence of obesity in U.S. children and youth. In 2000, childhood obesity was two to three times more common than in the early 1970s. Certain subpopulations of children, including those in several ethnic minority populations, in low-socioeconomic-status families, and in the southern region of the United States, tend to be most affected. Furthermore, there are particular concerns that the heaviest children are becoming heavier (i.e., a skewing of the population BMI distribution).

Obesity can have adverse impacts on a child's physical, social, and emotional well-being. It increases the incidence of type 2 diabetes and other chronic medical and psychosocial conditions. Furthermore, the metabolic and physiologic changes associated with childhood obesity, along with obesity itself, tend to track into adult life and eventually increase the individual's risk of disease, disability, and death.

Poor diet and physical inactivity contributed to an estimated 400,000 deaths that occurred in the U.S. population in 2000 (Mokdad et al., 2004); predictions indicate that diet and physical inactivity will ultimately overtake tobacco as the leading cause of death in the future. Obesity-associated annual hospital costs for children and youth were estimated to have more than tripled over a two-decade period, rising from $35 million (1979-1981) to $127 million (1997-1999).[7] Meanwhile, after adjusting for inflation and converting estimates to 2004 dollars, the national direct and indirect health-care expenditures related to adult obesity and overweight range from $98 billion to $129 billion. These figures clearly implicate obesity as a major determinant of health-care costs.

REFERENCES

ADA (American Diabetes Association). 2000. Type 2 diabetes in children and adolescents. *Pediatrics* 105(3):671-680.

ADA. 2003. Economic costs of diabetes in the U.S. in 2002. *Diabetes Care* 26(3):917-932.

Baughcum AE, Chamberlin LA, Deeks CM, Powers SW, Whitaker RC. 2000. Maternal perceptions of overweight preschool children. *Pediatrics* 106(6):1380-1386.

Berenson GS, Srinivasan SR, Bao W, Newman WP 3rd, Tracy RE, Wattigney WA. 1998. Association between multiple cardiovascular risk factors and atherosclerosis in children and young adults: The Bogalusa Heart Study. *N Engl J Med* 338(23):1650-1656.

Bjorntorp P. 2001. Do stress reactions cause abdominal obesity and comorbidities? *Obes Rev* 2(2):73-86.

Borra ST, Kelly L, Shirreffs MB, Neville K, Geiger CJ. 2003. Developing health messages: Qualitative studies with children, parents, and teachers help identify communications opportunities for healthful lifestyles and the prevention of obesity. *J Am Diet Assoc* 103(6):721-728.

Buchanan DR. 2000. *An Ethic for Health Promotion.* New York: Oxford University Press.

Caballero B, Himes JH, Lohman T, Davis SM, Stevens J, Evans M, Going S, Pablo J. 2003. Body composition and overweight prevalence in 1704 schoolchildren from 7 American Indian communities. *Am J Clin Nutr* 78:308-312.

---

[7]This estimate is based on 2001 dollars.

CDC (Centers for Disease Control and Prevention). 2002. *Behavioral Risk Factor Surveillance System Survey Data: Risk Factors and Calculated Variables–2002*. Atlanta, GA: U.S. Department of Health and Human Services, CDC. [Online]. Available: http://apps.nccd.cdc.gov/brfss/list.asp?cat=RF&yr=2002&qkey=4409&state=All   [accessed June 11 2004].

CDC. 2003. *Health, United States, 2003 with Chartbook on Trends in the Health of Americans*. [Online]. Available: http://www.cdc.gov/nchs/data/hus/hus03.pdf [accessed May 17, 2004].

Cook S, Weitzman M, Auinger P, Nguyen M, Dietz WH. 2003. Prevalence of a metabolic syndrome phenotype in adolescents: Findings from the Third National Health and Nutrition Examination Survey, 1988-1994. *Arch Pediatr Adolesc Med* 157(8):821-827.

Davis J, Busch J, Hammatt Z, Novotny R, Harrigan R, Grandinetti A, Easa D. 2004. The relationship between ethnicity and obesity in Asian and Pacific Islander populations: A literature review. *Eth Dis* 14(1):111-118.

Dean HJ, Flett B. 2002. Natural history of type 2 diabetes diagnosed in childhood: Long-term follow-up in young adult years. *Diabetes* 51:A24-A25.

Deckelbaum RJ, Williams CL. 2001. Childhood obesity: The health issue. *Obes Res* 9(S4):239S-243S.

DHHS (U.S. Department of Health and Human Services). 2001a. *The Surgeon General's Call to Action to Prevent and Decrease Overweight and Obesity*. Rockville, MD: Public Health Service, Office of the Surgeon General.

DHHS. 2001b. *Steps to a Healthier U.S.* Washington, DC: Office of Public Health Promotion. [Online]. Available: http://www.healthierus.gov/steps/steps_brochure.pdf [accessed June 18, 2004].

Dietz WH. 1998a. Childhood weight affects adult morbidity and mortality. *J Nutr* 128(2S):411S-414S.

Dietz WH. 1998b. Health consequences of obesity in youth: Childhood predictors of adult disease. *Pediatrics* 101(3):518-525.

Erickson SJ, Robinson TN, Haydel KF, Killen JD. 2000. Are overweight children unhappy? Body mass index, depressive symptoms, and overweight concerns in elementary school children. *Arch Pediatr Adolesc Med* 154(9):931-935.

Fagot-Campagna A, Saaddine JB, Engelgau MM. 2000. Is testing children for type 2 diabetes a lost battle? *Diabetes Care* 23(9):1442-1443.

Fagot-Campagna A, Saaddine JB, Flegal KM, Beckles GL. 2001. Diabetes, impaired fasting glucose, and elevated HbA1c in U.S. adolescents: The Third National Health and Nutrition Examination Survey. *Diabetes Care* 24(5):834-837.

Finkelstein EA, Fiebelkorn IC, Wang G. 2003. National medical spending attributable to overweight and obesity: How much, and who's paying? *Health Aff (Millwood)* 22:W3-219-226.

Finkelstein EA, Fiebelkorn IC, Wang G. 2004. State-level estimates of annual medical expenditures attributable to obesity. *Obes Res* 12(1):18-24.

Flegal KM, Troiano RP. 2000. Changes in the distribution of body mass index of adults and children in the US population. *Int J Obes Relat Metab Disord* 24(7):807-818.

Ford ES, Giles WH, Dietz WH. 2002. Prevalence of the metabolic syndrome among US adults: Findings from the Third National Health and Nutrition Examination Survey. *J Am Med Assoc* 287(3):356-359.

Freedman DS, Dietz WH, Srinivasan SR, Berenson GS. 1999. The relation of overweight to cardiovascular risk factors among children and adolescents: The Bogalusa Heart Study. *Pediatrics* 103(6):1175-1182.

French SA, Story M, Perry CL. 1995. Self-esteem and obesity in children and adolescents: A literature review. *Obes Res* 3(5):479-490.

Gascon F, Valle M, Martos R, Zafra M, Morales R, Castano MA. 2004. Childhood obesity and hormonal abnormalities associated with cancer risk. *Eur J Cancer Prev* 13(3):193-197.

Goodman E. 1999. The role of socioeconomic status gradients in explaining differences in US adolescents health. *Am J Public Health* 89(10):1522-1528.

Goodman E, Whitaker RC. 2002. A prospective study of the role of depression in the development and persistence of adolescent obesity. *Pediatrics* 109(3):497-504.

Goodman E, Slap GB, Huang B. 2003. The public health impact of socioeconomic status on adolescent depression and obesity. *Am J Public Health* 93(11):1844-1850.

Goran MI, Ball GD, Cruz ML. 2003. Obesity and risk of type 2 diabetes and cardiovascular disease in children and adolescents. *J Clin Endocrinol Metab* 88(4):1417-1427.

Gortmaker SL, Must A, Perrin JM, Sobol AM, Dietz WH. 1993. Social and economic consequences of overweight in adolescence and young adulthood. *N Engl J Med* 329(14):1008-1012.

Gunnar MR, Donzella B. 2002. Social regulation of the cortisol levels in early human development. *Psychoneuroendocrinology* 27(1-2):199-220.

Guo SS, Wu W, Chumlea WC, Roche AF. 2002. Predicting overweight and obesity in adulthood from body mass index values in childhood and adolescence. *Am J Clin Nutr* 76(3):653-658.

Haas JS, Lee LB, Kaplan CP, Sonneborn D, Phillips KA, Liang S-Y. 2003. The association of race, socioeconomic status, and health insurance status with the prevalence of overweight among children and adolescents. *Am J Public Health* 93(12):2105-2110.

Haffner SM, Valdez RA, Hazuda HP, Mitchell BD, Morales PA, Stern MP. 1992. Prospective analysis of the insulin-resistance syndrome (syndrome X). *Diabetes* 41(6):715-722.

Hedley AA, Ogden CL, Johnson CL, Carroll MD, Curtin LR, Flegal KM. 2004. Prevalence of overweight and obesity among US children, adolescents, and adults, 1999-2002. *J Am Med Assoc* 291(23):2847-2850.

Isomaa B, Almgren P, Tuomi T, Forsen B, Lahti K, Nissen M, Taskinen MR, Groop L. 2001. Cardiovascular morbidity and mortality associated with the metabolic syndrome. *Diabetes Care* 24(4):683-689.

Jain A, Sherman SN, Chamberlin DL, Carter Y, Powers SW, Whitaker RC. 2001. Why don't low-income mothers worry about their preschoolers being overweight? *Pediatrics* 107(5):1138-1146.

Keeler EB, Manning WG, Newhouse JP, Sloss EM, Wasserman J. 1989. The economic costs of a sedentary life-style. *Am J Public Health* 79(8):975-981.

Kelley E, Moy E, Kosiak B, McNeill D, Zhan C, Stryer D, Clancy C. 2004. Prevention health care quality in America: Findings from the First National Healthcare Quality and Disparities Reports. *Preventing Chronic Disease* 1(3). [Online]. Available: http://www.cdc.gov/pcd/issues/2004/jul/cover.htm [accessed June 18, 2004].

Kuczmarski RJ, Ogden CL, Grummer-Strawn LM, Flegal KM, Guo SS, Wei R, Mei Z, Curtin LR, Roche AF, Johnson CL. 2000. CDC growth charts: United States. *Adv Data* 8(314):1-27.

Kuczmarski RJ, Ogden CL, Guo SS, Grummer-Strawn LM, Flegal KM, Mei Z, Wei R, Curtin LR, Roche AF, Johnson CL. 2002. *Data from the National Health Survey. 2000 CDC Growth Charts for the United States: Methods and Development.* Hyattsville, MD: National Center for Health Statistics.

Lakka HM, Laaksonen DE, Lakka TA, Niskanen LK, Kumpusalo E, Tuomilehto J, Salonen JT. 2002. The metabolic syndrome and total and cardiovascular disease mortality in middle-aged men. *J Am Med Assoc* 288(21):2709-2716.

Latner JD, Stunkard AJ. 2003. Getting worse: The stigmatization of obese children. *Obes Res* 11(3):452-456.

Levin BE. 2000. The obesity epidemic: Metabolic imprinting on genetically susceptible neural circuits. *Obes Res* 8(4):342-347.

Lewin Group. 2000. *The Costs of Obesity.* Paper presented at Obesity: The Public Health Crisis Conference, Washington, DC, American Obesity Association, September 13, 2000.

Lumeng JC, Gannon K, Cabral HJ, Frank DA, Zuckerman B. 2003. Association between clinically meaningful behavior problems and overweight in children. *Pediatrics* 112(5):1138-1145.

Mahoney LT, Burns TL, Stanford W, Thompson BH, Witt JD, Rost CA, Lauer RM. 1996. Coronary risk factors measured in childhood and young adult life are associated with coronary artery calcification in young adults: The Muscatine Study. *J Am Coll Cardiol* 27(2):277-284.

Manning WG, Keeler EB, Newhouse JP, Sloss EM, Wasserman J. 1989. The taxes of sin. Do smokers and drinkers pay their way? *J Am Med Assoc* 261(11):1604-1609.

McGill HC Jr, McMahan CA, Herderick EE, Zieske AW, Malcom GT, Tracy RE, Strong JP. 2002. Obesity accelerates the progression of coronary atherosclerosis in young men. *Circulation* 105(23):2712-2718.

McGinnis JM, Foege WH. 1993. Actual causes of death in the United States. *J Am Med Assoc* 270(18):2207-2212.

McGinnis JM, Williams-Russo P, Knickman JR. 2002. The case for more active policy attention to health promotion: To succeed, we need leadership that informs and motivates, economic incentives that encourage change, and science that moves the frontiers. *Health Aff (Millwood)* 21(2):78-93.

Mokdad AH, Serdula MK, Dietz WH, Bowman BA, Marks JS, Koplan JP. 1999. The spread of the obesity epidemic in the United States, 1991-1998. *J Am Med Assoc* 282(16):1519-1522.

Mokdad AH, Ford ES, Bowman BA, Nelson DE, Engelgau MM, Vinicor F, Marks JS. 2000. Diabetes trends in the U.S.: 1990-1998. *Diabetes Care* 23(9):1278-1283.

Mokdad AH, Bowman BA, Ford ES, Vinicor F, Marks JS, Koplan JP. 2001. The continuing epidemics of obesity and diabetes in the United States. *J Am Med Assoc* 286(10):1195-1200.

Mokdad AH, Ford ES, Bowman BA, Dietz WH, Vinicor F, Bales VS, Marks JS. 2003. Prevalence of obesity, diabetes, and obesity-related health risk factors, 2001. *J Am Med Assoc* 289(1):76-79.

Mokdad AH, Marks JS, Stroup DF, Gerberding JL. 2004. Actual causes of death in the United States, 2000. *J Am Med Assoc* 291(10):1238-1245.

Must A, Anderson SE. 2003. Effects of obesity on morbidity in children and adolescents. *Nutr Clin Care* 6(1):4-12.

Must A, Strauss RS. 1999. Risks and consequences of childhood and adolescent obesity. *Int J Obes Relat Metab Disord* 23(2S):S2-S11.

Must A, Spadano J, Coakley EH, Field AE, Colditz G, Dietz WH. 1999. The disease burden associated with overweight and obesity. *J Am Med Assoc* 282(16):1523-1529.

Narayan KM, Boyle JP, Thompson TJ, Sorensen SW, Williamson DF. 2003. Lifetime risk for diabetes mellitus in the United States. *J Am Med Assoc* 290(14):1884-1890.

NHLBI (National Heart, Lung, and Blood Institute). 2002. *Third Report of the Expert Panel on Detection, Evaluation, and Treatment of High Blood Cholesterol in Adults (Adult Treatment Panel III).* Publication No. 02-5215. Rockville, MD: NIH.

OECD Health Data. 2003. *A Comparative Analysis of 30 Countries.* [Online]. Available: http://www.fedpubs.com/subject/health/oecdhealth.htm [accessed June 6, 2004].

Ogden CL, Flegal KM, Carroll MD, Johnson CL. 2002a. Prevalence and trends in overweight among US children and adolescents, 1999-2000. *J Am Med Assoc* 288(14):1728-1732.

Ogden CL, Kuczmarski RJ, Flegal KM, Mei Z, Guo S, Wei R, Grummer-Strawn LM, Curtin LR, Roche AF, Johnson CL. 2002b. Centers for Disease Control and Prevention 2000 growth charts for the United States: Improvements to the 1977 National Center for Health Statistics version. *Pediatrics* 109(1):45-60.

Ogden CL, Carroll MD, Flegal KM. 2003. Epidemiologic trends in overweight and obesity. *Endocrinol Metab Clin North Am* 32(4):741-760, vii.

Oken E, Gillman MW. 2003. Fetal origins of obesity. *Obes Res* 11(4):496-506.

Park YW, Zhu S, Palaniappan L, Heshka S, Carnethon MR, Heymsfield SB. 2003. The metabolic syndrome: Prevalence and associated risk factor findings in the US population from the Third National Health and Nutrition Examination Survey, 1988-1994. *Arch Intern Med* 163(4):427-436.

Pine DS, Goldstein RB, Wolk S, Weissman MM. 2001. The association between childhood depression and adulthood body mass index. *Pediatrics* 107(5):1049-1056.

Pinhas-Hamiel O, Dolan LM, Daniels SR, Standiford D, Khoury PR, Zeitler P. 1996. Increased incidence of non-insulin-dependent diabetes mellitus among adolescents. *J Pediatr* 128(5):608-615.

Pratt M, Macera CA, Wang G. 2000. Higher direct medical costs associated with physical inactivity. *Physician Sportsmed* 28(10):63-70.

Puhl R, Brownell KD. 2001. Bias, discrimination, and obesity. *Obes Res* 9(12):788-805.

Richardson LP, Davis R, Poulton R, McCauley E, Moffitt TE, Caspi A, Connell F. 2003. A longitudinal evaluation of adolescent depression and adult obesity. *Arch Pediatr Adolesc Med* 157(8):739-745.

Salinsky E, Scott W. 2003. *Obesity in America: A Growing Threat.* NHPF Background Paper. Washington, DC: The George Washington University.

Sargent JD, Blanchflower DG. 1994. Obesity and stature in adolescence and earnings in young adulthood: Analysis of a British birth cohort. *Arch Pediatr Adolesc Med* 148(7):681-687.

Schrank D, Lomax T. 2003. *The 2003 Urban Mobility Report.* Texas Transportation Institute. College Statation, TX: Texas A&M University System.

Schwartz MB, Puhl R. 2003. Childhood obesity: A societal problem to solve. *Obes Rev* 4(1).57-71.

Schwartz MW, Woods SC, Porte D Jr, Seeley RJ, Baskin DG. 2000. Central nervous system control of food intake. *Nature* 404(6778):661-671.

Seidell JC. 1995. The impact of obesity on health status: Some implications for health care costs. *Int J Obes Relat Metab Disord* 19(6S):S13-S16.

Silverman BL, Cho NH, Rizzo TA, Metzger BE. 1998. Long-term effects of the intrauterine environment: The Northwestern University Diabetes in Pregnancy Center. *Diabetes Care* 21(S2):B142-B149.

Solomon CG, Manson JE. 1997. Obesity and mortality: A review of the epidemiologic data. *Am J Clin Nutr* 66(4S):1044S-1050S.

Strauss CC, Smith K, Frame C, Forehand R. 1985. Personal and interpersonal characteristics associated with childhood obesity. *J Pediatr Psychol* 10(3):337-343.

Strauss RS. 2000. Childhood obesity and self-esteem. *Pediatrics* 105(1):E15.

Strauss RS, Knight J. 1999. Influence of the home environment on the development of obesity in children. *Pediatrics* 103(6):E85.

Strauss RS, Pollack HA. 2001. Epidemic increase in childhood overweight, 1986-1998. *J Am Med Assoc* 286(22):2845-2848.

Strauss RS, Pollack HA. 2003. Social marginalization of overweight children. *Arch Pediatr Adolesc Med* 157(8):746-752.

Sturm R. 2002. The effects of obesity, smoking, and drinking on medical problems and costs: Obesity outranks both smoking and drinking in its deleterious effects on health and health costs. *Health Aff (Millwood)* 21(2):245-253.

Sturm R, Wells KB. 2001. Does obesity contribute as much to morbidity as poverty or smoking? *Public Health* 115(3):229-235.

Styne DM. 2001. Childhood and adolescent obesity. Prevalence and significance. *Pediatr Clin North Am* 48(4):823-854.

Troiano RP, Flegal KM. 1998. Overweight children and adolescents: Description, epidemiology, and demographics. *Pediatrics* 101(3):497-504.

U.S. Bureau of Labor Statistics. 2004. *Consumer Price Indexes*. [Online]. Available: http://www.bls.gov/cpi/home.htm [accessed September 3, 2004].

Wang G, Dietz WH. 2002. Economic burden of obesity in youths aged 6 to 17 years: 1979-1999. *Pediatrics* 109(5):E81-E86.

Whitaker RC. 2004a. *Informational Report on Evidence-Based Literature for Development of a Childhood Obesity Interactive Tool*. Princeton, NJ: Mathematica Policy Research.

Whitaker RC. 2004b. Predicting preschooler obesity at birth: The role of maternal obesity in early pregnancy. *Pediatrics* 114(1):e29-e36.

Whitaker RC, Dietz WH. 1998. Role of the prenatal environment in the development of obesity. *J Pediatr* 132(5):768-776.

Whitaker RC, Wright JA, Pepe MS, Seidel KD, Dietz WH. 1997. Predicting obesity in young adulthood from childhood and parental obesity. *N Engl J Med* 337(13):869-873.

Williamson DF, Thompson TJ, Anda RF, Dietz WH, Felitti V. 2002. Body weight and obesity in adults and self-reported abuse in childhood. *Int J Obes Relat Metab Disord* 26(8):1075-1082.

Winkleby MA, Robinson TN, Sundquist J, Kraemer HC. 1999. Ethnic variation in cardiovascular disease risk factors among children and young adults: Findings from the Third National Health and Nutrition Examination Survey, 1988-1994. *J Am Med Assoc* 281(11):1006-1013.

Wolf AM, Colditz GA. 1998. Current estimates of the economic cost of obesity in the United States. *Obes Res* 6(2):97-106.

3

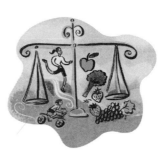

Developing an
Action Plan

The committee was charged with developing an action plan focused on preventing obesity in children and youth in the United States. The aim of the plan was to identify the most promising approaches for prevention, including policies and interventions for immediate action and in the longer term. The critical elements of the action plan's development, described in this and subsequent chapters, were as follows:

- Clarifying definitions related to key concepts
- Developing a framework to guide the type and scope of data gathered
- Articulating obesity prevention goals for children and youth
- Identifying criteria for conducting an in-depth review of the available evidence
- Translating the findings from the best available evidence into specific recommendations that comprise an integrated action plan.

DEFINITIONS AND TERMINOLOGY

Childhood and Adolescent Obesity

Body mass index (BMI) is an indirect measure of obesity based on the readily determined measures of height and weight. This report uses the term "obese" to refer to children and youth with BMIs equal to or greater than the 95th percentile of the age- and gender-specific BMI charts developed by the Centers for Disease Control and Prevention (CDC) (Kuczmarski et al., 2000). In most children, values at this level are known to indicate excess body fat, which itself is difficult to measure accurately in either clinical or population-based settings.

What constitutes "excess" is an amount of body fat (often expressed as a percentage of body mass) that is sufficient to cause adverse health consequences. The exact percentage of body fat at which adverse consequences occur can vary widely across individuals and the consequences themselves— ranging from low self-esteem or mild glucose intolerance to major depression or nephropathy—show considerable variation as well.

BMI—calculated as weight in kilograms divided by the square of height measured in meters (kg/m^2)—is the recommended indicator of obesity-related risks in both children and adults. For adults, overweight is defined as a BMI between 25 and 29.9 kg/m^2 and obesity is defined as a BMI equal to or greater than 30 kg/m^2 (NHLBI, 1998). The BMI cut-off points were based on epidemiological data that show increasing mortality above a BMI of 25 kg/m^2, with greater increases above 30 kg/m^2 (NHLBI, 1998).

Because children's development varies with age, and because boys and girls develop at different rates, the use of BMI to assess body weight in children requires growth and gender considerations. Thus, BMI values for children and youth are specific to both age and gender (Barlow and Dietz, 1998; Dietz and Robinson, 1998).

The committee recognizes that it has been customary to use the term "overweight" instead of "obese" to refer to children with BMIs above the age- and gender-specific 95th percentiles (Himes and Dietz, 1994; Barlow and Dietz, 1998; DHHS, 2001a; Kuczmarski et al., 2002; AAP, 2003). Obese has often been considered to be a pejorative term, despite having a specific medical meaning. There have also been concerns about misclassification, as BMI is only a surrogate measure of body fatness in children as in adults. Furthermore, children may experience functional impairment (physical or emotional) at different levels of body fatness.

However, the term "obese" more effectively conveys the seriousness, urgency, and medical nature of this concern than does the term "overweight," thereby reinforcing the importance of taking immediate action. Further, BMI in children correlates reasonably well to direct measures of body fatness (Mei et al., 2002), and high BMIs in children have been associated with many co-morbidities such as elevated blood pressure, insulin resistance, and increased lipids (Freedman et al., 2001). These are the same co-morbidities that often worsen in adult life and contribute to premature death from obesity.

The committee recognizes, however, that the term obese is probably not well suited for children younger than 2 years of age because the relationships among BMI, body fat, and morbidity are less clear at these ages.

Additionally, a high BMI in children younger than 2 years of age is less likely to persist than a high BMI in older children (Guo et al., 1994). BMI reference values are not established for children less than 2 years of age. Weight-for-length greater than the 95th percentile is used by CDC and the Special Supplemental Nutrition Program for Women, Infants, and Children to define overweight for children in this age group.

It is important that government agencies, researchers, health-care providers, insurers, and others agree on the same definition of childhood obesity. Although varying definitions have arisen from many uses of the term in public health, clinical medicine, insurance coverage, government programs and other settings, to the extent possible, there should be concurrence on definitions and terminology.

In this report, the term "obese" refers to children and youth between the ages of 2 and 18 years who have BMIs equal to or greater than the 95th percentile of the age- and gender-specific BMI charts developed by CDC.[1]

Prevention

To "prevent" means simply to take prior anticipatory action to hinder the occurrence of a course or event. Prevention efforts related to health traditionally have focused on preventing disease, particularly infectious disease. Conceptual frameworks have been developed that categorize health-related prevention efforts based on the segment of the population to which they are directed: the entire population (universal or population-based prevention); those who are at high risk of developing a disease (selective or high-risk prevention); or those who have a disease (targeted or indicated prevention) (Gordon, 1983; Rose, 1992; IOM, 1994; WHO, 2000).

Another traditional approach categorizes prevention according to disease progression: primary prevention involves avoiding the occurrence of a disease in a population; secondary prevention is aimed at early detection of the disease to limit its occurrence; and tertiary prevention is focused on limiting the consequences of the disease (DHHS, 2000).

A more recent framework conceptualizes a spectrum of prevention based on where—from the individual to the broader environment—the prevention actions are directed. Approaches include strengthening individual knowledge and skills, providing community education, educating

---

[1]This definition is consistent with current CDC recommendations with the exception of the terminology. International references such as the International Obesity Task Force or Cole BMI values allow for cross-cultural comparisons. These references use different populations and slightly differing techniques for developing cut-off points (Flegal et al., 2001).

providers, fostering coalitions and networks, changing institutional practices, and influencing policy (Cohen and Swift, 1999).

The prevention frameworks discussed lend themselves relatively easily
to infectious diseases in which there are clear endpoints and progressions.
But the frameworks can be more complex to apply to health outcomes (e.g.,
childhood obesity) in which the progression is a continuum and the condition is both a risk factor for other chronic diseases and a health outcome in
itself. The committee concluded that the well-established concept of primary prevention was most amenable to its assigned task of developing a
broad-based action plan that addresses the social, cultural, and environmental factors associated with childhood obesity.

A primary prevention approach emphasizes efforts that can help the
majority of children who are at a healthy weight to maintain that status and
not become obese. Within this approach, the committee developed the
majority of its recommendations as "population-based" actions—directed
to the entire population instead of high-risk individuals. However, the
committee acknowledges that obesity prevention will need to combine population-based efforts with targeted approaches for high-risk individuals and
subgroups. Consequently, the report also contains specific actions aimed at
high-risk populations affected by obesity, such as children and adolescents
in particular ethnic groups with higher than average obesity-prevalence
rates and communities in which there are recognizable social and economic
disparities. Subpopulations of children warranting special consideration
also include children with disabilities or special health-care needs. The
complex medical, psychological, physical, and psychosocial difficulties that
these children encounter may well put them at elevated risk for low physical
activity levels and unhealthful dietary behaviors.

The committee acknowledges that although population-based prevention approaches may be theoretically or conceptually the most useful approaches for addressing a society-wide problem, the practical challenge is in
determining how best to implement these interventions to achieve broad
outreach and maximal coverage. These issues will be discussed further in
the sections on local communities and evaluation of interventions (see Chapters 4 and 6).

The committee was not charged with, nor did it develop, recommendations directed specifically at obesity treatment or reducing excess weight in
children and youth. However, it is likely that many of the suggested actions
will also benefit children and youth who are already obese, even if the
interventions are insufficient to produce enough short-term weight loss for
achieving normal weight status. For example, obese children can benefit
from healthful choices in the school cafeteria.

Prevention of obesity, particularly among those at high risk, may seem
very similar to treatment in that screening is involved and individualized

intervention is often delivered in clinical settings. However, there are several important differences between prevention and treatment approaches (Kumanyika and Obarzanek, 2003). The targeted outcomes are different: prevention of weight gain is a satisfactory outcome for prevention approaches, whereas weight loss is the desired outcome for treatment. Motivations to maintain a healthful rate of weight gain for growing children may differ in nature and intensity from motivations to lose weight. Although treatment approaches may include relatively extreme behavioral changes over the short term, preventive strategies usually necessitate long-term continuation.

The committee's approach to obesity prevention is similar to the range of prevention efforts that have been used to address many other public health problems. Some efforts directly change the physical environment but require no purposeful action on the part of the target population (e.g., fluoridation of community drinking water and food fortification); others directly require behavior change in targeted high-risk populations (e.g., immunization of children); and some require environmental change to facilitate behavioral change (e.g., zoning and land-use regulations to encourage physical activity). The majority of efforts require multiple approaches; for example, efforts to reduce underage drinking and tobacco control have involved legislation, media campaigns, counseling, and many other mechanisms (NRC and IOM, 2003; Mensah et al., 2004).

Appendix B provides a glossary of terms used throughout this report.

FRAMEWORK FOR ACTION

●Using an ecological perspective, the committee developed a framework to depict the behavioral settings and leverage points that influence both sides of the energy balance[2] equation—energy intake and energy expenditure. An ecological systems theory model postulates that changes in individual characteristics are affected not only by personal factors (e.g., age, gender, genetic profile) but also by interactions with the larger social, cultural, and environmental contexts in which they live (e.g., family, school, community) (Figure 3-1) (Davison and Birch, 2001; Lobstein et al., 2004).

Building on this ecological model and drawing upon concepts from several relevant frameworks (Swinburn et al., 1999; Booth et al., 2001; Kumanyika et al., 2002; Swinburn and Egger, 2004), the committee developed a framework that shows layers of ecologic factors as influences on energy *im*balance, which is shown as the typical graphic in which energy

---

[2]Energy balance, as discussed in detail below, refers to a state in which energy intake is equivalent to energy expenditure, resulting in no net weight gain or weight loss.

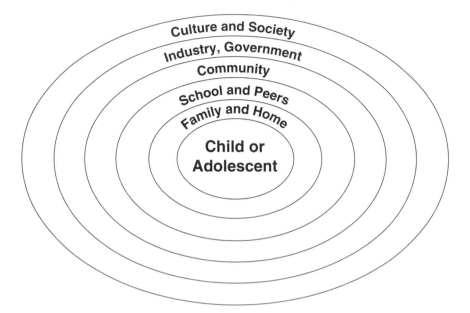

FIGURE 3-1 Simplified ecological systems theory model.

intake exceeds energy expenditure (Figure 3-2). Both aspects of energy imbalance (i.e., food and beverage intake and physical activity) interact with and are affected by multiple factors within each of the four ecological layers. The two innermost layers describe factors operating within the individual (including genetic factors, ethnic identity and culturally determined attitudes and beliefs, psychosocial factors, and current health status) and those operating within the physical and social locations and situations that define daily behavioral settings (Booth et al., 2001). The key behavioral settings for children and youth are the home, school, and community. As noted in the framework developed by the Partnership to Promote Healthy Eating and Active Living, behavioral settings are affected either directly or indirectly by a variety of other factors that potentially constitute primary and secondary leverage points for effecting changes (Booth et al., 2001). These leverage points include the major sectors that affect the food system, opportunities for physical activity or sedentary behavior, and information and education regarding dietary behaviors and physical activity. The outermost layer on the framework in Figure 3-2 reflects the critical concept of an overlay of social norms and values, that is, the social fabric that cuts across all the layers and processes below. Social norms and values both determine and respond to collective social and institutional processes within the con-

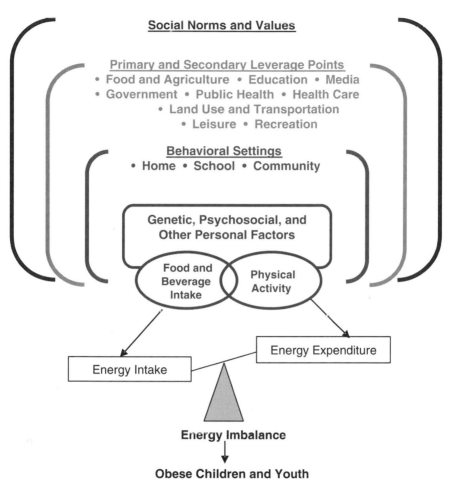

FIGURE 3-2 Framework for understanding obesity in children and youth.
NOTE: In this diagram energy intake is depicted as excessive when compared to energy expenditure, leading to a positive energy balance (or energy imbalance) resulting in obesity.

text of the larger U.S. culture. This framework, which emphasizes the need for obesity prevention efforts to leverage the interests and actions of a number of stakeholders working within and across multiple settings and sectors, guided the review of evidence and the development of recommendations in this report.

OBESITY PREVENTION GOALS

Clear specification of obesity prevention goals is essential in shaping an action plan and evaluating its success. Pertinent issues for setting obesity prevention goals for populations include concepts of optimum population BMI and healthy weight levels, potential effects on food intake and patterns of physical activity and inactivity (the primary modifiable determinants of obesity), as well as attitudes and social norms related to food and eating, physical activity and inactivity, body size, and dietary restrictions (WHO, 2000; Kumanyika et al., 2002). For children and youth, these considerations must be framed not only within the context of healthy physical, psychological, and cognitive development but in recognition that the increased prevalence of childhood obesity has broadened the emphasis of dietary guidance to address the overconsumption of energy-dense foods and beverages and physical activity patterns (ADA, 2003, 2004).

For individual children and youth, obesity prevention goals focus on maintaining energy balance (calories consumed versus calories expended). As discussed in greater detail later in the chapter, this involves engaging in healthful dietary behaviors and regular physical activity. Healthful dietary behaviors include choosing a balanced diet, eating moderate portion sizes, and heeding the body's own satiety cues that indicate physiological fullness. It is currently recommended that children and adolescents accumulate a minimum of 60 minutes of moderate to vigorous physical activity each day (see section on physical activity).

Children's food and beverage intake and their physical activity and sedentary behavior patterns can be influenced by a variety of environmental factors, including the availability and affordability of healthful foods, advertising messages, and opportunities to participate in physical activity within communities (Richter et al., 2000). Although individuals and families are embedded within broader social, economic, and political environments that influence their behaviors and may either promote or constrain the maintenance of health (IOM, 2001), such environments may also serve as contexts for change. These are the settings in which relationships are formed (e.g., home environment and support networks), and they represent a collection of formal and informal community institutions that monitor the behavior and safety of residents (Leventhal and Brooks-Gunn, 2001).

As will be noted throughout this report, changing the social, physical, and economic environments that contribute to the incidence and prevalence of childhood obesity—especially in populations in which the problem is longstanding and highly prevalent—may take many years to achieve. Therefore, the committee acknowledges that numerous intermediate goals, involving step-by-step improvements in diet patterns and physical activity levels of children and youth, are necessary for assessing progress. The ulti-

---

BOX 3-1
Goals of Obesity Prevention in Children and Youth

The goal of obesity prevention in children and youth is to create—through directed social change—an environmental-behavioral synergy that promotes:

- **For the *population* of children and youth**
  - Reduction in the incidence of childhood and adolescent obesity
  - Reduction in the prevalence of childhood and adolescent obesity
  - Reduction of mean population BMI levels
  - Improvement in the proportion of children meeting the Dietary Guidelines for Americans
  - Improvement in the proportion of children meeting physical activity guidelines
  - Achieving physical, psychological, and cognitive growth and developmental goals

- **For *individual* children and youth**
  - A healthy weight trajectory, as defined by the CDC BMI charts
  - A healthful diet (quality and quantity)
  - Appropriate amounts and types of physical activity
  - Achieving physical, psychosocial, and cognitive growth and developmental goals

Because it may take a number of years to achieve and sustain these goals, intermediate goals are needed to assess progress toward reduction of obesity through policy and system changes. Examples include:

- Increased number of children who safely walk and bike to school
- Improved access to and affordability of fruits and vegetables for low-income populations
- Increased availability and use of community recreational facilities
- Increased play and physical activity opportunities
- Increased number of new industry products and advertising messages that promote energy balance at a healthy weight
- Increased availability and affordability of healthful foods and beverages at supermarkets, grocery stores, and farmers markets located within walking distance of the communities they serve
- Changes in institutional and environmental policies that promote energy balance

---

mate aim of obesity prevention in children and youth, however, is to create, through directed social change, an environmental-behavioral synergy that promotes positive outcomes both at the population and individual levels. Box 3-1 summarizes these long-term and intermediate goals, which will be discussed in greater detail throughout the report.

Optimum BMI and Healthy Weight

The concept of optimum BMI can be applied to populations. For countries such as the United States, where undernutrition is not as common as in developing countries,[3] a BMI-distribution median of around 21 kg/m^2 may be optimal (WHO, 2000). Population weight goals for obesity prevention in adults can also be stated in terms of decreasing the proportion that exceed the threshold of 30 kg/m^2, although this goal includes both preventing new cases of obesity and reducing weight among those already over the threshold.

The same principles are appropriate for assessing the population of children in the United States in pursuit of the committee's primary objective: to stop, and eventually reverse, current trends toward higher BMI levels. Also, as discussed in Chapter 2, there are particular concerns about the population of obese children becoming heavier. Achieving this objective would have the effects of reducing the mean BMI as well as decreasing the proportion of children and youth in the population that exceeds the threshold definition of obesity.

Available research does not currently allow the committee to define an optimum BMI for children and youth. It suggests, however, that future research toward this aim should be focused on defining the associations between BMI and objective measures of concurrent and future growth and between BMI and physiological and psychological morbidity, mortality, and health (Robinson, 1993; Robinson and Killen, 2001).

Analogous to the current practice for adults, the committee recommends the use of BMI for assessing individual and population changes in children and youth over time and in response to interventions. Population weight goals for childhood obesity prevention should be stated in terms of changes in the mean BMI and in the shape of the entire BMI distribution. Alternatively, goals can be stated in terms of decreasing the proportion of children or youth who exceed particular thresholds—e.g., 75th, 85th, 90th, 95th, or 97th percentiles of BMI for age and gender on the CDC BMI charts. In the absence of an appropriate evidence base, however, threshold goals are necessarily somewhat arbitrary and sacrifice substantial information about the rest of the distribution as well as substantial statistical power to detect differences between groups and over time (Robinson and Killen, 2001).

---

[3]Hunger and food insecurity persist in the United States. In 2002, 35 million individuals including 13.1 million children lived in food insecure households (an estimated 11 percent of all U.S. households); 3.5 percent (3.8 million) of U.S. households were food insecure with hunger (Nord et al., 2003). Additionally, rates of micronutrient deficiencies remain unacceptably high in certain subgroups of the U.S. population (Wright et al., 1998; Ballew et al., 2001; Ganji et al., 2003; Hampl et al., 2004).

The current CDC guidelines for healthy weight in children and youth are in the range of the 5th to 85th percentiles of the age- and gender-specific BMI charts. Therefore, a child whose weight tracks in that range—that is, he or she does not cross to lower than the 5th or higher than the 85th percentiles—would be considered to be in the healthy weight range according to these definitions.

The CDC BMI charts are mathematically smoothed curves of the pooled growth parameters of children and adolescents sampled in cross-sectional national health surveys conducted from 1963 to 1994. An analogy would be to consider the curves as compiled from a series of "snapshots" of large national samples made at different times over three decades. But because the sample sizes at each age level get much smaller at the extremes of the distributions, the growth curves may be more prone to errors at the upper and lower ends.

Because of the increases in body weight that occurred in the 1980s and 1990s—after the second National Health and Nutrition Examination Survey (NHANES II) conducted in 1976-1980—a decision was made not to include the NHANES III (1988-1994) body-weight data in the revised 2000 BMI charts for children aged 6 years or older. The NHANES III data would have shifted the affected curves (weight-for-age and BMI-for-age) upward, which was considered to be biologically and medically undesirable. However, the fact that the CDC BMI charts were developed from data for a prior time period in which children were leaner, on average, leads to an occasionally confusing situation—for example, where more than 5 percent of the population is above the 95th percentile—but this is readily clarified in the context of the charts' historical source.

The CDC BMI charts are derived from cross-sectional samples of children (data for different age groups are based on different children). That is, they do not directly represent the longitudinal growth trajectory for the same set of children who have been measured as they age.[4] Therefore, it is not known whether an individual child's height, weight, or BMI should be expected to follow along the same percentile curve over time in order to maintain health or whether there are health implications of variations throughout childhood (e.g., crossing percentiles by going from the 20th percentile at age 1 to the 60th percentile at age 5 to the 40th percentile at age 12). Mei and colleagues (2004) found that shifts in growth rates were

---

[4]The latter approach has been used to develop longitudinal growth charts that are used in several other countries (Tanner and Davies, 1985; Cameron, 2002). These types of charts are generally developed from smaller, and potentially less representative, samples.

common during birth to 6 months and less common in children aged 2 to 5 years. More research is needed to determine whether there is an increased prevalence of "crossing" percentiles in different populations or during different age intervals and whether there are associations between crossing percentiles and health-related outcomes.

The problem is how to proceed despite this lack of certainty. The committee concluded that because the CDC BMI charts are based on large national samples of the U.S. population of children and youth, they are the best available tools for assessing growth in clinical and public health settings. Although there are many unknowns about how to apply this information to individual children, and clinicians face difficulties in making generalizations regarding normal growth trajectories, experience suggests that children who demonstrate rapid changes—that is, frequently crossing up or down percentiles—may require special health-care attention. Health- and medical-care professionals should be consulted regarding growth-related questions for individual children as they can assess a child's own growth trajectory in context (see Chapter 6).

ENERGY BALANCE

Obesity prevention involves maintaining energy balance at a healthy weight while protecting overall health, growth and development, and nutritional status. **Energy balance refers to the state in which energy intake is equivalent to energy expenditure, resulting in no net weight gain or weight loss.** In adults, who have stopped growing, this relationship between energy intake and output must be equal and reach a zero net energy balance to prevent body storage of extra calories[5] from food as fat and result in weight gain, which represents a positive energy balance. **Strictly speaking, growing children, even those at a healthy body weight, must be in a slightly positive energy balance to satisfy the additional energy needs of tissue deposition for normal growth. However, for the purpose of simplicity in this report, the committee uses the term "energy balance" in children to indicate an equality between energy intake and energy expenditure that supports normal growth without promoting excess weight gain.**

In children, energy expenditure constitutes the calories used for basal metabolism, processing of food, maintenance and repair of the body, and daily physical activity—in addition to the calories required for normal growth and development. Inappropriate weight gain (excess fat storage) results when energy expenditure is consistently exceeded by energy intake over time.

---

[5]In this report the term "calories" is used synonymously with "kilocalories."

Energy intake is the calories ingested in the form of food and beverages. Children require a dietary pattern consisting of a variety of foods that provide all the necessary nutrients to support normal growth and development, as well as regular physical activity. Thus, a balanced diet refers to the consumption of appropriate amounts of a wide variety of nutrient-dense foods that provide adequate amounts and proportions of macronutrients (protein, fat, and carbohydrates) as well as sufficient essential micronutrients (vitamins, minerals) and dietary fiber, in addition to providing adequate energy to meet the needs of maintenance, growth, and development.

Although "energy intake = energy expenditure" looks like a fairly basic equation, in reality it is extraordinarily complex when considering the multitude of genetic, biological, psychological, sociocultural, and environmental factors that affect both sides of the energy balance equation and the interrelationships among these factors (Figure 3-2). For example, the amount, type, and intensity of physical activity influence body composition and physical fitness, which in turn influence the energy cost of physical activity (Hill et al., 2004).

There are several concepts regarding energy balance and weight gain in children and youth that the committee determined were important to clarify:

• Genetics is a factor in excess weight but it is not the explanation for the recent epidemic of obesity (Koplan and Dietz, 1999). Although inherited tendencies toward weight gain may be a partial explanation for excess weight in children, as discussed below, there have been no measurable changes in the genetic composition of the population during the recent decades that could explain the significant increases in obesity.

• Growth spurts do occur at several points throughout childhood and adolescence, but it cannot be assumed that a child will lose his or her excess weight at those times. Many experienced clinicians assess an individual child's relative weight status by examining the consistency of that child's weight or BMI percentiles over time. Thus, for example, after the age of about 4 years, normally growing children who are in the 20th or 50th or 65th percentile for weight would be expected to remain around these same percentiles for weight, during the remainder of their childhood. However, what can be considered normal variation to that pattern is not yet known, and is an important research question.

• Physiological reasons for a child's excess weight should be carefully explored by health-care professionals. However, the identifiable medical conditions that cause childhood obesity are rare and are not the principal underlying causes of the current obesity epidemic in the population.

• The perceptions of what healthy children should "look like" differ among generations, cultures, and individuals. However, it is important that obesity not become the norm in society for children and youth as it poses

---

BOX 3-2
Balancing Food Intake and Physical Activity

• One small chocolate chip cookie (50 calories) is equivalent to walking brisk-
ly for 10 minutes.
• The difference between a large chocolate chip cookie and a small chocolate
chip cookie is estimated to be about 200 calories or about 40 minutes of raking
leaves.
• One hour of walking at a moderate pace (20 minutes/mile) uses about the
same amount of energy that is in one jelly-filled doughnut (300 calories).
• A fast food meal containing a double patty cheeseburger, extra-large fries,
and a 24 ounce soft drink is equal to running $2^1/_2$ hours at a 10 minute/mile pace
(1500 calories).

SOURCE: DHHS, 2001b.

---

serious health risks during childhood that can continue throughout adult
life.

In the simplest terms, energy balance represents calories consumed
versus calories expended, although as noted above, many individual variables can affect that balance. The discretionary variables under an
individual's control on a daily basis are dietary energy intake and the
energy expended during physical activity.[6] Daily energy intake is determined by the calorie content of the specific food and beverages consumed.
Energy expenditure above resting metabolism is largely dependent on the
nature and intensity of the activity and is often measured in calories per
minute of activity (e.g., walking at a moderate or brisk pace of 3 to 4.5
miles per hour on a level surface expends between 3.5 and 7 calories per
minute as measured in adults [CDC, 2004]). Knowing this, it is possible to
determine the amount of physical activity that would be required to "burn
off" the energy contained in a given food (Box 3-2). The relatively high
amount of physical activity required to balance the calories in many preferred foods highlights the challenges of maintaining energy balance under
conditions of a sedentary lifestyle and when surrounded by abundant food
in large portions at relatively low cost. Much remains to be learned regarding the interactive effects of diet and physical activity—for example, the

---

[6]Resting metabolism also contributes to daily energy expenditure but it is not subject to
modification by the individual in the short term. Resting metabolic rate changes as a function
of body mass and composition which generally takes weeks or months to change under an
applied regimen.

extent to which increased physical activity or decreased dietary intake might improve the body's own ability to regulate energy balance.

Furthermore, greater understanding is needed regarding the relative contribution of energy intake and energy expenditure to the energy imbalance that is driving the obesity epidemic. The increasing prevalence of obesity among children and youth in the United States could be the result of an upward shift in energy intake, a downward shift in energy expenditure, or the occurrence of both trends concurrently (Hill and Peters, 1998; Harnack et al., 2000; Hill et al., 2003). Some researchers have suggested that most of the effect is attributable to excessive energy intake (Sturm, 2005), while others have focused on the decline in regular physical activity and the increase in sedentary behaviors (Cutler et al., 2003).

It has been hypothesized that obesity can result from very small excesses in energy intake relative to expenditure and that the average weight gain in U.S. adults could be prevented if chronic energy expenditure exceeded intake by only 100 calories per day (Hill and Peters, 1998; Hill et al., 2003). However, estimates in a population of Hispanic children have shown greater potential energy gaps, ranging from approximately 200 to 500 calories per day (Butte and Ellis, 2003). This is an area requiring further research.

The following sections provide a brief overview of the context for energy balance and the complexities that researchers and policy makers face in these areas.

Genetic Variation and Biological Considerations

Obesity has long been recognized to occur in families, and having overweight or obese parents increases a child's risk of being obese. After age 3, parental obesity is a stronger predictor of a child's future obesity as an adult than is the child's current weight (Whitaker et al., 1997).

Nonetheless, the familial clustering of obese individuals does not alone predict an individual's weight characteristics, which reflect the combined effects of genetic variations, the common or shared environmental variations within family (which may include both intrauterine and infant feeding factors), and the environmental variations external to the family (Bouchard et al., 2003).

Quantifying with any precision the specific contributions of each of these factors to the development of obesity has been difficult, despite a variety of studies in nuclear families, in families with identical twins reared together or reared apart, and in families with adopted children. Bouchard and colleagues (2003) reviewed approximately 50 such studies and concluded that heritability accounts for about 25 to 40 percent of an individual's expressed variation in weight and body fat mass. Specific maternal or paternal effects could not be identified. Using a new approach to twin studies, Segal and Allison (2002) concluded that common environmental effects might account for approximately 25 percent of the BMI variance in twins. It is important to note the difficulty in assigning proportionality to what is a gene-person-environment interaction.

Similarly, despite its intensity, the search for the specific genes responsible for an individual's obese status has also been difficult. More than 400 genes, markers, and chromosomal regions have been linked to obesity phenotypes, 208 quantitative trait loci for human obesity have been identified, and 41 Mendelian disorders manifesting obesity have been genomically mapped (Snyder et al., 2004). However, only six single-gene defects resulting in obesity have been found, and in fewer than 150 individuals (Snyder et al., 2004). Thus, even though these monogenetic disorders have provided significant insight into the pathophysiology of obesity (Cummings and Schwartz, 2003; O'Rahilly et al., 2003), with few exceptions, human obesity appears to be a complex genetic trait. Nonetheless, genome-wide scans in widely varying populations have identified several genomic regions containing common quantitative trait loci for obesity phenotypes, suggesting that there may be shared genetic factors predisposing individuals of different ethnic origins to excessive storage of body fat (Bouchard et al., 2003). **What is clear, however, is that the genetic characteristics of human populations have not changed in the last three decades, while the prevalence of obesity has approximately doubled. Thus, the recent population rise in body weight reflects the interaction of genotypes that predispose individuals to obesity with detrimental behavioral and environmental factors.**

In animals, the evidence is strong for such gene-environment interactions affecting body weight and energy balance (Barsh et al., 2000), with the responsible genes orchestrating a complex system of biological feedback. In this system, central nervous system signals integrate messages about energy intake sent from the gastrointestinal tract with information about the current status of fuel reserves received from the energy-storing adipose tissue. The result is the direction of ingested food either into storage as fat or dissipation as energy, depending on the body's status and needs at the time (Rosenbaum and Leibel, 1998; Havel, 2000, 2004; Druce and Bloom, 2003; Gale et al., 2004). What now seems clear is that this system evolved to defend the body from excessive energy deficit, a defense mechanism that has far less relevance today, when many humans are exposed to situations of food excess (Schwartz et al., 2003; Havel, 2004). Furthermore, although the system has now been characterized extensively in rodents and in adult humans, little is known about its development during the fetal period, infancy, or childhood (Box 3-3).

BOX 3-3
Food Intake Regulatory Systems

In 1994, it was discovered that a peptide hormone—leptin—is manufactured and secreted by fat cells, travels through the circulatory system, crosses the blood-brain barrier, and acts on the brain's hypothalamus to influence appetite (Zhang et al., 1994). This finding has led to the concept of a "fat-brain axis" (Elmquist and Flier, 2004), a pathway by which events in the periphery of the body are communicated to the brain. As a result, the brain may "monitor" the body's energy or adipose stores and, when indicated, start a chain of events that either initiates or terminates feeding.

There is now evidence that leptin affects both neuronal activity (Pinto et al., 2004) and synaptic plasticity (Bouret et al., 2004) in the arcuate nucleus of the hypothalamus, which is home to two distinct populations of neurons with opposing actions—one group that stimulates food intake and another that suppresses it (Elmquist and Flier, 2004). Furthermore, Bouret and colleagues (2004) suggest that leptin plays a neurotrophic role during the development of the hypothalamus that is restricted to a "neonatal critical period"—that is, the plasticity present early in life is apparently lost by adulthood. Although it is widely appreciated that good nutrition and a healthful lifestyle during the pregnancy period are important for producing healthy babies, these findings raise the possibility that the baby's food-intake and body fat regulatory systems may be permanently shaped during this period.

Future research undoubtedly will be directed to determining whether this communication system is indeed fundamental to the mechanisms of food-intake and body fat regulation in humans, and whether its timing is so narrowly focused.

Psychosocial and Behavioral Considerations

Dietary Intake

Everyone needs to eat food and consume beverages for daily sustenance. But beyond the physical necessities are the complex social, cultural, and emotional nuances that involve food and permeate many facets of daily life. Children and adults alike consume food and beverages in part because they are hungry but also because eating and drinking are pleasurable and are an integral part of family life, celebrations, recreational events, and other social occasions. Food is also important in the psychosocial well-being, emotional expression, and coping responses of many people. It is, therefore, unrealistic to base recommended eating patterns solely on the chemical composition of foods without taking cultural, social, economic, and emotional drivers of food consumption into account. Furthermore, while few would dispute the negative aspects of individual substances such as tobacco, alcohol, or illegal drugs, there have been strong debates over

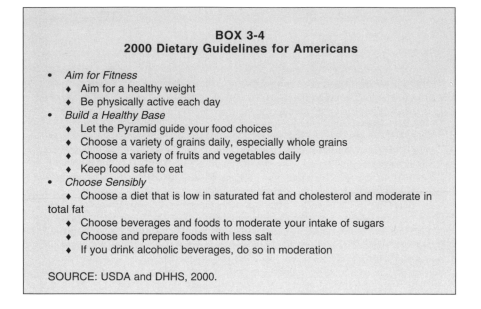

BOX 3-4
2000 Dietary Guidelines for Americans

- *Aim for Fitness*
  - ◆ Aim for a healthy weight
  - ◆ Be physically active each day
- *Build a Healthy Base*
  - ◆ Let the Pyramid guide your food choices
  - ◆ Choose a variety of grains daily, especially whole grains
  - ◆ Choose a variety of fruits and vegetables daily
  - ◆ Keep food safe to eat
- *Choose Sensibly*
  - ◆ Choose a diet that is low in saturated fat and cholesterol and moderate in
total fat
  - ◆ Choose beverages and foods to moderate your intake of sugars
  - ◆ Choose and prepare foods with less salt
  - ◆ If you drink alcoholic beverages, do so in moderation

SOURCE: USDA and DHHS, 2000.

"good foods" versus "bad foods, even taking a purely nutritional perspective. Energy intake and dietary quality are determined by the total amounts and combination of foods consumed. A given food or beverage may have multiple nutritional quality dimensions and will have a differential impact on the overall eating pattern depending on what other foods are eaten. Nevertheless, the frequency of consuming certain types of foods is an indicator of the likelihood that the overall quantity and quality of foods will be appropriate, particularly in growing children for whom the nutrient density of diets (i.e., adequacy of vitamins and minerals per unit of energy intake) is important.

Based on current scientific evidence, the Dietary Guidelines for Americans provide nutritional advice to the American public on how to attain a balanced diet (defined in this report as an overall dietary pattern that provides all the essential nutrients in the appropriate amounts to meet nutritional needs and support life processes such as growth in children without promoting excess weight gain[7]) (Boxes 3-4 and 3-5; also see Chapter 5 and Appendix B).

Based on the Dietary Guidelines for Americans, the Healthy Eating

---

[7]The U.S. Dietary Guidelines for Americans are currently under revision and the sixth edition will be released in 2005. The Food Guide Pyramid is an educational tool that depicts qualitative dietary guidance based on the principles of balance, proportionality, and moderation.

BOX 3-5
Benefits Associated with a Healthful Diet

- **A low-fat, low-saturated-fat, and low-cholesterol diet** is associated with reduced risk of coronary heart disease.
- **Fruits and vegetables** supply fiber which binds to lipids such as cholesterol and decreases their concentration in the blood, thereby decreasing the risk of coronary heart disease. Increased consumption is also associated with lower caloric intake, lower percentage of calories from fat, and a lower BMI. Fruits and vegetables provide vitamins A, C, and E that are essential for normal metabolism and may act as antioxidants, thus reducing the risk of developing certain cancers (including stomach, esophageal, lung, and colorectal cancers).
  - Diets that are **moderate in salt** help prevent high blood pressure.
  - Diets that are **moderate in sugar** help prevent tooth decay.
- **Calcium** maintains healthy bones and teeth and plays a vital role in nerve conduction, muscle contraction, and blood coagulation. Adequate calcium intake during childhood and adolescence is key to peak bone-mass development and the prevention of osteoporosis later in life.

SOURCES: IOM, 1997, 2002, 2004; USDA and DHHS, 2000.

Index (HEI) is a tool developed by the U.S. Department of Agriculture to assess diet quality in order to provide a comprehensive assessment of diet in the U.S. population. A low HEI score suggests a poor diet and is also associated with overweight and obesity (Guo et al., 2004). Thus, the use of the HEI and the Dietary Guidelines for Americans as a way to improve health should be emphasized. However, the overall effectiveness of the Dietary Guidelines for Americans in disease prevention requires further research (Guo et al., 2004).

There are some indications of a small but significant increase in the average number of calories consumed daily by children over the last 15 to 20 years. The Continuing Survey of Food Intakes by Individuals, which examined changes between two time periods—1989-1991 and 1994-1996—in nationally representative samples of school-aged children, found an increase from 88 to 94 percent of the recommended energy allowance (Gleason and Suitor, 2001). Because no changes were seen in the energy intake from breakfast or lunch, the authors suggest that the increase was due to increased food consumption at dinner or in the form of snacks. Subsequent analyses of trends in energy intakes of children and youth have produced mixed findings (Enns et al., 2002; Nielsen et al., 2002; Sturm, 2005), and much remains to be learned about the dietary factors that contribute to the obesity epidemic in these groups.

Many challenges remain in conducting research on children's dietary intake. They include difficulties in children accurately recalling and quantifying foods consumed, the accuracy of third-party reports (usually parents or caregivers), and varying estimations of portion size. Use of the 24-hour recall method is common, but the need to collect information for multiple days to determine typical intake of foods or nutrients makes it a time- and labor-consuming process (Goran, 1998). Furthermore, the energy requirements for children vary, depending on the timing of growth and developmental spurts, and may be highly individualized.

Physical Activity

Physical activity, which has been defined as "any bodily movement produced by skeletal muscles that results in energy expenditure" (Caspersen et al., 1985), is in many respects synonymous with childhood. One of the joys and benefits of childhood is that being physically active is often a natural and fun part of playing and interacting with family and friends and does not generally involve a conscious decision to exercise. This play time is also developmentally important for children's cognitive, motor-skill, and social development (NRC and IOM, 2000). Physical activity—not only in free play time, but in school, organized sports, and other activities—is an integral part of many children's daily routines. However, as children grow, they generally become less physically active in adolescence and adulthood (Caspersen et al., 2000; Sallis, 2000). Additionally, children's patterns of physical activity often differ from those of older adolescents and adults. Children often engage in intermittent activity mixed with brief periods of rest rather than in prolonged exercise (Goran et al., 1999).

Current recommendations are for children and adolescents to accumulate a minimum of 60 minutes of moderate to vigorous physical activity each day (Biddle et al., 1998; USDA and DHHS, 2000; Cavill et al., 2001; IOM, 2002; NASPE, 2004). The National Association for Sport and Physical Education recommends that children aged 5 through 12 years be involved in age-appropriate physical activity (including moderate to vigorous physical activity, most of it intermittent) that adds up to at least 60 minutes—and as much as several hours—per day on most days of the week (NASPE, 2004). Furthermore, long periods (two hours or more) of inactivity during the day time are discouraged in this age group. One of the strongest correlates of physical activity in children is time spent outside (Klesges et al., 1990; Baranowski et al., 1993; Sallis et al., 1993).

The health and quality-of-life benefits associated with regular moderate physical activity extend beyond the prevention of obesity (CDC, 1997) (Box 3-6). One of the major research challenges in this area is how to accurately measure physical activity, particularly in young children. Tools and techniques vary in terms of their intrusiveness into normal daily rou-

---

BOX 3-6
Benefits Associated with Physical Activity
for Children and Adolescents

Cardiovascular System
- Improves plasma lipid/lipoprotein profile, including reduction of low-density lipoproteins (LDLs) and increase of high-density lipoproteins (HDLs) in children and youth with at-risk levels. Elevated plasma LDL and lowered HDL are risk factors for the development of coronary heart disease (CHD) and evidence indicates that atherosclerosis begins in childhood.
- Prevents or delays the development of hypertension and decreases blood pressure.

Musculoskeletal System
- Develops higher peak bone masses (which have been linked with reduced risk of osteoporosis in adulthood), increases bone-mineral density and bone size (which confers bone strength), and decreases the likelihood of fractures.
- Increases muscular strength and aerobic endurance
- Maintains joint structure and function
- Increases fat-free mass, reduces body-fat percentage

Mental Health, Psychological and Emotional Well-Being
- Reduces stress and symptoms of depression and anxiety
- Improves self-esteem and body image

Chronic Disease Prevention
- Helps prevent chronic diseases such as hypertension, type 2 diabetes, obesity, and cardiovascular diseases.
- Improves overall health and improves adult health status

SOURCES: DHHS, 1996; Sothern et al., 1999; Boreham and Riddock, 2001; Maziekas et al., 2003.

---

tines (perhaps affecting activity level) and in the cost and time needed to collect and monitor the results. Questionnaires of parents and children are often confounded by recall problems and varying assessments of the type, intensity, and duration of the activity (Saris, 1986; Goran, 1998; Sirard and Pate, 2001). Measures of motion (e.g., pedometers and accelerometers) have come into wide use as research tools in recent years, but additional work is needed to ensure the validity of these methods in diverse groups of children and youth and in diverse settings. Additionally, research is needed to establish better methods of measurement of energy expenditure in children going through their normal daily activities in their home and school environments.

Sociocultural and Other Environmental Considerations

The specific types and levels of environmental factors to be considered as influences on food intake and physical activity are numerous. Tables 3-1 and 3-2 provide an illustrative listing of factors operating within different ecological layers (Swinburn et al., 1999). What is available with respect to food intake and physical activity opportunities (physical environment) is influenced by policies and financial inputs (political and economic environments) and is also targeted to the sociocultural milieu. Availability affects the range of possible individual choices, but personal choice is also mediated through a range of sociocultural variables that differ by age, gender, ethnicity, region, neighborhood characteristics, and socioeconomic status.

This matrix of environmental levels and types can also be developed to facilitate consideration of influences on obesity-related variables such as the availability of education and counseling and broader health promotion about weight gain prevention (physical environment), cost of preventive services (economic), and coverage of preventive services by third-party payers (policy environment). As discussed in the following sections, in the sociocultural domain, attitudes about body size and obesity are also critical contextual considerations when designing obesity prevention interventions.

Considerations Regarding Stigmatization

One of the concerns that arises in discussions regarding the prevention of childhood obesity is how to effectively focus on the behaviors that contribute to obesity without stigmatizing obese children and youth. As noted in Chapter 2, there is a body of research indicating that obese children and youth are stigmatized and experience negative stereotyping and discrimination by their peers, with adverse social and emotional consequences (Schwartz and Puhl, 2003).

Given that the stigmatization of obese children appears to have increased over a 40-year period from 1961 to 2001, there is a need to focus on the sensitivities regarding this issue and to explicitly reduce negative attitudes and behaviors such as teasing and discrimination directed toward obese children and youth (Latner and Stunkard, 2003; Schwartz and Puhl, 2003). This focus needs to be a consideration in the design of the range of interventions discussed throughout this report.

There is also the need to consider the adverse effects of normalization when discussing stigmatization. In many ways, American society has become more accepting of larger sizes in the products and portions we consume. Furthermore, our society often accommodates obesity as the social norm, for example, by resizing clothing, expanding the width of seating in public areas, and retrofitting ambulances to accommodate larger girth

TABLE 3-1 Examples of Environmental Influences on Food Intake, by Type of Environment

Size or Level of the Environment	Type of Environment: Food-Related Influences			
	Physical	Economic	Policy/Political	Sociocultural
Microenvironments (e.g., behavioral settings such as homes, schools, and communities)	• Location and type of food stores • Vending machine placement and products • Point-of-purchase information • Local food production	• Locally imposed taxes • Vendor pricing policies • Financial support for health promotion programs • Sponsorship of healthful food policies and practices	• Family rules related to food purchasing and consumption • Food policies of local schools or school districts	• "Ethos" or climate related to food and eating in the home, school, and neighborhood • Role models for eating behaviors at home, in school, and in community settings (e.g., churches)
Macroenvironments (e.g., societal sectors such as food and agriculture, education, medical, government, public health, or health care)	• Food production/ importing • Food manufacturing • Food marketing • Federal nutrition labeling guidelines	• Costs of food production, manufacturing, and distribution • Taxes, pricing policies, subsidies • Wage structure and other factors that influence personal and household income	• National food and nutrition policies, regulations, and laws, including food labeling • Food industry standards and practices • Regulations and guidelines on advertising to children	• Mass media influences on food selections and eating behaviors • General consumer trends in food and eating

SOURCE: Adapted from Swinburn et al., 1999.

TABLE 3-2 Examples of Environmental Influences on Physical Activity, by Type of Environment

Size or Level of the Environment	Type of Environment			
	Physical	Economic	Policy/Political	Sociocultural
Microenvironments (e.g., behavioral settings such as homes, schools, and communities)	• Sidewalks and footpaths • Cycle paths • Public transportation • Street lights • Recreational facilities and clubs	• Cost of gym memberships • Budget allocations for recreation centers or walking and cycling paths • Funding for improved public transport • Sponsorship of physical activity-related health promotion • Influences on household income and time expenditures	• Family rules about television watching • Family rules about household chores • Restrictions on automobile traffic • Restrictions on bicycle or pedestrian traffic • Zoning for protection of open spaces • Building codes	• "Ethos" or climate related to physical activity and inactivity in the home, school, and neighborhood • Role models for physical activity and inactivity in the home, at school, and in the neighborhood
Macroenvironments (e.g. societal sectors such as food and agriculture, education, medical, government, public health or health care)	• Automobile industry	• Public transport funding and subsidies	• State-level policies on physical education in schools	• Mass media influences on physical activity and inactivity • General consumer trends in patterns of physical activity and inactivity

SOURCE: Adapted from Swinburn et al., 1999.

(Newman, 2004). Just as there are social and emotional consequences of stigmatization, there are also social and health consequences for obesity becoming the accepted social norm. This tension between stigmatization and normalization can be addressed, as it has been for other public health concerns, by focusing on the behaviors that can be changed to promote health rather than on the individual and his or her appearance.

It is important to note that the lessons learned from tobacco prevention and control efforts are not entirely applicable to obesity prevention. Bans against smoking in public buildings, on airplanes, and at other locations have encouraged some people to quit smoking due to the added inconvenience and public disapproval of this behavior. However, foods and beverages are necessary for sustenance and the issue is not "whether or not" to eat but rather what to eat, how much, and how often.

Areas of further research on this issue include how to encourage children to accept peers of all sizes and shapes and how to assist and support parents, teachers, children, and youth in addressing and coping with social stigma.

Body Image

A community's norms, values, and expectations also affect the way that children in the normal or overweight (but not obese) range view their bodies. There is also concern that obesity prevention efforts will lead to inappropriate weight concern, dieting preoccupation, or unhealthful weight control practices among children and youth. Attitudes toward body size differ across cultures and especially affect females. Standards of attractiveness in males are less weight-dependent. Consistent with the stigma associated with being obese, the dominant attitudes in the United States and many similar societies favor a thin or lean body type in females, although as discussed below there is cultural variation in the degree of fatness or thinness that is acceptable as well as in preferred body shapes (Brown and Bentley-Condit, 1998). Attitudes about acceptable body size and shape also change over time and may apply differently to people of different ages.

The potential importance of this issue is underscored by reports of weight concerns in young children and in adolescents, in numerous ethnic groups, and in both low and high socioeconomic strata (see Chapter 2). Studies of children as young as the first grade have reported that a substantial proportion of children (about 50 percent of girls and 30 to 40 percent of boys), when given a choice of silhouettes will choose a thinner body size than their own as the "ideal" body size (Thompson et al., 1997). Robinson and colleagues (2001) studied a multiethnic and socioeconomically diverse sample of third graders (mean age was 8.5 years) in 13 northern California elementary schools, and reported that concerns about being obese and dissatisfaction with body size were highly prevalent, increased with increasing BMI, and present—although to varying degrees—in all socioeconomic strata and ethnic groups. Furthermore, a study of 4,700 adolescents in Minnesota public schools (grades 7 through 12; mean age was 15 years) found high body satisfaction (versus low or moderate) in only 20 percent of girls and 34 percent of boys (Neumark-Sztainer et al., 2002).

Several studies have examined potential correlates of body image dissatisfaction and weight concerns or dieting practices, particularly gender, ethnicity, and socioeconomic status. Most of the studies that have examined ethnic differences consistently find less weight concern, less body size dissatisfaction, and a heavier ideal body size in African-American girls compared with white girls, but not necessarily boys, and sometimes demonstrate significant differences within African Americans across different socioeconomic levels (e.g., concern was greater at higher levels) (Thompson et al., 1997; Brown et al., 1998; Halpern et al., 1999; Adams et al., 2000; Neumark-Sztainer et al., 2002). These findings in children and adolescents are generally parallel to the numerous studies in adults indicating a relatively lower level of weight concern and higher level of body satisfaction in black women compared to white women; even considering the higher weight levels of the black women (Flynn and Fitzgibbon, 1998).

In contrast to the data for African Americans, available studies suggest that weight concerns in Hispanic and Asian girls are comparable to or exceed those in non-Hispanic white girls (Robinson et al., 2001; Neumark-Sztainer et al., 2002). The finding in Hispanic girls is consistent with data in adults (Serdula et al., 1999). Data for Native Americans in the Minnesota study (which were adjusted for grade level, socioeconomic status, and BMI) indicated a similar level of body satisfaction to that in white girls, but a significantly lower level of concern about controlling their weight (Neumark-Sztainer et al., 2002).

Socioeconomic Status

Socioeconomic status has generally been inversely associated with obesity prevalence (see Chapter 2) and children with obese mothers and low family income were found to have significantly elevated risks of becoming obese, independent of other demographic and socioeconomic factors (Strauss and Knight, 1999). When compared with food-insufficient households of higher income, low-income food-insufficient households had more obese children; however, food insufficiency by itself was not associated with self-reported measures of childhood obesity (Casey et al., 2001). Other studies have not been able to show a clear relationship between childhood obesity and food insufficiency or food insecurity[8] after adjusting for other confounding variables (Alaimo et al., 2001b; Kaiser et al., 2002; Matheson et al., 2002). However, food insecurity is associated with adverse health outcomes in infants and toddlers below 36 months of age (Cook et al., 2004) and with negative academic and psychosocial outcomes including depression in older children (Alaimo et al., 2001a, 2002).

Many of the variables in Tables 3-1 and 3-2 may be potential mediators of the relationship between socioeconomic inequities and childhood obesity. Both food and physical activity options are more likely to be periodically inadequate, unpredictable, or of lower quality for those with low personal incomes or those living in low-income neighborhoods (Travers, 1996; Morland et al., 2002a,b; Addy et al., 2004; Fitzgibbon and Stolley, 2004; Molnar et al., 2004). Poverty and living in low-income neighborhoods limit access to healthful foods. Some types of leisure-time physical activity are theoretically available at low or no cost, but these options may be less available to children in low-income neighborhoods because of neighborhood safety concerns, lack of adult supervision, or limited community recreational or other resources. Addressing childhood obesity in these contexts will require attention to root causes, and attempts to mitigate the underlying social and environmental adversity will be needed (Travers, 1997).

Racial and Ethnic Disparities

The substantially higher prevalence of obesity in adults, children, and youth in some African-American, Hispanic, American-Indian, and Pacific Islander populations (see Chapter 2) generates considerations across the entire ecologic framework (see Figure 3-2). A relatively high obesity prevalence in some Hispanic and American-Indian groups was noted prior to the obesity epidemic (Kumanyika, 1993); the pattern of excess weight gain and accelerated rates of obesity prevalence in African-American children and youth is a more recent development. It is now understood that issues of race are much more complex than the traditional U.S. Census Bureau racial and ethnic groupings often used in epidemiological research (Cooper, 2003; Cooper et al., 2003). However, the different historical and geographical

---

[8]*Food insufficiency* is defined as inadequacy in the amount of food intake because of limited money or resources. *Food insecurity* is the limited or uncertain availability of nutritionally adequate and safe foods, or the inability to acquire such foods in a socially acceptable way. Although these definitions are similar, food insecurity describes a broader condition that not only encompasses food insufficiency but also the psychological and other dimensions of the food system (Cook et al., 2004).

trajectories of these social and politically defined groups are associated with some differences in gene frequencies that may be linked with obesity development. Regardless, as discussed earlier in this chapter, the predominant factors responsible for the expression of obesity as a general population phenomenon are the linked behavioral and environmental factors outlined in the framework in Figure 3-2.

Many factors that potentially mediate racial and ethnic differences and predispose minority children and youth to high obesity risks can be postulated across physical, economic, sociocultural, and policy/political environments (Tables 3-1 and 3-2). Socioeconomic inequities are disproportionately common in minority populations and some of the excess risk may be mediated through economic and physical environmental factors related to low income or living in low-income communities. Other factors may affect individuals and communities on the basis of sociocultural factors that are not dependent upon socioeconomic status. Eating and physical activity patterns in some minority communities are less favorable to weight control than those in the general population, and these differences are observed within socioeconomic strata (Kumanyika and Krebs-Smith, 2001). For example, targeted marketing of high-calorie, low-nutrient-dense foods on black-oriented television has been reported (Tirodkar and Jain, 2003). Less access to supermarkets or to good quality food in supermarkets has been associated with black neighborhoods (Morland et al., 2002a) (see Chapter 6).

Sociocultural variables that need to be considered when approaching obesity prevention to reduce racial and ethnic disparities include traditional cuisines and any aspect of the attitudes, beliefs, and values (referred to in Tables 3-1 and Table 3-2 as the ethos or climate) that may facilitate or inhibit the promotion of healthful eating, physical activity, and weight control patterns in children and youth in these communities (Kumanyika and Morssink, 1997; Kumanyika, 2002, 2004). This ethos may include cultural values of responsiveness to or harmonization with the existing environmental context, as opposed to assumptions that the context can (or should) necessarily be changed. Included in the sociocultural environment are the high prevalence of obesity (e.g., the normative presence of the problem) as well as high levels of obesity-related health problems. In addition, to the extent that a history of discrimination or marginalization based on race or ethnicity becomes intertwined with other sociocultural factors, a certain level of skepticism or distrust relative to mainstream information and initiatives, including health information, may influence the receptivity to obesity prevention messages—particularly when these messages seem to conflict with pre-existing attitudes and beliefs.

REVIEW OF THE EVIDENCE

The committee identified a primary prevention, population-based approach to be the most viable long-term strategy for reducing obesity and its chronic disease burdens. Examples of the effectiveness of primary prevention interventions include smoking cessation to reduce lung cancer incidence, condom use to lower HIV transmission, and fruit and vegetable consumption to prevent cancer and cardiovascular diseases (CVDs) (Kroke et al., 2003; WHO, 2003).

There is no single acceptable standard, however, for assessing the entire range of prevention interventions and programs (Kellam and Langevin, 2003). Each phase of prevention research involves specific criteria for evidence and a variety of possible research designs. This is often a process whereby the preceding phase of research informs the subsequent generation of research—from efficacy to effectiveness, sustainability, going-to-scale, and, finally, sustaining system-wide[9] (Figure 3-3). Numerous evidence-based prevention strategies are currently being used, though their focus—whether on individuals, institutions, or societal structures—can vary (Kellam and Langevin, 2003).

An Evidence-Based Medicine Approach

Evidence-based medicine is a valuable concept for informing clinical medicine that provides universally accepted standards for testing the scientific method and developing clinical practice guidelines (Harris et al., 2001; Heller and Page, 2002). This approach uses an accepted hierarchy of evidence—in accordance with its type, quality, and strength—to support recommendations (Table 3-3) (Harris et al., 2001; Kroke et al., 2003), and it establishes a cause-and-effect relationship guided by the principles of predictability, replicability, generalizability, and falsifiability. Predictability depends on a properly implemented intervention producing expected outcomes, a clear understanding of the intervention's elements, and a cause-and-effect interaction among those elements (Tang et al., 2003). Replicability and generalizability rely on an intervention's potential for

---

[9]*Efficacy* research addresses whether an intervention produces a beneficial impact under optimal conditions of implementation and scientific rigor. *Effectiveness* research tests an intervention under normal conditions such as those in which the intervention may be employed. *Sustainability* research assesses whether the training and support structures developed for effectiveness trials can work to continue the implementation of the intervention by other implementers and with other cohorts of the population. *Going-to-scale* research designs and tests methods of training, support, and assessment that can be implemented across an entire system. *Sustaining system-wide* research determines how to maintain high-quality standards for an entire program over the long term (Kellam and Langevin, 2003).

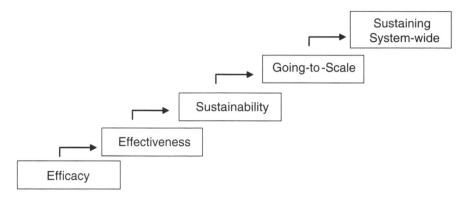

FIGURE 3-3 Five phases of prevention research.
SOURCE: Reprinted with permission, from Kellam and Langevin, 2003. Copyright 2003 by *Prevention Science.*

universal application that is independent of time, place, or context (Tang et al., 2003). Falsifiability refers to the possibility that an evaluation could determine, if relevant, that the intervention is ineffective (Tang et al., 2003).

An evidence-based medicine approach has been adopted by federal and scientific institutions to guide obesity treatment in adults (NHLBI, 1998). However, efforts to apply its principles to identifying effective interventions for other areas of disease prevention and health promotion have met with varying degrees of success (Osaka Declaration, 2001; McQueen, 2002; WHO, 2003; Victora et al., 2004). Indeed, it has been suggested that clinical decisions may have a relatively small impact on health outcomes compared to changes in the social environment, and that broadening evidence-based medicine beyond clinical policy decision-making—to public health decision-making—often has the potential to produce a larger beneficial impact on the health of populations (Heller and Page, 2002).

An Evidence-Based Public Health Approach

As the public health and health promotion disciplines have evolved, *evidence-based public health* has become the goal with a knowledge base that includes disease frequency and distribution; correlates, determinants and consequences of disease; and the safety, efficacy, effectiveness, and cost-effectiveness of a range of interventions (Victora et al., 2004). But given the complex environment in which multiple social, economic, cultural, and political elements interact to produce change in population-wide problems such as obesity, causality may not always be established for the

TABLE 3-3 Hierarchy of Research Design Used for Evidence-Based Clinical Medicine

Level of Evidence	Type of Study
I	Evidence obtained from at least one properly designed randomized controlled trial (RCT) that provides a consistent pattern of findings in the population for which a recommendation is made.
II-1	Evidence obtained from well-designed controlled trials without randomization.
II-2	Evidence obtained from well-designed cohort or case-controlled analytical studies, preferably from more than one center or research group.
II-3	Evidence obtained from multiple time-series or correlational studies with or without then intervention.
III	Evidence obtained from opinions of respected authorities, based on clinical experience, descriptive studies and case reports, or reports of expert committees.

SOURCES: Harris et al., 2001; Kroke et al., 2003.

relationships among the various interventions (McQueen, 2002; Tang et al., 2003).

Several factors complicate the task. The first is complexity in the causal sequences, including mediating factors, multiple causes acting simultaneously (some independently, others interactively), and the potential for unintended consequences from well-intended interventions. The second factor is that scientific uncertainty is associated with many or most of the causal links, which can vary across different social contexts and be constrained by current methods and ethical limitations (NRC, 1994). A third factor is that individuals and groups differ in the benefits and costs they attach to each of the causes, potential solutions, intended outcomes, and unintended consequences (Slovic, 1987, 2000). It has been suggested that there can be no purely scientific answer to the question of what should be done because the answer depends on social values (NRC, 1978). A fourth factor is that individuals and groups vary in how much uncertainty they are willing to tolerate before acting to address a problem (NRC, 1989).

The conclusion that results from these well-established principles is that while scientists can strive to clarify causal relations and reduce uncertainty, they are incapable of recommending specific actions (or inaction) without making implicit value judgments (NRC, 1978, 1996). The solution to this dilemma ideally lies in the development and application of new approaches for integrating scientific considerations with social and normative considerations in a transparent, fair, and competent manner (Renn et al., 1995; NRC, 1996; Klinke and Renn, 2002).

Although randomized controlled trials (RCTs) are the gold standard for testing interventions in clinical and public health research, it is not always feasible, appropriate, or ethical to use that methodology in conducting population-based research; furthermore, RCTs may not always illuminate the complexity of some population-based prevention strategies (Robinson et al., 1998; Briss et al., 2000).

Therefore, the evidence base regarding public health prevention efforts often involves the integration of a range of research methodologies. Several health promotion and disease prevention initiatives have implemented comprehensive population health programs using a broader integrated approach to the evidence. For example, Table 3-4 illustrates the different approaches required for guiding the design of individual and community-based approaches to CVD prevention (Osaka Declaration, 2001).

TABLE 3-4 Comparison of Individual and Community Approaches for CVD Prevention

Clinical Practice Approaches for Individuals	Community and Population-Based Approaches for Health Promotion
The evidence standards are RCTs	The evidence standards are RCTs and outcome and process evaluations that use both quantitative and qualitative methods
The focus is on individual patients	The focus is on the community
Less than a therapeutic dose is unacceptable	Preventive dose rarely applies
Easier to treat an individual	Difficult to scale up health promotion programs that reach the entire population
Outcomes of interventions are individual change	Outcomes are to change social norms, environments, and the behavior of entire populations
Interventions can focus on most factors relevant to outcomes	Interventions rarely take on social determinants external to the community

SOURCE: Adapted from Osaka Declaration, 2001.

Developing Recommendations Based on an Integrated
Approach to the Evidence

The committee faced a significant challenge in deciding what types of evidence to use in formulating recommendations for obesity prevention in children and youth. A review of randomized controlled interventions for obesity prevention and treatment among children and adolescents identified only 35 such studies (Campbell et al., 2002). Due to the limited number of RCTs in obesity prevention efforts and methodological issues, including small sample sizes and high attrition rates of study participants, there is a paucity of RCT data from which to generalize results to broader populations (NHS Centre for Reviews and Dissemination, 2002).

The committee, therefore, developed guidelines for an integrated use of the available evidence to inform population-based obesity prevention interventions and on which to base its recommendations. This was deemed necessary to enhance the biological, psychosocial, and environmental plausibility of its inferences and identify consistency and congruency of information due to the paucity of causal research. Such an integrated-evidence approach has been used successfully to apply science-based principles to other public health efforts (Appendix D), such as in establishing a framework for evaluating the safety of dietary-supplement ingredients (IOM and NRC, 2004).

As childhood obesity is a serious public health problem calling for immediate reductions in obesity prevalence and in its health and social consequences, the committee strongly believed that actions should be based on the best *available* evidence—as opposed to waiting for the best *possible* evidence.

The different types of evidence that the committee used in developing the report's recommendations are illustrated in Table 3-5, and the following principles guided the committee's process:

- Evidence is needed to inform and guide policy and programmatic decisions, justify a course of action, and evaluate the effectiveness of interventions that support obesity prevention.
- Although the strength of the evidence is a basis for policy development, other considerations—including the fiscal and sociopolitical climate within which governments, institutions, and communities operate—must also be taken into account (Tang et al., 2003).
- Absence of experimental evidence does not indicate a lack of causation or the ineffectiveness of an obesity prevention intervention. Given the methodological challenges, as well as the complexities in linkages between different elements and in their environments, certain interventions may prove effective even though their mechanisms for success are not known.

TABLE 3-5 Proposed Components of Evidence-Based Obesity Prevention

Objective	Policy or Program Relevance	Relevant Evidence and Information	Types of Outputs
Estimate the Health Burden Why should we do something about obesity?	• Show urgency of taking action on obesity • Compare costs, health burden, and gains from prevention with other risk factors and diseases • Address prioritization of obesity relative to other issues • Identify populations of special interest • Benchmarks for goal setting	• Monitoring and surveillance data (e.g., prevalence, trends) • Observational studies (e.g., relative risks, occurrence rates in different populations) • Economic analyses (e.g., costs of obesity, disability-adjusted life years [DALYs] lost) • Informed opinion (e.g., for modeling assumptions)	• Prevalence estimates including projected trends • Estimates of the costs of obesity (direct, indirect, intangible) • Comparative health burdens in terms of years of life or DALYs lost • Estimated possible reductions in burden with interventions
Identify the Determinants What are the causative and protective factors that could potentially be targeted by interventions?	• Identify targets for intervening • Relate obesity issues to other existing agendas • Identify congruent and conflicting policies and activities • Identify the key government, nongovernmental organization, and private sector stakeholders that are central to obesity prevention	• Observational studies • Experimental studies • Indirect evidence • Monitoring and surveillance data • Informed opinion (e.g., on current policies and activities that influence obesity)	• Evidence reviews of specific modifiable determinants of obesity and its pathways including levels of certainty and likely size of impact • Identified important stakeholder groups and areas of congruence and conflict

Step	Objectives	Sources of Evidence	Outputs
Describe the Framework for Action How and where should we intervene?	• Links to and compatibility with existing plans, policies, and programs • Specification of the comprehensive and multi-dimensional nature of the action needed • Persuasion of stakeholders of the feasibility and necessity of a comprehensive approach • Evidence of precedence	• Parallel evidence from other public health initiatives • Pre-existing frameworks for action (e.g., Ottawa Charter) • Informed opinion (e.g., about other successful frameworks and feasible strategies) • Information on current relevant initiatives • Program logic and theory	• Comprehensive obesity prevention in a standalone framework or as part of a broader plan of action for nutrition and physical activity, and/or noncommunicable diseases • Identified settings, sectors, and support actions, and short- and long-term population goals
Evaluate Potential Interventions What are the specific and potential interventions and their likely effectiveness?	• Consensus on potential concrete actions • Move obesity initiatives through the agenda-setting process • Identify resource implications	• Experimental studies • Observational studies • Effectiveness analyses • Economic analyses • Program logic and theory • Process evaluation (e.g., of existing community or demonstration interventions)	• Specific descriptions of interventions and support actions • Effectiveness, cost-effectiveness, or cost-utility estimates for the interventions
Select a Portfolio of Policies, Programs, and Actions What is a comprehensive portfolio of initiatives that is sufficient to prevent increases in obesity?	• Gain stakeholder input into judgments on policy and implementation implications • Gain stakeholder support for priority interventions	• Informed opinion on specific interventions and actions regarding their feasibility and sustainability; potential other positive or negative potential impacts; effects on equity; and acceptability to stakeholders	• Specific portfolio of policies, programs, and other actions to prevent obesity

SOURCE: Adapted from Swinburn et al., 2005.

This has been exemplified by programs that reduce television viewing time and decrease BMI in children (Robinson, 1999).

• Given the significant shortage at present of experimental evidence to guide programs and policies, and the fact that many societal variables of interest have not been well addressed in controlled experimental studies as moderating or mediating factors, obesity prevention will require an evidence-based public health approach that continues to draw on RCTs, quasi-experiments, and observational studies as important sources of information (Victora et al., 2004).

• Given that obesity is a serious health risk, preventive actions should be taken even if there is as-yet-incomplete scientific evidence on the interventions to address specific causes and correlates of obesity. However, there is an obligation to accumulate appropriate evidence not only to justify a course of action but to assess whether it has made a difference.

• Finally, for interventions that have minimal potential risk and require few resources, formative and process evaluations may be sufficient to provide a "preponderance" of evidence (Robinson et al., 1998).

As described in Appendix C, the committee conducted a thorough bibliographic search of the relevant scientific databases and benefited from the expertise of academic, industry, government, and nonprofit sector experts during its deliberations. In examining the literature, the committee focused on studies that examined weight and body composition outcomes, but it also broadened its scope to include studies that looked at changes in physical activity (or sedentary behavior) levels and in dietary intake patterns.

In examining the evidence on obesity-related prevention interventions, the committee considered the methodologies used by individual studies. Evaluating such studies involves characterizing the appropriateness of their designs for measuring target outcomes (e.g., increasing physical activity) as well as assessing the quality and generalizability of the study execution. The committee also considered the strength of the overall body of available evidence. Other factors considered by the committee included the feasibility of implementing the recommended actions, the opportunities for making changes, and the past success of parallel public health and social change efforts. Where trends of social, dietary, and other factors and health outcomes ran in parallel, the committee believes these trends merit further study and concern while acknowledging the possible occurrence of confounding.

It is also important to note that the committee focused on areas for improvement rather than on specific products, mechanisms for distribution, or industries. For example, the report emphasizes the nutritional evaluation of the contents of vending machines in schools rather than the removal of vending machines (Chapter 7); considers the nutrient quality and energy density of foods and beverages rather than focusing on specific types of products (e.g., soft drinks, chips, candy); and highlights the improvements needed and actions that can promote energy balance rather than addressing any one industry (e.g., fast food restaurants).

SUMMARY

This report uses the term "obese" to refer to children and youth between the ages of 2 and 18 years who have BMIs equal to or greater than the 95th percentile of the age- and gender-specific BMI charts developed by CDC. For individuals, obesity prevention involves maintaining energy balance at a healthy weight while protecting overall health, growth and development, and nutritional status. Energy balance (calories consumed versus calories expended) is an extraordinarily complex concept when considering the multitude of genetic, biological, psychological, sociocultural, and environmental factors that affect both sides of the energy balance equation and the interrelationships among these factors.

Clear specification of obesity prevention goals is essential in shaping an action plan and evaluating its success. Relevant issues for setting obesity prevention goals for populations include concepts of optimum population BMI and healthy weight levels, potential effects on food intake and patterns of physical activity and inactivity, as well as attitudes and social norms related to food and eating, physical activity, inactivity, body size, and dietary restrictions. This chapter discusses a variety of influences on children's diets and physical activity patterns including genetic variation and biological considerations, and sociocultural and other environmental factors.

Using an ecological systems theory model and a primary prevention evidence-based public health approach, this report focuses on how changes in the individual child's behaviors are affected not only by individual factors but also through interactions with the larger social, cultural, and environmental contexts in which he or she lives (e.g., family, school, community, social and physical environments).

REFERENCES

AAP (American Academy of Pediatrics), Committee on Nutrition. 2003. Prevention of pediatric overweight and obesity. *Pediatrics* 112(2):424-430.
ADA (American Dietetic Association). 2003. Position of the American Dietetic Association: Child and adolescent food and nutrition programs. *J Am Diet Assoc* 103(7):887-893.
ADA. 2004. Position of the American Dietetic Association: Dietary guidance for healthy children ages 2 to 11 years. *J Am Diet Assoc* 104(4):660-677.

Adams K, Sargent RG, Thompson SH, Richter D, Corwin SJ, Rogan TJ. 2000. A study of body weight concerns and weight control practices of 4th and 7th grade adolescents. *Ethn Health* 5(1):79-94.

Addy CL, Wilson DK, Kirtland KA, Ainsworth BE, Sharpe P, Kimsey D. 2004. Associations of perceived social and physical environmental supports with physical activity and walking behavior. *Am J Public Health* 94(3):440-443.

Alaimo K, Olson CM, Frongillo EA Jr. 2001a. Food insufficiency and American school-aged children's cognitive, academic, and psychosocial development. *Pediatrics* 108(1):44-53.

Alaimo K, Olson CM, Frongillo EA Jr. 2001b. Low family income and food insufficiency in relation to overweight in US children: Is there a paradox? *Arch Pediatr Adolesc Med* 155(10):1161-1167.

Alaimo K, Olson CM, Frongillo EA. 2002. Family food insufficiency, but not low family income, is positively associated with dysthymia and suicide symptoms in adolescents. *J Nutr* 132(4):719-725.

Ballew C, Bowman BA, Sowell AL, Gillespie C. 2001. Serum retinol distributions in residents of the United States: Third National Health and Nutrition Examination Survey, 1988-1994. *Am J Clin Nutr* 73(3):586-593.

Baranowski T, Thompson WO, DuRant RH, Baranowski J, Puhl J. 1993. Observations on physical activity in physical locations: Age, gender, ethnicity, and month effects. *Res Q Exerc Sport* 64(2):127-133.

Barlow SE, Dietz WH. 1998. Obesity evaluation and treatment: Expert committee recommendations. The Maternal and Child Health Bureau, Health Resources and Services Administration and the Department of Health and Human Services. *Pediatrics* 102(3):E29.

Barsh GS, Farooqi IS, O'Rahilly S. 2000. Genetics of body-weight regulation. *Nature* 404(6778):644-651.

Biddle S, Sallis JF, Cavill NA. 1998. *Young and Active? Young People and Health Enhancing Physical Activity. Evidence and Implication.* London: Health Education Authority.

Booth SL, Sallis JF, Ritenbaugh C, Hill JO, Birch LL, Frank LD, Glanz K, Himmelgreen DA, Mudd M, Popkin BM, Rickard KA, St Jeor S, Hays NP. 2001. Environmental and societal factors affect food choice and physical activity: Rationale, influences, and leverage points. *Nutr Rev* 59(3 Pt 2):S21-S39.

Boreham C, Riddock C. 2001. The physical activity, fitness and health of children. *J Sports Sci* 19(12):915-929.

Bouchard C, Pérusse L, Rice T, Rao DC. 2003. Genetics of human obesity. In: Bray GA, Bouchard C, eds. *Handbook of Obesity. Etiology and Pathophysiology.* 2nd ed. New York: Marcel Dekker.

Bouret SG, Draper SJ, Simerly RB. 2004. Trophic action of leptin on hypothalamic neurons that regulate feeding. *Science* 304(5667):108-110.

Briss PA, Zaza S, Pappaioanou M, Fielding J, Wright-De Aguero L, Truman BI, Hopkins DP, Mullen PD, Thompson RS, Woolf SH, Carande-Kulis VG, Anderson L, Hinman AR, McQueen DV, Teutsch SM, Harris JR, Task Force on Community Preventive Services. 2000. Developing an evidence-based guide to community preventive services: Methods. *Am J Prev Med* 18(1S):35-43.

Brown KM, McMahon RP, Biro FM, Crawford P, Schreiber GB, Similo SL, Waclawiw M, Striegel-Moore R. 1998. Changes in self-esteem in black and white girls between the ages of 9 and 14 years. The NHLBI Growth and Health Study. *J Adolesc Health* 23(1):7-19.

Brown PJ, Bentley-Condit VK. 1998. Culture, evolution, and obesity. In: Bray GA, Bouchard C, James WPT, eds. *Handbook of Obesity.* New York: Marcel Dekker. Pp. 143-156.

Butte NF, Ellis KJ. 2003. Comment on "Obesity and the environment: Where do we go from here?" *Science* 301(5633):598b.

Cameron N. 2002. British growth charts for height and weight with recommendations concerning their use in auxological assessment. *Ann Hum Biol* 29(1):1-10.

Campbell K, Waters E, O'Meara S, Kelly S, Summerbell C. 2002. *Interventions for Preventing Obesity in Children.* Oxford, U.K.: Cochrane Library.

Casey PH, Szeto K, Lensing S, Bogle M, Weber J. 2001. Children in food-insufficient, low-income families: Prevalence, health, and nutrition status. *Arch Pediatr Adolesc Med* 155(4):508-514.

Caspersen CJ, Powell KE, Christenson GM. 1985. Physical activity, exercise, and physical fitness: Definitions and distinctions for health-related research. *Public Health Rep* 100(2):126-131.

Caspersen CJ, Pereira MA, Curran KM. 2000. Changes in physical activity patterns in the United States, by sex and cross-sectional age. *Med Sci Sports Exerc* 32(9):1601-1609.

Cavill N, Biddle S, Sallis JF. 2001. Health enhancing physical activity for young people: Statement of the United Kingdom Expert Consensus Conference. *Pediatr Exer Sci* 13:12-25.

CDC (Centers for Disease Control and Prevention). 1997. Guidelines for school and community programs to promote lifelong physical activity among young people. *MMWR Recomm Rep* 46(RR-6):1-36.

CDC. 2004. *Measuring Physical Activity.* [Online]. Available: http://www.cdc.gov/nccdphp/dnpa/physical/measuring/index.htm [accessed August 18, 2004].

Cohen L, Swift S. 1999. The spectrum of prevention: Developing a comprehensive approach to injury prevention. *Inj Prev* 5(3):203-207.

Cook JT, Frank DA, Berkowitz C, Black MM, Casey PH, Cutts DB, Meyers AF, Zaldivar N, Skalicky A, Levenson S, Heeren T, Nord M. 2004. Food insecurity is associated with adverse health outcomes among human infants and toddlers. *J Nutr* 134(6):1432-1438.

Cooper RS. 2003. Race, genes, and health: New wine in old bottles? *Int J Epidemiol* 32:23-25.

Cooper RS, Kaufman JS, Ward R. 2003. Race and genomics. *N Engl J Med* 348(12):1166-1170.

Cummings DE, Schwartz MW. 2003. Genetics and pathophysiology of human obesity. *Annu Rev Med* 54(1):453-471.

Cutler D, Glaeser E, Shapiro J. 2003. *Why Have Americans Become More Fat?* NBER Working Paper No. W9446. Cambridge, MA: National Bureau of Economic Research.

Davison KK, Birch LL. 2001. Childhood overweight: A contextual model and recommendations for future research. *Obes Rev* 2(3):159-171.

DHHS (U.S. Department of Health and Human Services). 1996. *Physical Activity and Health: A Report of the Surgeon General.* Atlanta, GA: CDC.

DHHS. 2000. *Healthy People 2010: Understanding and Improving Health.* 2nd edition. Washington, DC: U.S. Government Printing Office. [Online]. Available: http://www.healthypeople.gov/document/tableofcontents.htm [accessed April 9, 2004].

DHHS. 2001a. *The Surgeon General's Call to Action to Prevent and Decrease Overweight and Obesity.* Rockville, MD: Public Health Service, Office of the Surgeon General.

DHHS. 2001b. *Overweight and Obesity: What You Can Do. Being Physically Active Can Help You Attain or Maintain a Healthy Weight.* [Online]. Available: http://www.surgeongeneral.gov/topics/obesity/calltoaction/fact_whatcanyoudo.htm [accessed August 9, 2004].

Dietz WH, Robinson TN. 1998. Use of the body mass index (BMI) as a measure of overweight in children and adolescents. *J Pediatr* 132(2):191-193.

Druce M, Bloom SR. 2003. Central regulators of food intake. *Curr Opin Clin Nutr Metab Care* 6(4):361-367.

Elmquist JK, Flier JS. 2004. Neuroscience. The fat-brain axis enters a new dimension. *Science* 304(5667):63-64.

Enns CW, Mickle SJ, Goldman JD. 2002. Trends in food and nutrient intakes by children in the United States. *Fam Econ Nutr Rev* 14(2):56-68.

Fitzgibbon ML, Stolley MR. 2004. Environmental changes may be needed for prevention of overweight in minority children. *Pediatr Ann* 33(1):45-49.

Flegal KM, Ogden CL, Wei R, Kuczmarski RL, Johnson CL. 2001. Prevalence of overweight in US children: Comparison of US growth charts from the Centers for Disease Control and Prevention with other reference values for body mass index. *Am J Clin Nutr* 73(6):1086-1093.

Flynn KJ, Fitzgibbon M. 1998. Body images and obesity risk among black females: A review of the literature. *Ann Behav Med* 20(1):13-24.

Freedman DS, Khan LK, Dietz WH, Srinivasan SR, Berenson GS. 2001. Relationship of childhood obesity to coronary heart disease risk factors in adulthood: The Bogalusa Heart Study. *Pediatrics* 108(3):712-718.

Gale SM, Castracane VD, Mantzoros CS. 2004. Energy homeostasis, obesity and eating disorders: Recent advances in endocrinology. *J Nutr* 134(2):295-298.

Ganji V, Hampl JS, Betts NM. 2003. Race-, gender- and age-specific differences in dietary micronutrient intakes of US children. *Int J Food Sci Nutr* 54(6):485-490.

Gleason P, Suitor C. 2001. *Children's Diets in the Mid-1990's: Dietary Intake and Its Relationship with School Meal Participation.* Report No. CN-01-CD1. Alexandria, VA: USDA.

Goran MI. 1998. Measurement issues related to studies of childhood obesity: Assessment of body composition, body fat distribution, physical activity, and food intake. *Pediatrics* 101(3 Pt 2):505-518.

Goran MI, Reynolds KD, Lindquist CH. 1999. Role of physical activity in the prevention of obesity in children. *Int J Obesity* 23(S3):S18-S33.

Gordon R. 1983. An operational classification of disease prevention. *Public Health Reports* 98:107-109.

Guo SS, Roche AF, Chumlea WC, Gardner JD, Siervogel RM. 1994. The predictive value of childhood body mass index values for overweight at age 35 y. *Am J Clin Nutr* 59(4):810-819.

Guo X, Warden BA, Paeratakul S, Bray GA. 2004. Healthy Eating Index and obesity. *Eur J Clin Nutr* May 19 [Online]. Available: http://dx.doi.org/10.1038/sj.ejcn.1601989 [accessed September 8, 2004].

Halpern CT, Udry JR, Campbell B, Suchindran C. 1999. Effects of body fat on weight concerns, dating, and sexual activity: A longitudinal analysis of black and white adolescent girls. *Dev Psychol* 35(3):721-736.

Hampl JS, Taylor CA, Johnston CS. 2004. Vitamin C deficiency and depletion in the United States: The Third National Health and Nutrition Examination Survey, 1988 to 1994. *Am J Public Health* 94(5):870-875.

Harnack L, Snyder P, Story M, Holliday R, Lytle L, Neumark-Sztainer D. 2000. Availability of a la carte food items in junior and senior high schools: A needs assessment. *J Am Diet Assoc* 100(6):701-703.

Harris RP, Helfand M, Woolf SH, Lohr KN, Mulrow CD, Teutsch SM, Atkins D, Methods Work Group, Third US Preventive Services Task Force. 2001. Current methods of the U.S. Preventive Services Task Force: A review of the process. *Am J Prev Med* 20(3S):21-35.

Havel PJ. 2000. Role of adipose tissue in body-weight regulation: Mechanisms regulating leptin production and energy balance. *Proc Nutr Soc* 59(3):359-371.

Havel PJ. 2004. Update on adipocyte hormones: Regulation of energy balance and carbohydrate/lipid metabolism. *Diabetes* 53(S1):S143-S151.

Heller RF, Page J. 2002. A population perspective to evidence based medicine: "Evidence for population health." *J Epidemiol Community Health* 56(1):45-47.

Hill JO, Peters JC. 1998. Environmental contributions to the obesity epidemic. *Science* 280(5368):1371-1374.

Hill JO, Wyatt HR, Reed GW, Peters JC. 2003. Obesity and the environment: Where do we go from here? *Science* 299(5608):853-855.

Hill JO, Saris WHM, Levine JA. 2004. Energy expenditure in physical activity. In: Bray GA, Bouchard C, eds. *Handbook of Obesity: Etiology and Pathophysiology*. 2nd ed. New York: Marcel Dekker.

Himes JH, Dietz WH. 1994. Guidelines for overweight in adolescent preventive services: Recommendations from an expert committee. The Expert Committee on Clinical Guidelines for Overweight in Adolescent Preventive Services. *Am J Clin Nutr* 59(2):307-316.

IOM (Institute of Medicine). 1994. *Reducing Risks for Mental Disorders*. Washington, DC: National Academy Press.

IOM. 1997. *Dietary Reference Intakes for Calcium, Phosphorus, Magnesium, Vitamin D, and Fluoride*. Washington, DC: National Academy Press.

IOM. 2001. *Health and Behavior: The Interplay of Biological, Behavioral, and Societal Influences*. Washington, DC: National Academy Press.

IOM. 2002. *Dietary Reference Intakes for Energy, Carbohydrate, Fiber, Fat, Fatty Acids, Cholesterol, Protein, and Amino Acids*. Washington, DC: The National Academies Press.

IOM. 2004. *Dietary Reference Intakes for Water, Potassium, Sodium, Chloride, and Sulfate*. Washington, DC: The National Academies Press.

IOM, NRC (National Research Council). 2004. *Dietary Supplements: A Framework for Evaluating Safety*. Washington, DC: The National Academies Press.

Kaiser LL, Melgar-Quinonez HR, Lamp CL, Johns MC, Sutherlin JM, Harwood JO. 2002. Food security and nutritional outcomes of preschool-age Mexican-American children. *J Am Diet Assoc* 102(7):924-929.

Kellam SG, Langevin DJ. 2003. A framework for understanding "evidence" in prevention research and programs. *Prevention Science* 4(3):137-153.

Klesges RC, Eck LH, Hanson CL, Haddock CK, Klesges LM. 1990. Effects of obesity, social interactions, and physical environment on physical activity in preschoolers. *Health Psychol* 9(4):435-449.

Klinke A, Renn O. 2002. A new approach to risk evaluation and management: Risk-based, precaution-based, and discourse-based strategies. *Risk Anal* 22(6):1071-1093.

Koplan JP, Dietz WH. 1999. Caloric imbalance and public health policy. *J Am Med Assoc* 282(16):1579-1582.

Kroke A, Boeing H, Rossnagel K, Willich SN. 2003. History of the concept of 'levels of evidence' and their current status in relation to primary prevention through lifestyle intervention. *Public Health Nutr* 7(2):279-284.

Kuczmarski RJ, Ogden CL, Grummer-Strawn LM, Flegal KM, Guo SS, Wei R, Mei Z, Curtin LR, Roche AF, Johnson CL. 2000. CDC growth charts: United States. *Adv Data* (314):1-27.

Kuczmarski RJ, Ogden CL, Guo SS, Grummer-Strawn LM, Flegal KM, Mei Z, Wei R, Curtin LR, Roche AF, Johnson CL. 2002. *Data From the National Health Survey. 2000 CDC Growth Charts for the United States: Methods and Development*. Hyattsville, MD: National Center for Health Statistics.

Kumanyika SK. 1993. Ethnicity and obesity development in children. *Ann NY Acad Sci* 699:81-92.

Kumanyika SK. 2002. Obesity treatment in minorities. In: Wadden TA, Stunkard AJ, eds. *Handbook of Obesity Treatment*. 3rd ed. New York: Guilford Publications. Pp. 416-446.

Kumanyika SK. 2004. Cultural differences as influences on approaches to obesity treatment. In: Bray GA, Bouchard C, eds. *Handbook of Obesity: Clinical Applications.* 2nd ed. New York: Marcel Dekker.

Kumanyika SK, Krebs-Smith SM. 2001. Preventive nutrition issues in ethnic and socioeconomic groups in the United States. In: Bendich A, Deckelbaum RJ, eds. *Primary and Secondary Preventive Nutrition.* Totowa, NJ: Humana Press. Pp. 325-356.

Kumanyika SK, Morssink CB. 1997. Cultural appropriateness of weight management programs. In: Dalton S, ed. *Overweight and Weight Management.* Gaithersburg, MD: Aspen. Pp. 69-106.

Kumanyika SK, Obarzanek E. 2003. Pathways to obesity prevention: Report of a National Institutes of Health Workshop. *Obes Res* 11(10):1263-1274.

Kumanyika S, Jeffery RW, Morabia A, Ritenbaugh C, Antipatis VJ, Public Health Approaches to the Prevention of Obesity (PHAPO) Working Group of the International Obesity Task Force (IOTF). 2002. Obesity prevention: The case for action. *Int J Obes Relat Metab Disord* 26(3):425-436.

Latner JD, Stunkard AJ. 2003. Getting worse: The stigmatization of obese children. *Obes Res* 11(3):452-456.

Leventhal T, Brooks-Gunn J. 2001. Changing neighborhoods and child well-being: Understanding how children may be affected in the coming century. In: Owens T, Hofferth S, eds. *Children at the Millennium: Where Have We Come From, Where Are We Going?* Advances in Life Course Research. New York: Elsevier Science.

Lobstein T, Baur L, Uauy R, IASO International Obesity TaskForce. 2004. Obesity in children and young people: A crisis in public health. *Obes Rev* 5(Suppl 1):4-85.

Matheson DM, Varady J, Varady A, Killen JD. 2002. Household food security and nutritional status of Hispanic children in the fifth grade. *Am J Clin Nutr* 76(1):210-217.

Maziekas MT, LeMura LM, Stoddard NM, Kaercher S, Martucci T. 2003. Follow up exercise studies in pediatric obesity: Implications for long term effectiveness. *Br J Sports Med* 37(5):425-429.

McQueen DV. 2002. Strengthening the evidence base for health promotion. *Health Promotion International* 16(3):261-268.

Mei Z, Grummer-Strawn LM, Pietrobelli A, Goulding A, Goran MI, Dietz WH. 2002. Validity of body mass index compared with other body-composition screening indexes for the assessment of body fatness in children and adolescents. *Am J Clin Nutr* 75(6):978-985.

Mei Z, Grummer-Strawn LM, Thompson D, Dietz WH. 2004. Shifts in percentiles of growth during early childhood: Analysis of longitudinal data from the California Child Health and Development Study. *Pediatrics* 113(6):e617-e627.

Mensah GA, Goodman RA, Zaza S, Moulton AD, Kocher PL, Dietz WH, Pechacek TF, Marks JS. 2004. (April). Law as a tool for preventing chronic diseases: Expanding the spectrum of effective public health strategies [Part 1 and 2]. *Preventing Chronic Disease* [Online]. Available: http://www.cdc.gov/pcd/issues/2004/apr/04_0009.htm [accessed April 20, 2004].

Molnar BE, Gortmaker SL, Bull FC, Buka SL. 2004. Unsafe to play? Neighborhood disorder and lack of safety predict reduced physical activity among urban children and adolescents. *Am J Health Promot* 18(5):378-386.

Morland K, Wing S, Diez Roux A, Poole C. 2002a. Neighborhood characteristics associated with the location of food stores and food service places. *Am J Prev Med* 22(1):23-29.

Morland K, Wing S, Diez Roux A. 2002b. The contextual effect of the local food environment on residents' diets: The atherosclerosis risk in communities study. *Am J Public Health* 92(11):1761-1767.

NASPE (National Association for Sport and Physical Education). 2004. *Physical Activity for Children: A Statement of Guidelines for Children Ages 5-12.* 2nd edition. Reston, VA: NASPE.

Neumark-Sztainer D, Croll J, Story M, Hannan PJ, French SA, Perry C. 2002. Ethnic/racial differences in weight-related concerns and behaviors among adolescent girls and boys: Findings from Project EAT. *J Psychosom Res* 53(5):963-974.

Newman C. 2004. Why are we so fat? *National Geographic* (August):46-61.

NHLBI (National Heart, Lung, and Blood Institute). 1998. *Clinical Guidelines on the Identification, Evaluation, and Treatment of Overweight and Obesity in Adults: The Evidence Report.* NIH Publication No. 98-4083. Rockville, MD: NIH. [Online]. Available: http://www.nhlbi.nih.gov/guidelines/obesity/ob_gdlns.pdf [accessed November 21, 2003].

NHS Centre for Reviews and Dissemination. 2002. The prevention and treatment of childhood obesity. *Eff Health Care* 7(6):1-12.

Nielsen SJ, Siega-Riz AM, Popkin BM. 2002. Trends in energy intake in U.S. between 1977 and 1996: Similar shifts seen across age groups. *Obes Res* 10(5):370-378.

Nord M, Andrews M, Carlson S. 2003. *Household Food Security in the United States, 2002.* Alexandria, VA: USDA Economic Research Service. Food Assistance and Nutrition Research Report 35.

NRC (National Research Council). 1978. *Knowledge and Policy: The Uncertain Connection.* Washington, DC: National Academy Press.

NRC. 1989. *Improving Risk Communication.* Washington, DC: National Academy Press.

NRC. 1994. *Science and Judgment in Risk Assessment.* Washington, DC: National Academy Press.

NRC. 1996. *Understanding Risk: Informing Decisions in a Democratic Society.* Washington, DC: National Academy Press.

NRC, IOM. 2000. *From Neurons to Neighborhoods: The Science of Early Childhood Development.* Washington, DC: National Academy Press.

NRC, IOM. 2003. *Reducing Underage Drinking: A Collective Responsibility.* Washington, DC: The National Academies Press.

O'Rahilly S, Farooqi IS, Yeo GS, Challis BG. 2003. Minireview: Human obesity—Lessons from monogenic disorders. *Endocrinology* 144(9):3757-3764.

Osaka Declaration. 2001 (May). *Health, Economics and Political Action: Stemming the Global Tide of Cardiovascular Disease.* Declaration of the Fourth International Heart Health Conference, Osaka, Japan.

Pinto S, Roseberry AG, Liu H, Diano S, Shanabrough M, Cai X, Friedman JM, Horvath TL. 2004. Rapid rewiring of arcuate nucleus feeding circuits by leptin. *Science* 304(5667):110-115.

Renn O, Webler T, Wiedemann P, eds. 1995. *Fairness and Competence in Citizen Participation: Evaluating Models for Environmental Discourse.* Boston, MA: Kluwer Academic Publishers.

Richter KP, Harris KJ, Paine-Andrews A, Fawcett SB, Schmid TL, Lankenau BH, Johnston J. 2000. Measuring the health environment for physical activity and nutrition among youth: A review of the literature and applications for community initiatives. *Prev Med* 31(2 Part 2):S98-S111.

Robinson TN. 1993. Defining obesity in children and adolescents: Clinical approaches. *Crit Rev Food Sci Nutr* 33(4-5):313-320.

Robinson TN. 1999. Reducing children's television viewing to prevent obesity: A randomized controlled trial. *J Am Med Assoc* 282(16):1561-1567.

Robinson TN, Killen JD. 2001. Obesity prevention for children and adolescents. In: Thompson JK, Smolak L, eds. *Body Image, Eating Disorders, and Obesity in Youth: Assessment, Prevention, and Treatment*. Washington, DC: American Psychological Association. Pp. 261-292.

Robinson TN, Patrick K, Eng TR, Gustafson D. 1998. An evidence-based approach to interactive health communication: A challenge to medicine in the information age. Science Panel on Interactive Communication and Health. *J Am Med Assoc* 280(14):1264-1269.

Robinson TN, Chang JY, Haydel KF, Killen JD. 2001. Overweight concerns and body dissatisfaction among third-grade children: The impacts of ethnicity and socioeconomic status. *J Pediatr* 138(2):181-187.

Rose G. 1992. *The Strategy of Preventive Medicine*. New York: Oxford University Press.

Rosenbaum M, Leibel RL. 1998. The physiology of body weight regulation: Relevance to the etiology of obesity in children. *Pediatrics* 101(3 Part 2):525-539.

Sallis JF. 2000. Age-related decline in physical activity: A synthesis of human and animal studies. *Med Sci Sports Exerc* 32(9):1598-1600.

Sallis JF, Nader PR, Broyles SL, Berry CC, Elder JP, McKenzie TL, Nelson JA. 1993. Correlates of physical activity at home in Mexican-American and Anglo-American preschool children. *Health Psychol* 12(5):390-398.

Saris WH. 1986. Habitual physical activity in children: Methodology and findings in health and disease. *Med Sci Sports Exerc* 18(3):253-263.

Schwartz MB, Puhl R. 2003. Childhood obesity: A societal problem to solve. *Obes Rev* 4(1):57-71.

Schwartz MW, Woods SC, Seeley RJ, Barsh GS, Baskin DG, Leibel RL. 2003. Is the energy homeostasis system inherently biased toward weight gain? *Diabetes* 52(2):232-238.

Segal NL, Allison DB. 2002. Twins and virtual twins: Bases of relative body weight revisited. *Int J Obes Relat Metab Disord* 26(4):437-441.

Serdula MK, Mokdad AH, Williamson DF, Galuska DA, Mendlein JM, Heath GW. 1999. Prevalence of attempting weight loss and strategies for controlling weight. *J Am Med Assoc* 282(14):1353-1358.

Sirard JR, Pate RR. 2001. Physical activity assessment in children and adolescents. *Sports Med* 31(6):439-454.

Slovic P. 1987. Perception of risk. *Science* 236(4799):280-285.

Slovic P. 2000. Perceived risk, trust, and democracy. In: Connolly T, Arkes H, Hammond K, eds. *Judgment and Decision Making: An Interdisciplinary Reader*. New York: Cambridge University Press. Pp. 500-516.

Snyder EE, Walts B, Perusse L, Chagnon YC, Weisnagel SJ, Rankinen T, Bouchard C. 2004. The human obesity gene map: The 2003 update. *Obes Res* 12(3):369-439.

Sothern MS, Loftin M, Suskind RM, Udall JN, Blecker U. 1999. The health benefits of physical activity in children and adolescents and implications for chronic disease prevention. *Eur J Pediatr* 158(4):271-274.

Strauss RS, Knight J. 1999. Influence of the home environment on the development of obesity in children. *Pediatrics* 103(6):E85.

Sturm R. 2005 (in press). Childhood obesity – What can we learn from existing data on societal trends. Part 2. *Preventing Chronic Disease* [Online]. Available: http://www.cdc.gov/pcd/issues/2005/apr/04_0039.htm [access after March 15, 2005].

Swinburn BA, Egger GJ. 2004. Influence of obesity-producing environments. In: Bray GA, Bouchard C, eds. *Handbook of Obesity. Clinical Applications*. 2nd ed. New York: Marcel Dekker.

Swinburn BA, Egger G, Raza F. 1999. Dissecting obesogenic environments: The development and application of a framework for identifying and prioritizing environmental interventions for obesity. *Prev Med* 29(6 Pt 1):563-570.

Swinburn B, Gill T, Kumanyika S. 2005 (in press). Obesity prevention: A proposed framework for translating evidence into action. *Obes Rev* 6(1).

Tang KC, Ehsani JP, McQueen DV. 2003. Evidence-based health promotion: Recollections, reflections, and reconsiderations. *J Epidemiol Community Health* 57(11):841-843.

Tanner JM, Davies PS. 1985. Clinical longitudinal standards for height and height velocity for North American children. *J Pediatr* 107(3):317-329.

Thompson SH, Corwin SJ, Sargent RG. 1997. Ideal body size beliefs and weight concerns of fourth-grade children. *Int J Eat Disord* 21(3):279-284.

Tirodkar MA, Jain A. 2003. Food messages on African American television shows. *Am J Public Health* 93(3):439-441.

Travers KD. 1996. The social organization of nutritional inequities. *Soc Sci Med* 43(4):543-553.

Travers KD. 1997. Reducing inequities through participatory research and community empowerment. *Health Educ Behav* 24(3):344-356.

USDA (U.S. Department of Agriculture), DHHS (U.S. Department of Health and Human Services). 2000. *Nutrition and Your Health: Dietary Guidelines for Americans.* Home and Garden Bulletin No. 232, 5th ed. Washington, DC: Government Printing Office.

Victora CG, Habicht JP, Bryce J. 2004. Evidence-based public health: Moving beyond randomized trials. *Am J Public Health* 94(3):400-405.

Whitaker RC, Wright JA, Pepe MS, Seidel KD, Dietz WH. 1997. Predicting obesity in young adulthood from childhood and parental obesity. *N Engl J Med* 337(13):869-873.

WHO (World Health Organization). 2000. *Obesity: Preventing and Managing the Global Epidemic.* WHO Technical Report Series 894. Geneva. WHO.

WHO. 2003. *Diet, Nutrition and the Prevention of Chronic Diseases.* WHO Technical Report Series 916. Geneva: WHO.

Wright JD, Bialostosky K, Gunter EW, Carroll MD, Najjar MF, Bowman BA, Johnson CL. 1998. Blood folate and vitamin B12: United States, 1988-1994. *Vital Health Stat* 11(243):1-78.

Zhang Y, Proenca R, Maffei M, Barone M, Leopold L, Friedman JM. 1994. Positional cloning of the mouse obese gene and its human homologue. *Nature* 372(6505):425-432.

4

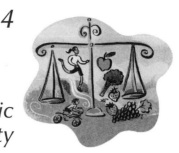

A National Public Health Priority

Although the general public has become increasingly aware of the personal health consequences of obesity, what may not yet be generally apparent is the *public* health nature of the obesity epidemic and the consequent need for population-based approaches to address it.

Obesity prevention should be public health in action at its broadest and most inclusive level, as is true for the ongoing efforts to prevent youth from smoking. For example, local communities are passing ordinances that ban or limit cigarette vending machines, schools and community youth organizations are discouraging or banning smoking, states are passing excise taxes to raise tobacco prices, the federal government is providing national leadership and the resources for research and programs, and the private sector is restricting smoking in workplaces (Box 4-1) (Economos et al., 2001; IOM, 2003). In addition, a broad, complementary, and continuing campaign aimed at reducing adult smoking continues to be conducted. The 2004 Surgeon General's report on tobacco use emphasized that "a comprehensive approach—one that optimizes synergy from a mix of educational, clinical, regulatory, economic, and social strategies—has emerged as the guiding principle for effective efforts to reduce tobacco use" (DHHS, 2004).

A similarly broad-based approach is needed for childhood obesity prevention. Across the country these efforts are beginning. As discussed throughout this report, current efforts range from new school board policies and state legislation regarding school physical education requirements and nutrition standards for beverages and foods sold in schools to community initiatives to expand bike paths and improve recreational facilities.

BOX 4-1
Comprehensive Efforts to Address Public Health Concerns

Highway Safety:
- **Federal government:** Safety regulations for new vehicles; highway design and safety regulations; establishment of the National Highway Traffic Safety Administration; state and community grant programs; research funding
- **State and local governments:** Highway safety offices; primary enforcement of safety belt laws; alcohol-impaired-driving laws; requirements for licensing and driver education; motor vehicle inspections
- **Public support and advocacy:** Citizen advocacy groups (e.g., Mothers Against Drunk Driving)
- **Research**
- **Media campaigns**
- **Education:** Driver education; parent education regarding safety seats

Tobacco:
- **Federal government:** Airline smoking ban; warnings on tobacco packages; research funding; Surgeon Generals' reports; establishment of the Office on Smoking and Health
- **State and local governments:** Excise taxes, laws that establish smoke-free workplaces and public locations
- **Public support and advocacy:** Grassroots efforts to prevent exposure to second hand smoke; community coalitions (e.g., ASSIST)
- **Research**
- **Media campaigns**
- **Education:** School-based programs

NOTE: This box denotes only selected examples of the multiple approaches used to address each public health problem.
SOURCES: IOM, 1999, 2003; Economos et al., 2001.

Parallel and synergistic efforts to prevent adult obesity, which will contribute to improvements in health for the U.S. population at all ages, are also beginning. Grassroots efforts made by citizens and organizations will likely drive many of the obesity prevention efforts at the local level and can be instrumental in driving policies and legislation at the state and national levels (Economos et al., 2001).

A policy analysis by Kersh and Morone (2002) shows that three of the seven common triggers for strong public action in response to a public health problem are beginning to be activated with respect to the U.S. obesity epidemic: social disapproval that shifts the social norm, evidence-based medical research, and self-help movements for overweight and obese individuals. Other triggers that have worked successfully for public health problems such as tobacco, alcohol, and illicit-drug use (a widespread coordinated movement or campaign; fear of problem-related behaviors or related culture, such as the drug culture; coordinated interest group advocacy; and targeting of groups or industries contributing to the problem) are not yet fully in place for obesity prevention or may not be relevant to this issue (Kersh and Morone, 2002; Haddad, 2003).

The additional impetus that is needed is the political will to make childhood obesity prevention a national public health priority. Effective prevention efforts on a nationwide basis will require federal, state, and local governments to commit sufficient resources for surveillance, research, programs, evaluation, and dissemination.

As the nation focuses on obesity as a health problem and begins to address the societal and cultural issues that contribute to excess weight, poor food choices, and inactivity, many different stakeholders will need to make difficult trade-offs and choices. Industries and businesses must re-examine many of their products and marketing strategies. Governments at the local, state, and national levels must consider this issue in setting priorities for programs and resources. Schools need to ensure that consistent messages regarding energy balance are a basic part of the school environment. Community organizations and numerous other stakeholders must examine the ways in which local opportunities for a healthful diet and physical activity are made accessible, available, affordable, and acceptable to children, youth, and their parents. Families need to make their homes more conducive to a healthful diet and daily physical activity. Many of these changes will be challenging because they present Americans with difficult trade-offs. However, as institutions, organizations, and individuals across the nation begin to make changes, societal norms are likely to change as well; in the long term, we may become a nation where proper nutrition and physical activity that support energy balance at a healthy weight will become the standard.

Within the United States and globally, attention is being focused on obesity prevention efforts. A number of interest groups, coalitions, national governments, and intergovernmental organizations have examined the rising obesity and chronic disease problems in a variety of contexts, recognized its complicated nature, and proposed actions to reduce its prevalence both nationally and globally (e.g., WHO, 2000, 2003; DHHS, 2001; Health Council of the Netherlands, 2003; National Board of Health, 2003; New South Wales Department of Health, 2003; Canadian Institute for Health Information, 2004; Lobstein et al., 2004; Raine, 2004; United Kingdom Parliament, 2004; Willett and Domolky, 2004). Many of the strategies and action plans that have been developed from these efforts do not differ greatly from the recommendations in this report. The committee has gained insights from these efforts, and in this report draws together the evidence on obesity prevention, nutrition, and physical activity with the lessons learned from other public health issues (Box 4-2) to develop an action plan for childhood obesity prevention that is as informed, responsive, and realis-

BOX 4-2
Lessons Learned from Other Public Health Issues and
Potential Applicability to Obesity Prevention
(see Appendix D)

- **Advertising**—Although obesity prevention does not involve restricted products to minors as is pertinent for tobacco and alcohol product advertising, there are similar concerns regarding young children's inability to detect persuasive intent.
- **Consumer information**—Providing information to consumers has many parallels including the need for label information on tobacco, food, and drug products.
- **Public education campaigns** to convey public health messages such as those regarding youth smoking, and seat belt and child car seat use provide examples for obesity prevention media campaigns.
- **Grassroots efforts and coalition building**—Community organizations (including youth and civic organizations) are active in health promotion efforts and coalitions resulting from grassroots efforts have been successful in legislative and social changes (e.g., drunk driving laws).
- **School environment**—Changes to promoting a healthier overall school environment have parallels in smoking bans in schools. Further, classroom education and particularly health education efforts focus on a number of health promotion topics including safety, HIV prevention, and violence prevention.
- **Health-care system**—As with numerous other health promotion issues, the health-care system provides opportunities for parent and child education as well as for prevention interventions such as administering vaccines.
- **Changes in the physical environment**—Modifications of highways, roads, and intersections to enhance pedestrian and traveler safety provide parallel examples for the funding, regulatory, and prioritization efforts required to enhance opportunities for physical activity.
- **Government support and funding**—The long-term commitment from both federal and state governments for research, surveillance, and program efforts on a number of public health issues (e.g., highway improvements, research centers, surveys) provides parallels for sustained efforts on obesity prevention.
- **Industry involvement**—Numerous health-promoting products such as sunscreens are developed and marketed by industry.
- **Comprehensive approach**—As indicated in Box 4-1, comprehensive approaches have been used in enhancing highway safety and in preventing tobacco use by youth. A similar comprehensive effort is suggested for obesity prevention.
- **Taxation and pricing**—Obesity prevention efforts do not involve access to a restricted product for youth (as do tobacco and alcohol prevention efforts). Excise taxes and pricing strategies have played an important role in tobacco control efforts. However, it is more difficult to identify specific food and beverage products on which to impose taxes or tax breaks.
- **Litigation** changed the tobacco control environment including the public's view of the issue. It is unclear whether the same issues that led to litigation for tobacco are relevant to obesity prevention.
- **Access and opportunity**—For restricted products, laws and regulations to restrict access to tobacco and alcohol have decreased availability. The ubiquitous nature of foods and beverages makes that a less feasible option for obesity prevention.

tic as possible. The committee acknowledges, as have many other similar efforts, that obesity prevention is a complex issue, that a thorough understanding of the causes and determinants of the obesity epidemic is lacking, and that progress will require changes not only in individual and family behaviors but also in the marketplace and the social and built environments. No simple solutions are anticipated; therefore, multiple stakeholders need to make a long-term commitment to improve opportunities for healthful nutrition and physical activity.

Although this chapter focuses on actions that need to be taken by the federal, state, and local governments, it is essential to mobilize and involve the numerous private organizations that fund obesity prevention programs and initiatives. It is in the best interest of the nation's children for all relevant stakeholders to make obesity prevention efforts a priority.

The committee recognizes the importance of combined social deliberation, problem analysis, and social mobilization around the issue of childhood obesity prevention at different levels and in various settings. This report and others that follow can set forth recommendations and broadly outline suggested actions; however, many of the next steps for progress on this issue will involve discussions and interactions of the implementers and innovators—the people, agencies, and organizations concerned about this issue and ready to work together to develop, implement, and evaluate approaches to prevent childhood obesity that fit the needs of their state, county, community, school, or neighborhood.

LEADERSHIP, COORDINATION, AND PRIORITY SETTING

A National Priority

The federal government has a long-standing commitment to programs that address nutritional deficiencies (beginning in the 1930s) and encourage physical fitness, but only recently has obesity been targeted. Physical activity and overweight/obesity are now designated as priority areas and leading health indicators in the nation's health objectives, *Healthy People 2010*, developed by the Department of Health and Human Services (DHHS) in collaboration with state and territorial health officials and numerous national membership organizations. The goal set by *Healthy People 2010* is to reduce the proportion of children and adolescents who are obese to 5 percent by 2010 (DHHS, 2000).

Obesity prevention is a cross-cutting issue that does not naturally fall under the purview of any one federal department. It encompasses health concerns central to the mission of DHHS; nutrition, nutrition education, and food-related issues for which the U.S. Department of Agriculture (USDA) has responsibilities; and school curriculum and school environment concerns that the Department of Education addresses. In addition, the agendas of numerous other federal departments include transportation, housing, and many other issues that are key to increasing physical activity levels and improving dietary quality and patterns.

Given the importance of obesity prevention for the health of American children, and given the overarching nature of this issue, prevention efforts need to be coordinated at the highest federal levels. **The committee recommends that the President request that the Secretary of DHHS convene a high-level task force that includes the Secretaries or senior officials from DHHS, Agriculture, Education, Transportation, Housing and Urban Development, Interior, Defense, and other relevant federal agencies.** The goal of the task force would be to ensure coordinated budgets, policies, research efforts, and program requirements and establish effective interdepartmental collaboration and priorities for action. It would be important for the task force to meet on a regular basis with local and state officials, representatives from nongovernmental organizations including foundations and advocacy groups, industry representatives, civic and youth-related organizations, and other relevant stakeholders.

It is expected that high-level focused attention on this issue will result in fostering interdisciplinary and interdepartmental research collaborations that span agriculture, health, behavioral sciences, economics, urban planning, and other relevant disciplines. Given the public health nature of the childhood obesity epidemic, it is the committee's judgment that the Secretary of Health and Human Services should chair this coordinating task force.

To maintain the momentum over the long term, the committee urges that the coordinating task force consider periodic reassessments of its organization and its goals. In the initial work of the task force, participation of the Secretaries of the departments or senior officials will be needed to give high-level visibility, authority, and credence to the coordinating efforts. However, it is unrealistic to expect such high-level participation to continue indefinitely. After 2 to 3 years, an assessment may be needed to determine the best way to continue the collaboration and keep the research partnerships energized. In any case, sustained coordination will be primary to addressing this health issue, and it is up to the federal departments to ensure that it is a long-term priority.

As part of its focus on obesity prevention in children and youth, the federal government should document its efforts and progress through an annual report to the nation. This report, which would include updates on the new and recently evaluated efforts in each of the cabinet departments as well as on cross-cutting efforts, could be coordinated through the Centers for Disease Control and Prevention (CDC). Content would include up-to-date epidemiologic data on childhood obesity trends, the amount and sources of government funds that are targeted to childhood obesity prevention, information on programs and research, and the results of program evaluations. It would also be informative to have an overview of federal, state, and local policy measures that have been taken to address the issue, as well as profiles of model programs that show promise.

Meanwhile, it will be important to continue the current intra- and interdepartmental collaboration efforts, including the National Institutes of Health (NIH) Task Force on Obesity Prevention (which coordinates efforts between the NIH institutes on this issue), and the 2005 Dietary Guidelines Advisory Committee (which is conducting a review of the current scientific and medical knowledge on childhood obesity in order to provide a technical report of recommendations to the Secretaries of DHHS and USDA that will inform the 2005 edition of the Dietary Guidelines for Americans; see Chapter 3). This review will ensure consistency of dietary recommendations across DHHS and USDA agencies regarding national dietary recommendations for the American public.

Just as it has done with automobile and highway safety initiatives (Box 4-1), efforts to curb youth smoking, and current efforts to defend against potential bioterrorist threats, the federal government should set forth obesity prevention as a national health priority—one that is acted upon through extensive and sustained funding and a long-term commitment of resources (IOM, 2003).

Congressional support will be crucial in ensuring that funding is made available for pilot programs and for research, public education, and program efforts. Furthermore, congressional leadership is needed on issues such as nutritional standards for foods and beverages sold in schools and in other areas that need legislative authorization.

The federal government should take a leadership role in the prevention of obesity in children and youth by making this issue a top priority for the U.S. Departments of Health and Human Services, Agriculture, and Education. This priority should be reflected in the departments' public statements, programs, research priorities, and budgets. These departments along with other relevant federal entities (e.g., the Departments of Transportation, Housing and Urban Development, Interior, and Defense) should together pursue an integrated approach that promotes healthful eating and regular physical activity to achieve energy balance.

STATE AND LOCAL PRIORITIES

State and local governments have important roles to play in obesity prevention because they can focus on the specific needs of their communities' populations (see Chapter 6). Many of the issues involved in preventing childhood obesity require decisions by county, city, or town officials. Actions on street and neighborhood design, planning for parks and community recreational facilities, and locations of new schools and retail food facilities are usually up to the local zoning boards, planning commissions, and similar entities. Efforts can be tailored to local residents and institutions, and can be more quickly adapted and revised to meet changing demands and integrate new approaches.

State governments and agencies, including state departments of health, education, and transportation, are also key to ensuring that obesity prevention policies are developed and programs are implemented. Further, state governments are responsible for programs that provide food assistance, address the consequences of obesity (e.g., diabetes and heart disease), and influence health spending and policy (such as Medicaid, Title V [Maternal and Child Health], and direct funding for community development/housing and transportation). In some states, major policy decisions for school systems are made at the community or county level, but in others it is the state department of education that makes most of these decisions.

As numerous and diverse programs and initiatives are being planned or under way in states and communities, organizations that bring together state and local leaders—such as the National Governors Association, the U.S. Conference of Mayors, the National Association of County and City Health Officials, the Association of State and Territorial Health Officials, and the American Public Health Association—can each raise awareness of obesity issues, facilitate the sharing of lessons learned, and help coordinate obesity prevention efforts.

One avenue for expanding state-based obesity prevention efforts is through CDC's grants program that focuses on local capacity building and implementation of programs to prevent obesity and other chronic diseases (CDC, 2004a). As discussed in Chapter 6, expansion of this grant program could be instrumental in establishing community demonstration projects. Twenty states received funding through these grants in fiscal year (FY) 2003. **By expanding the total funding for the state grant programs, needed resources could be allocated to support additional states, particularly those with the highest prevalence of childhood and youth obesity.** For example, the committee notes the critical role that the federal government has played in highway safety by providing states with grant funding (the Section 402 State and Community Highway Safety Grant program); these funds have been used for the development and evaluation of new innovative programs to increase the use of seat belts and child safety seats (IOM, 1999).

Another recent initiative to provide funds for city- and community-based health efforts is the DHHS Steps to a Healthier U.S. Initiative (see Chapter 5). In 2003, DHHS provided 12 grants to promote community and tribal initiatives focused on reducing the burden of diabetes, overweight, obesity, and asthma and emphasizing efforts to address physical inactivity, poor nutrition, and tobacco use. Evaluation and further funding of this program is encouraged.

State and local governments should make childhood obesity prevention a priority by devoting resources to this issue and providing leadership in launching and evaluating prevention efforts.

State and Local Public Health Agencies

Government public health agencies are critical components of the nation's response to childhood obesity at national, state, and local levels, not only because the public health workforce has the needed expertise, but also because it has access to a large number of children, youth, and families; the ability to galvanize community efforts; and the resources to implement prevention programs. As the only institutions with the mission and legal mandate to protect the health of the public-at-large, federal, state, and local government public health agencies are the most publicly accountable entities within the health system. Public health has a long record of remarkable achievement despite modest resources, and the recent infusion of federal support to bolster preparedness for biological terrorism has strengthened the infrastructure to respond to disease emergencies (IOM, 2003).

The state and local public health agencies in particular comprise the front line of the public health system. Although they are in an ideal position to assess the childhood obesity epidemic and the local conditions that are fueling it, these agencies need to be restructured for collaborative approaches that address behavioral, social, and environmental factors and that involve diverse community stakeholders and engage even the most disenfranchised communities. Such partners can include schools, child-care centers, nutrition services, parks and recreation departments, civic and ethnic organizations, faith-based groups, businesses, and community planning and transportation boards (see Chapter 6).

As noted above, the committee urges increased funding for CDC's program of state-based obesity prevention grants to provide the resources needed by state and local departments of health and others for improved surveillance efforts to identify specific community, state, and regional issues; training of public health professionals on obesity prevention; planning, implementing, and evaluating obesity prevention efforts including support for community coalitions and other collaborative efforts with community stakeholders, schools, and other key partners; and development of better tools for public communication.

Health departments have the added dimension of serving as regulator or educator of standards for practice. Immunization programs, tobacco control efforts, and food service or restaurant inspection are all examples of public health (or environmental health) agencies overseeing and informing private-sector entities in order to protect health. With sufficient resources and staff training, public health and environmental health agencies may be able to develop complementary obesity-related programs to educate food service workers on nutritional values and portion size, for example, and to monitor and sanction institutional compliance with nutrition and physical activity standards for children.

State and local public health agencies should make childhood obesity prevention a priority and work collaboratively with families, communities, schools, health- and medical-care providers, and industry to ensure that outcome. Further, state and local governments should increase funding for their health agencies so that they can more fully implement and evaluate obesity prevention efforts. State and local public health agencies should work with other state and local agencies, such as planning and public works departments, in establishing an interagency and multisectoral coordinating task force to facilitate collaborative planning, implementation, and assessment; coordinate and leverage governmental and nongovernmental resources; assure the capacity, workforce skills, standards, and resources necessary to achieve obesity prevention goals; support community coalitions (see Chapter 6); and work with community partners.

RESEARCH AND EVALUATION

Much remains to be learned about the causes and correlates of childhood obesity, as well as the optimum measures for preventing it. Experimental behavioral research and community-based research are key to learning more about changes in dietary and physical activity behaviors in individuals and populations (see Chapter 9). Moreover, as discussed elsewhere in this report, the funding and evaluation of a wide variety of obesity prevention intervention approaches are critical, given that there is a dearth of knowledge on this subject. Interventions focused on high-risk populations are particularly important. Such programs should be culturally relevant and designed to address the barriers to healthy lifestyles in these populations' physical and social environments.

An interdisciplinary research effort is greatly needed. Topics as diverse as the impacts of the built environment on health and behavior, gene-environment interactions, and the social underpinnings of healthful lifestyles require a research approach that embraces and encourages interdisciplinary research in agricultural and food sciences, nutritional sciences, economics, public health, marketing, behavioral and social sciences, policy sciences, urban planning, physiology, and health care. Innovative intervention designs, collaborative research efforts, and rigorous evaluation are key. A frequently overlooked component of the research cycle—the rapid translation and diffusion of effective programs and policies to community settings—is especially vital for making needed headway in obesity prevention efforts. Such transfer necessarily involves innovative intervention design and rigorous evaluation (see Chapter 3).

Because nutrition, physical activity, and obesity research encompass broad areas of investigation, federally funded research efforts are now dispersed amongst a number of U.S. agencies, including NIH, CDC, and USDA. In FY 2003, NIH spent $379 million on obesity-related research (NIH, 2004b). The NIH Obesity Research Task Force recently developed a strategic plan, focused primarily on the biobehavioral causes of obesity, for coordinating the NIH efforts (NIH, 2004a). CDC funds a range of state-based nutrition and physical activity grants, in addition to its own extensive epidemiologic efforts, to study the correlates of the obesity epidemic. USDA conducts extensive nutrition research and funds six human nutrition research centers across the country, one of them specifically devoted to children's nutrition (including childhood obesity).

The interdisciplinary nature of obesity-related research, however, offers exciting opportunities for strengthening and expanding intra- and interdepartmental research efforts. USDA, for example, could link land grant institutions and other higher education entities with federal nutrition assistance programs and could field multidisciplinary teams to evaluate program changes (NRC, 2004).

The federal investment in research on the prevention of childhood obesity must be strengthened. Further, foundations and other health-related organizations that fund research should consider designating childhood obesity prevention as a key area for funding. Interdisciplinary efforts should emphasize behavioral and community-based research, particularly in addressing childhood obesity prevention in high-risk populations.

A top research priority is the evaluation of obesity prevention interventions (see Chapter 9). Despite broad acknowledgement of the importance of the obesity crisis and the urgent need for effective prevention approaches, systematic reviews of the literature find few high-quality studies of the efficacy and/or effectiveness of various interventions to prevent weight gain and obesity in children (Campbell et al., 2002). As discussed throughout the report, there are many studies on correlates of obesity, physical activity, sedentary behavior, and various dietary intake patterns, many of which conclude that their findings will be useful in designing effective prevention programs. However, much of this research does not bear directly on understanding how best to manipulate these correlates to achieve changes in children's physical activity, sedentary behavior, diet, or weight. As a result, there are gaps in knowledge regarding how to successfully apply current understandings of causes and correlates into feasible and efficacious interventions and, subsequently, effective public health programs. Thus there is a need for more experimental research—studying purposeful manipulations

---

BOX 4-3
Evaluation Framework

Steps for designing and evaluating programs in public health:

• Engage stakeholders—include those involved in program operations, those served or affected by the programs, and primary users of the evaluation
• Describe the program
• Focus the evaluation design
• Gather credible evidence
• Justify conclusions
• Ensure use and share lessons learned

SOURCE: CDC, 1999.

---

of biological, behavioral, environmental, and policy factors—in tightly controlled laboratory studies, in randomized clinical trials, in quasi-experimental trials, and in natural experiments of environmental and policy changes. What distinguishes this research from nonexperimental research is the ability to reasonably make causal inferences and to translate the results into policies or programs for either further testing or clinical or public health practice.

One opportunity for obtaining needed information is to incorporate evaluation into the planning and implementation of programs and initiatives already being put forward (Box 4-3). As noted throughout this report, numerous relevant policies and programs are currently being planned or implemented at all levels of society. However, often the evaluation component is not considered an integral part of the implementation plan or time or funding constraints limit or negate evaluation efforts. When evaluations of these policies and programs are absent or inadequate, neither the policy nor the program sponsor and others will ever know whether or not the programs were successful. Until a sufficient evidence base is built, therefore, attention must be given to ensuring that careful evaluation research is conducted as part of all new policy and program initiatives. Through these evaluation efforts, interventions can be refined; those that are unsuccessful can be discontinued or refocused, and those that are successful can be identified, replicated, and disseminated.

Furthermore, cost-benefit and cost-effectiveness analyses must become a central component of prevention research because these assessments can guide appropriate policy making on the best use of limited resources (Kellam and Langevin, 2003). CDC is currently working on Project MOVE (Measurement of the Value of Exercise) which is calculating cost-effectiveness of previously conducted physical activity interventions based on published data. One of the literature's few cost-effectiveness studies on this topic examined Planet Health, a middle-school-based obesity prevention intervention with nutrition and physical activity components; the researchers calculated that the intervention (cost of $33,677 or $14 per student per year) would prevent 1.9 percent of the female students from becoming overweight as adults, thereby saving an estimated 4.1 quality-adjusted life years. The estimated savings in medical care costs ($15,887) and loss of productivity costs ($25,104) would result in a net savings to society of $7,313 (Wang et al., 2003). Assessments of the cost-effectiveness of other interventions are needed. **Increased funding is needed to ensure rigorous evaluation of the net benefit and cost-effectiveness of childhood obesity prevention interventions that are being implemented at local, state, and national levels.**

SURVEILLANCE AND MONITORING

National, state, and regional surveillance systems monitor the childhood obesity problem and contribute information on its prevalence (Table 4-1). For example, CDC's Youth Risk Behavior Surveillance System (YRBSS) surveys examine a variety of obesity-related factors, including physical activity and nutrition, in 12- to 19-year-olds. The School Health Policies and Programs Study (SHPPS), a national survey of states, school districts, schools, and classrooms, which has been conducted twice (1994 and 2000), examines policies for school health services, food services, and physical education (CDC, 2004b).

The National Health and Nutrition Examination Survey (NHANES) monitors the population—through home interviews and health examinations of representative samples of U.S. households with participants as young as 2 months of age—to gather a wealth of information relevant to obesity prevention efforts (see Chapter 2). The current NHANES measures many factors that relate to energy balance: dietary intake, physical activity, body mass index, body composition, cardiovascular fitness, and biochemical indicators such as blood pressure and serum glucose. Furthermore, collaborations between DHHS and USDA have facilitated the recent integration of the Continuing Survey of Food Intakes by Individuals (CSFII) and NHANES, so that dietary intake and health data can be more accurately correlated. Efforts are ongoing to incorporate the diet and health knowledge segment (previously in CSFII) into NHANES as well, providing further insights into knowledge and attitudes about diet and nutrition.

The health examination segment of NHANES includes fitness tests and questions regarding physical activity for 12- to 49-year-old participants. The current NHANES assessments of body composition include the use of

TABLE 4-1 Selected Surveillance Systems

Surveillance System	Primary Sponsor	Frequency	Description
CSFII Continuing Survey of Food Intakes by Individuals	USDA	1989-1991; 1994-1996; 1998; now part of NHANES	Nationally representative survey of dietary intake. Respondents were asked to provide 2 to 3 days of food intake data. CSFII is now incorporated into NHANES.
NHANES National Health and Nutrition Examination Survey	CDC	Previously conducted periodically, now continuous survey	Ongoing nationally representative survey assessing the health and nutritional status of adults and children in the United States through interviews and direct physical examinations. Currently, in partnership with USDA, NHANES incorporates the CSFII.
NHTS National Household Travel Survey	BTS and FHWA	2001	Survey of long-distance and local travel by the American public. The survey information includes mode of transportation, duration, distance and purpose of trip. Prior related surveys include the Nationwide Personal Transportation Survey conducted in 1969, 1977, 1983, 1990, and 1995 and the American Travel Survey conducted in 1977 and 1995.
National Longitudinal Study of Adolescent Health	NICHD	1994, 1996, and 2001-2002	Nationally representative study that explores health-related behaviors by following a sample of adolescents who were in grades 7 through 12 in 1994-1995 into young adulthood.

NLSY National Longitudinal Survey of Youth	BLS	Annual interviews	Nationally representative study of youths who were 12 to 16 years old in 1996. Initial interviews were with the youth and one parent. Subsequent annual interviews with the youth. Topics range from education and employment to health issues and time use.
PedNSS Pediatric Nutrition Surveillance System	CDC	Compiled from ongoing reports	Program-based surveillance system that examines nutritional status of children in low-income households. The system uses data collected from health, nutrition, and food assistance programs for infants and children, such as WIC.
SHPPS School Health Policies and Programs Study	CDC	1994 and 2000; to be conducted in 2006	Periodic collection of information on school health-related policies and programs at the state, district, school, and classroom levels.
YRBSS Youth Risk Behavior Surveillance System	CDC	1991-present; every 2 years	Monitors health risk behavior in adolescents through national, state, and local school-based surveys of representative samples of 9th through 12th grade students.

NOTE: BLS = Bureau of Labor Statistics; BTS = Bureau of Transportation Statistics; CDC = Centers for Disease Control and Prevention; CSFII = Continuing Survey of Food Intakes by Individuals; FHWA = Federal Highway Administration; NICHD = National Institute of Child Health and Human Development; USDA = U.S. Department of Agriculture.

multifrequency bioelectrical impedance analysis data on participants aged 8 to 49 years and dual energy x-ray absorptiometry measures on participants older than 8 years of age. This information allows greater accuracy in determining body-weight status and in examining correlates of nutrition and physical activity. NHANES data are used to track trends in obesity prevalence. But it is critical that additional information be collected and analyzed to provide insights into obesity prevention efforts.

Many of the current surveillance efforts collect data on only one age range (most often adolescents) and usually lack the resources to focus on high-risk populations at the state and regional levels. More detailed information is needed on weight status; physical activity; nutrition; social, environmental, and behavioral risk factors for obesity; and economic and medical consequences of obesity (such as type 2 diabetes in children and youth). Information on children's physical activity levels is particularly scant because most national surveys focus on adolescents. Additional information is needed at the state and regional level to provide more in-depth information on specific geographic areas or high-risk populations. Further efforts should also be made to monitor community-level variables in order to assess the impact of environmental-level changes and policies. Examples include the number of school districts requiring daily physical education in schools, the number of grocery stores selling fresh fruits and vegetables within low-income neighborhoods, or the percentage of children living within a mile of school who commute by walking or biking. Innovative approaches should be explored and evaluated that would monitor the impact of changes at the local level and feed that information back to national sources so that successful programs could be refined and expanded.

Relevant surveillance and monitoring efforts should be supported and strengthened by increased federal funding; this applies particularly to NHANES, as it is a valuable information resource for obesity prevention programs. Special efforts should be made to identify those populations most at risk of childhood obesity, and to monitor the social, environmental, and behavioral factors contributing to that elevated risk.

Further efforts to collect longitudinal data would be useful, as longitudinal studies can examine potential risk factors associated with the development of obesity and normal weight, which is not possible from cross-sectional studies. Discussions are ongoing about initiating a new national longitudinal study on U.S. children that would follow a large cohort over time to examine health and well-being issues. As this national study is being considered, the committee urges that weight status, as well as nutrition- and physical activity-related measures, be included in such an effort's basic set of questions. A precedent is the Avon Longitudinal Study of Pregnancy and Childhood (ALSPAC), based in England and involving other European collaboration centers. ALSPAC is examining nutrition and other antecedents as well as growth outcomes. Any national longitudinal cohort study of children that is established should examine antecedents and outcomes, including physical activity levels, dietary patterns, eating behaviors, and weight status, related to the development of obesity during childhood.

NUTRITION AND PHYSICAL ACTIVITY PROGRAMS

A number of public- and private-sector programs educate consumers of all ages about proper nutrition and regular physical activity. For example, the USDA's Expanded Food and Nutrition Education Program (EFNEP) uses the resources of county Cooperative Extension System services and other local agencies to reach low-income families and youth, and both the Special Supplemental Nutrition Program for Women, Infants, and Children (WIC) and the Food Stamp Program (FSP) have nutrition education components. Team Nutrition has been developed by USDA to improve school nutrition and nutrition education, and it has components for students, parents, teachers, and food service personnel. The Five-A-Day media campaigns, the result of an extensive public-private partnership, promote the consumption of fruits and vegetables. These programs still face challenges, however. A recent assessment of several USDA nutrition education efforts revealed limited resources, competing program requirements, and a lack of systematic data collection on the types of nutrition education offered (GAO, 2004). Actions are therefore needed that clearly identify program goals, tailor nutrition education to meet the needs of participants, and collect data on program results (GAO, 2004).

Increasingly, more public- and private-sector programs are focusing on physical activity, or they are working to promote both good nutrition and physical activity. The President's Council on Physical Fitness and Sports is developing a Fit 'n Active Kids program. The Partnership for a Walkable America is an extensive public-private collaboration to promote walking and improve conditions for walking. The America on the Move initiative sponsored by the Partnership to Promote Healthy Eating and Active Living (an organization of nonprofit and private-sector partners) targets prevention of adult weight gain as a first step toward combating obesity; the initiative specifically advocates increasing physical activity by 100 calories per day and decreasing caloric intake by 100 calories per day (America on the Move, 2004). CDC's VERB campaign (see Chapter 5) focuses on media messages on physical activity for 9- to 13-year-olds and involves collaborations with schools, youth organizations, and other organizations.

The existing infrastructure and capabilities of these and other relevant federal programs and public-private collaborations can provide an avenue to raise awareness of the health consequences of childhood obesity and to convey, through well-evaluated interventions, information on energy balance and the benefits to children of healthful food choices and regular physical activity. Some of these programs were developed to accomplish goals other than obesity prevention, and evaluation of how to best use them to respond to the current information needs for obesity prevention may be needed. Children, youth, and their families need to have the information to make positive lifestyle decisions just as they need access to nutritious foods and recreational facilities in order to implement these choices (see Chapter 8). Providing obesity-related information to parents and families is often quite a challenge, because there is no one source or avenue throughout the United States for parent education. Several options are available at present, including federal and state nutrition education programs, parenting magazines and other media, health-care visits, and school-based programs. However, other innovative approaches need to be explored.

Program implementation efforts should particularly address childhood obesity prevention in high-risk populations. Some of the ongoing federal food and nutrition efforts—including EFNEP, FSP, WIC, the National School Lunch Program (NSLP), the School Breakfast Program (SBP), the Summer Food Service Program, and the Child and Adult Care Food Program (CACFP)—address the needs of low-income, high-risk populations that have significant health disparities. But these programs could do more, even within their existing infrastructure, through a sustained commitment to funding for obesity prevention research and intervention development, implementation, and evaluation.

Federal support is needed for programs that emphasize improved nutrition and physical activity in children, youth, and their families, with particular attention paid to populations at high risk of obesity. These programs should be required to have strong evaluation components, and the evaluation results should consequently be reflected in program refinements that strengthen their evidence-based approaches. Programs should also explore and evaluate new approaches to educating children and their families about concepts related to energy balance.

NUTRITION ASSISTANCE PROGRAMS

One in five Americans utilizes one or more of the 15 federal nutrition assistance programs (USDA, 2003a). Many of these programs provide food to children either directly, through the school breakfast and lunch programs, or indirectly, through vouchers that may be used by the family to supplement household food resources (Table 4-2).

In FY 2001, approximately 4 million children were served each month by the FSP, 28 million were served daily by the NSLP, and 8.1 million were served daily by the SBP. Although the FSP includes a nutrition education component in selected states, the program is designed as a food equity

TABLE 4-2 Selected Federal Food and Nutrition Assistance Programs

		FY 2002
Food Stamp Program	Average monthly participation (millions)	19.1
	Average benefit per person (dollars/month)	79.68
	Total expenditures ($ billions)	20.7
WIC	Average monthly participation (millions)	7.5
	Total expenditures ($ billions)	4.3
National School Lunch Program	Average daily participation (millions)	28.0
	Total expenditures ($ billions)	6.9
School Breakfast Program	Average daily participation (millions)	8.1
	Total expenditures ($ billions)	1.6
Child and Adult Care Food Program	Meals served in:	
	• Child care centers (millions)	984
	• Family child care homes (millions)	708
	• Adult day care centers (millions)	45
	Total annual expenditures ($ billions)	1.9

SOURCE: USDA, 2003a.

program to alleviate hunger and food insecurity; thus it does not have guidelines on the specific types of food that recipients may purchase with their benefits. There has been growing interest, however, in examining the relationships among food insecurity, federal nutrition assistance program participation, and the risk of obesity among children and youth. Because resource-constrained families are more likely to participate in nutrition programs, any association of program participation with obesity must be evaluated within the context of poverty and food insecurity (Frongillo, 2003).

As noted in Chapter 3, food insecurity in children has not been associated with obesity, except in white girls aged 8 to 16 years (Alaimo et al., 2001; Casey et al., 2001; Frongillo, 2003). In fact, existing empirical data suggests that there is a lower risk of overweight and obesity in school-aged food-insecure girls who participated in the FSP, NSLP, and the SBP (Jones et al., 2003).

The WIC program provides nutrition information, supplemental foods, and referrals to health care for low-income women, infants, and children up to age 5 who are at nutritional risk. Approximately half of all infants and 25 percent of all 1- to 4-year-old children in the United States participate in the WIC program (Oliveira et al., 2002). A study of low-income preschool children in 18 states and Washington, DC (most were WIC recipients) found that one in ten was overweight in 1995, a relative increase of 20 percent from 1983 (Mei et al., 1998). Two studies examining potential associations between the WIC food package and overweight status in children found that WIC foods did not contribute to overweight (CDC, 1996) and that the weight status of children in the WIC program was comparable to that of other low-income children (Burstein et al., 2000). The Institute of Medicine is currently conducting a study to review the nutritional needs of the populations served by the WIC Program, assess their supplemental nutritional needs, and propose recommendations for the contents of the WIC food packages.

Given that a great deal is known about good nutrition and the dietary composition of balanced diets, it would be advantageous to the health of children participating in federal nutrition assistance programs if nutrient-rich foods were made available and if there was access to ethnically and culturally appropriate foods. The committee is particularly interested in urging USDA to expand pilot programs that focus on increasing the availability of fresh fruits and vegetables and other nutritious foods or provide incentives for the purchase of these items. Ideas for such programs have included double or specifically designated fruit and vegetable vouchers; coupons or other discount promotions; and the ability to use electronic benefit transfer cards at farmers' markets or community-supported agricultural markets (GAO, 2002). Additionally, a systematic study should examine potential strategies for improving the community food environment to ensure that FSP recipients have access to supermarkets, farmers' markets, and other venues that provide fresh, high-quality, and affordable produce and other healthful foods (see Chapter 6).

In addition to their current objectives to improve food access and dietary quality, the federal nutrition assistance programs (e.g., WIC, FSP) should include obesity prevention as an explicit goal for the populations served. Congress should request independent assessments of these programs to ensure that each provides adequate access to healthful dietary choices (including fruits, vegetables, and whole grains) for the populations served. USDA should also continue to explore pilot programs within the nutrition assistance programs that encourage diet and physical activity behaviors that promote energy balance at a healthy weight in children and youth.

AGRICULTURAL POLICIES

As the traditional paradigm of "farm to table" shifts to one of "table to farm," driven by consumer demand and an awareness of the connections between diet and health, decision makers in the United States should take a new look at the impact of agricultural and food policies (NRC, 2004). The committee acknowledges that the nation's food supply is part of a global food system, and that many food-related issues lie outside of any one nation's purview. However, the committee also realizes that the global implications of domestic solutions to the childhood obesity epidemic should be thoughtfully considered so that new problems are not created that may produce adverse consequences (Appendix D).

There are a number of mechanisms by which U.S. federal agricultural policies may potentially affect the types of foods available to and marketed to children. For example, schools participating in the NSLP may choose to receive entitlement commodities purchased by USDA specifically for the program or receive bonus commodities from USDA to bolster the agricultural markets for particular products (to address temporary surpluses or to help stabilize farm prices) (USDA, 2002, 2004b). In the 2001-2002 school year, USDA's Agricultural Marketing Service and Farm Service Agency together spent more than $765 million on school lunch entitlement purchases and approximately $58 million in providing bonus commodities (USDA, 2004b). These included beef, fish, poultry, eggs, fruits, vegetables, flours, grains, dairy products, and peanut products. As discussed in Chapter 7, there are several federal, state, and local programs at present, such as the Department of Defense's Fresh Produce Program, that provide the distribution mechanisms for delivering fresh produce from farms to schools.

A second set of policies to examine involves the check-off programs, used for agriculture products such as beef, pork, and dairy, in which producers are required to donate money—a fixed amount for each unit sold—to a fund established by federal legislation but run by a national private-sector board (Dairy Management, 2004; National Pork Board, 2004; USDA, 2004a). For example, the National Pork Board reports that pork producers and importers pay 40 cents on each $100 when pigs or pork products are sold; these funds generated $47.8 million in 2003 (National Pork Board, 2004) for use in advertising, marketing, education, research, and other programs that promoted the commodity.

Concerns have been raised about the many factors that influence food demand and food consumption behaviors of Americans—the types and prices of available foods, technological advances, time pressures, and government policies on agriculture, taxes, and exports/imports—which are outside of consumer control (NRC, 2004).

A review of agricultural policies could identify unintended effects of U.S. agricultural subsidies on human health. For example, Americans' per capita consumption of caloric sweeteners—primarily sucrose derived from cane, beets, and corn (notably high fructose corn syrup)—increased by 43 pounds, or 39 percent, between 1950-1959 and 2000 (USDA, 2003b). In 2000, the average American consumed 152 pounds of caloric sweeteners, which was equivalent to 52 teaspoons of added sugars per person per day

(USDA, 2003b), more than 40 percent of which came from high fructose corn syrup (Bray et al., 2004). The possible relationships among agricultural policies (such as corn subsidies and the production and use of high fructose corn syrup in the U.S. food supply), the obesity epidemic (Bray et al., 2004), and the marked increase in type 2 diabetes (Gross et al., 2004; Schulze et al., 2004) warrant further investigation.

An independent assessment should be conducted of U.S. agricultural policies, including agricultural subsidies and commodity programs, that may affect the types and quantities of foods available to children through the federal food assistance programs. Further, other efforts (such as check-off programs) that have involved federal legislation should be examined to ensure that they work to promote a healthful dietary intake among children. Policies and programs should be revised as necessary to promote a U.S. food system that supports energy balance at a healthy weight.

OTHER POLICY CONSIDERATIONS

The imposition of taxes on certain foods or beverages, particularly high-calorie food items or those with low nutrient density, has been discussed with regard to the obesity epidemic. Several states including Arkansas, Tennessee, Virginia, and Washington, currently impose excise taxes on soft drinks. Although the tax rates have been found to be too small to affect sales, in certain jurisdictions the revenues generated are substantial but generally have not been used to fund obesity prevention activities (Jacobson and Brownell, 2000). It is not known whether imposing a sales tax on designated foods such as soft drinks would have a significant effect on beverage sales (Jacobson and Brownell, 2000). Moreover, there is the difficulty of determining which foods would be taxable—for example, how to define soft drink and snack foods (Jacobson and Brownell, 2000). Taxation and pricing strategies have been found to contribute to tobacco prevention and control efforts (Levy et al., 2004). Pricing policies for food are much more complex than tobacco and there is limited evidence about the price elasticity of high-energy-dense foods (Yach et al., 2003). It is notable that other countries, such as Norway, have effectively used agricultural policies such as consumer and producer subsidies to encourage the consumption of healthful foods (Milio, 1998).

The committee has carefully considered the issues regarding taxes on specific foods, particularly soft drinks and energy-dense snack foods, but at this time, it is the committee's judgment that there is not sufficient evidence to make a strong recommendation either for or against taxing these foods. More research is needed to determine objective methods for defining and characterizing foods based on nutritional considerations such as the quality and quantity of nutrients or the energy density. Additionally, because low-income families spend a greater proportion of their household income on food than do higher-income families (Nord et al., 2003), taxes on foods may have the effect of being regressive and may lead to unintended consequences such as increasing food insecurity. In any case, taxation may not address the main issue, that many people will not consume greater amounts of healthful foods, even if their relative prices are lower, simply because they prefer energy-dense foods.

Because some states are already taxing specific types of food or beverage products, studying these examples may prove useful. The committee suggests that research into the effects of taxation and pricing strategies be considered a priority to help shed light on the potential outcomes of more broadly applying taxation as a public health strategy for promoting improved dietary behaviors, more physical activity, and reduced sedentary behaviors.

RECOMMENDATION

Childhood obesity is a serious nationwide health problem requiring urgent attention and a population-based prevention approach. Innovative ideas, commitments of time and resources by diverse sectors and stakeholders, and sustained efforts involving individual, institutional, and societal changes are needed to ensure that all children grow up physically and emotionally healthy.

Also needed is national leadership that elevates childhood obesity prevention to a top national health priority and dedicates the funding and resources required to make this goal a long-term commitment. Only through policies, legislation, programs, and research will meaningful changes be made. Steady monitoring and evaluation of those changes will inform and refine future efforts. **Prevention of obesity in children and youth should be a national public health priority.**

Recommendation 1: *National Priority*
Government at all levels should provide coordinated leadership for the prevention of obesity in children and youth. The President should request that the Secretary of the DHHS convene a high-level task force to ensure coordinated budgets, policies, and program requirements and to establish effective interdepartmental collaboration and priorities for action. An increased level and sustained commitment of federal and state funds and resources are needed.

To implement this recommendation, the federal government should:

• Strengthen research and program efforts addressing obesity prevention, with a focus on experimental behavioral research and community-based intervention research and on the rigorous evaluation of the effectiveness, cost-effectiveness, sustainability, and scaling up of effective prevention interventions

• Support extensive program and research efforts to prevent childhood obesity in high-risk populations with health disparities, with a focus both on behavioral and environmental approaches

• Support nutrition and physical activity grant programs, particularly in states with the highest prevalence of childhood obesity

• Strengthen support for relevant surveillance and monitoring efforts, particularly NHANES

• Undertake an independent assessment of federal nutrition assistance programs and agricultural policies to ensure that they promote healthful dietary intake and physical activity levels for all children and youth

• Develop and evaluate pilot projects within the nutrition assistance programs that would promote healthful dietary intake and physical activity and scale up those found to be successful

To implement this recommendation, state and local governments should:

• Provide coordinated leadership and support for childhood obesity prevention efforts, particularly those focused on high-risk populations, by increasing resources and strengthening policies that promote opportunities for physical activity and healthful eating in communities, neighborhoods, and schools

• Support public health agencies and community coalitions in their collaborative efforts to promote and evaluate obesity prevention interventions

REFERENCES

Alaimo K, Olson CM, Frongillo EA Jr. 2001. Low family income and food insufficiency in relation to overweight in US children: Is there a paradox? *Arch Pediatric Adolesc Med* 155(10):1161-1167.

America on the Move. 2004. *America on the Move*. [Online]. Available: http://www.americaonthemove.org [accessed May 15, 2004].

Bray GA, Nielsen SJ, Popkin BM. 2004. Consumption of high-fructose corn syrup in beverages may play a role in the epidemic of obesity. *Am J Clin Nutr* 79(4):537-543.

Burstein NR, Fox MK, Hiller JB, Kornfeld R, Lam K, Price C, Rodda DT. 2000. *Profile of WIC Children*. Cambridge, MA. Prepared by Abt Associates for USDA, FNS, Office of Analysis, Nutrition, and Evaluation.

Campbell K, Waters E, O'Meara S, Kelly S, Summerbell C. 2002. *Interventions for Preventing Obesity in Children*. Oxford, U.K.: Cochrane Library.

Canadian Institute for Health Information. 2004. Obesity. In: *Improving the Health of Canadians*. Ottawa, Ontario: CIHI. Pp. 105-142.

Casey PH, Szeto K, Lensing S, Bogle M, Weber J. 2001. Children in food-insufficient, low-income families: Prevalence, health, and nutrition status. *Arch Pediatr Adolesc Med* 155(4):508-514.

CDC (U.S. Centers for Disease Control and Prevention). 1996. Nutritional status of children participating in the Special Supplemental Nutrition Program for Women, Infants, and Children—United States, 1998-1991. *MMWR* 45(3):65-69.

CDC. 1999. Framework for program evaluation in public health. *MMWR Recomm Rep* 48(RR11):1-40.

CDC. 2004a. *CDC's State-Based Nutrition and Physical Activity Program to Prevent Obesity and Other Chronic Diseases*. [Online]. Available: http://www.cdc.gov/nccdphp/dnpa/obesity/state_programs/index.htm [accessed April 21, 2004].

CDC. 2004b. *School Health Policies and Programs Study*. [Online]. Available: http://www.cdc.gov/nccdphp/dash/shpps/index.htm [accessed May 26, 2004].

Dairy Management, Inc. 2004. *About the Dairy Checkoff*. [Online]. Available: http://www.dairycheckoff.com/ [accessed March 15, 2004].

DHHS (U.S. Department of Health and Human Services). 2000. *Healthy People 2010: Objectives for Improving Health*. Washington, DC: DHHS.

DHHS. 2001. *The Surgeon General's Call to Action to Prevent and Decrease Overweight and Obesity*. Rockville, MD: Public Health Service, Office of the Surgeon General.

DHHS. 2004. *The Health Consequences of Smoking: A Report from the Surgeon General*. Washington, DC: DHHS. [Online]. Available: http://www.cdc.gov/tobacco/sgr/sgr_2004/index.htm [accessed June 8, 2004].

Economos CD, Brownson RC, DeAngelis MA, Foerster SB, Foreman CT, Gregson J, Kumanyika SK, Pate RR. 2001. What lessons have been learned from other attempts to guide social change? *Nutr Rev* 59(3 Pt 2):S40-S56.

Frongillo EA. 2003. Understanding obesity and program participation in the context of poverty and food insecurity. *J Nutr* 133(7):2117-2118.

GAO (U.S. General Accounting Office). 2002. *Fruits and Vegetables: Enhanced Federal Efforts to Increase Consumption Could Yield Health Benefits for Americans*. GAO-02-657. Washington, DC: GAO.

GAO. 2004. *Nutrition Education: USDA Provides Services Through Multiple Programs, but Stronger Linkages Among Efforts are Needed*. GAO-04-528. Washington, DC: GAO.

Gross LS, Li L, Ford ES, Liu S. 2004. Increased consumption of refined carbohydrates and the epidemic of type 2 diabetes in the United States: An ecologic assessment. *Am J Clin Nutr* 79(5):774-779.

Haddad L. 2003. *What Can Food Policy Do to Redirect the Diet Transition?* FCND Discussion Paper No. 165. Washington, DC: International Food Policy Research Institute.

Health Council of The Netherlands. 2003. *Overweight and Obesity*. Publication 2003/07. The Hague, Netherlands: Health Council of The Netherlands.

IOM (Institute of Medicine). 1999. *Reducing the Burden of Injury: Advancing Prevention and Treatment*. Washington, DC: National Academy Press.

IOM. 2003. *The Future of the Public's Health in the 21st Century*. Washington, DC: The National Academies Press.

Jacobson MF, Brownell KD. 2000. Small taxes on soft drinks and snack foods to promote health. *Am J Public Health* 90(6):854-857.

Jones SJ, Jahns L, Laraia BA, Haughton B. 2003. Lower risk of overweight in school-aged food insecure girls who participate in food assistance: Results from the panel study of income dynamics child development supplement. *Arch Pediatr Adolesc Med* 157(8):780-784.

Kellam SG, Langevin DJ. 2003. A framework for understanding "evidence" in prevention research and programs. *Prev Sci* 4 (3):137-153.

Kersh R, Morone J. 2002. How the personal becomes political: Prohibitions, public health, and obesity. *Stud Am Polit Dev* 16:162-175.

Levy DT, Chaloupka F, Gitchell J. 2004. The effects of tobacco control policies on smoking rates: A tobacco control scorecard. *J Public Health Manag Pract* 10(4):338-353.

Lobstein T, Baur L, Uauy R, IASO International Obesity Task Force. 2004. Obesity in children and young people: A crisis in public health. *Obes Rev* 5(Suppl 1):4-85.

Mei Z, Scanlon KS, Grummer-Strawn LM, Freedman DS, Yip R, Trowbridge FL. 1998. Increasing prevalence of overweight among U.S. low-income preschool children: The Centers for Disease Control and Prevention Pediatric Nutrition Surveillance, 1983 to 1995. *Pediatrics* 101:E12.

Milio N. 1998. Norwegian nutition policy: Progress, problems and prospects. In: Milio N, Helsing E, eds. *European Food and Nutrition Policies in Action.* WHO Regional Publications, European Series, No. 73. Copenhagen, Denmark: Regional Office for Europe.

National Board of Health. 2003. *National Action Plan Against Obesity. Recommendations and Perspectives. Short Version.* Copenhagen, Denmark: National Board of Health, Center for Health Promotion and Prevention.

National Pork Board. 2004. *About Pork Checkoff.* [Online]. Available: http://www.porkboard.org/about/ [accessed March 15, 2004].

New South Wales Department of Health. 2003. *Prevention of Obesity in Children and Young People. NSW Government Action Plan 2003-2007.* North Sydney, NSW, Australia: NSW Department of Health.

NIH (National Institutes of Health). 2004a. *Strategic Plan for NIH Obesity Research.* [Online]. Available: http://obesityresearch.nih.gov/About/ObesityEntireDocument.pdf [accessed August 24, 2004].

NIH. 2004b. *Estimates of Funding for Various Diseases, Conditions, Research Areas.* [Online]. Available: http://www.nih.gov/news/fundingresearchareas.htm [accessed June 22, 2004].

Nord M, Andrews M, Carlson S. 2003. *Household Food Security in the United States, 2002.* Food Assistance and Nutrition Research Report 35. Alexandria, VA: Economic Research Service.

NRC (National Research Council). 2004. *Exploring a Vision: Integrating Knowledge for Food and Health.* Washington, DC: The National Academies Press.

Oliveira V, Racine E, Olmsted J, Ghelfi LM. 2002. *The WIC Program: Background, Trends, and Issues.* Food Assistance and Nutrition Research Report, Number 27. Washington, DC: USDA, Economic Research Service.

Raine KD. 2004. *Overweight and Obesity in Canada: A Population Health Perspective.* Ottawa, Ontario: Canadian Institute for Health Information.

Schulze MB, Manson JE, Ludwig DS, Colditz GA, Stampfer MJ, Willett WC, Hu FB. 2004. Sugar-sweetened beverages, weight gain, and incidence of type 2 diabetes in young and middle-aged women. *J Am Med Assoc* 292(8):927-934.

United Kingdom Parliament. 2004. *Health–Third Report.* House of Commons: Select Committee on Health. [Online]. Available: http://www.parliament.the-stationery-office.co.uk/pa/cm200304/cmselect/cmhealth/23/2302.htm [accessed June 10, 2004].

USDA (U.S. Department of Agriculture). 2002. *Availability of Fresh Produce in Nutrition Assistance Programs*. Nutrition Assistance Program Report Series, No. CN-02-FV. Alexandria, VA: USDA Food and Nutrition Service, Office of Analysis, Nutrition, and Evaluation.

USDA. 2003a. *The Food Assistance Landscape*. Food Assistance and Nutrition Research Report Number 28-3. Washington, DC: Economic Research Service.

USDA. 2003b. Profiling food consumption in America. In: *Agriculture Fact Book 2001-2002*. Washington, DC: USDA. U.S. Government Printing Office.

USDA. 2004a. *Beef Promotion and Research Order*. Agricultural Marketing Service. Livestock and Seed Program. [Online]. Available: http://www.ams.usda.gov/lsg/mpb/beef/beefchk.htm [accessed March 15, 2004].

USDA. 2004b. *National School Lunch Program*. Agricultural Marketing Service. [Online]. Available: http://www.ams.usda.gov/nslpfact.htm [accessed March 15, 2004].

Wang LY, Yang Q, Lowry R, Wechsler H. 2003. Economic analysis of a school-based obesity prevention program. *Obes Res* 11(11):1313-1324.

WHO (World Health Organization). 2000. *Obesity: Preventing and Managing the Global Epidemic*. Report of a WHO Consultation: WHO Technical Report Series 894. Geneva: WHO.

WHO. 2003. *Diet, Nutrition and the Prevention of Chronic Diseases*. Technical Report Series No. 916. Geneva: WHO.

Willett WC, Domolky S. 2004. *Strategic Plan for the Prevention and Control of Overweight and Obesity in New England*. Providence, RI: New England Coalition for Health Promotion and Disease Prevention. [Online]. Available: http://www.ncconinfo.org/Strategic_Plan_02-11-03.pdf [accessed June 6, 2004].

Yach D, Hawkes C, Epping-Jordan JE, Galbraith S. 2003. The World Health Organization's framework convention on tobacco control: Implications for global epidemics of food-related deaths and disease. *J Public Health Policy* 24(3/4):274-290.

5

Industry, Advertising, Media, and Public Education

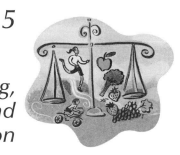

To lead a healthier and more active lifestyle, many young consumers and their parents will need to alter their food and beverage preferences and engage in fewer sedentary pursuits in order to achieve energy balance. Market forces may be very influential in changing both consumer and industry behaviors. The food, beverage, restaurant, entertainment, leisure, and recreation industries must share responsibility for childhood obesity prevention and can be instrumental in supporting this goal. Federal agencies such as the U.S. Department of Health and Human Services (DHHS), the U.S. Department of Agriculture (USDA), and the Federal Trade Commission (FTC) all have the potential to strengthen industry efforts through general support, technical assistance, research expertise, and regulatory guidance. In addition, government is an important source of positive reinforcement. It can recognize industry stakeholders who are willing to take the financial risks of developing new products and services consistent with the goals of healthful eating behaviors and regular physical activity, thereby setting examples for other private-sector entities to follow.

INDUSTRY

American children and youth represent dynamic and lucrative markets. For example, food and beverage sales to young consumers exceeded $27 billion in 2002 (*U.S. Market for Kids' Foods and Beverages*, 2003). Similarly, young people are major consumers of the products and services of the entertainment, leisure, and recreation industries.

Providing young consumers and their families with the knowledge and skills to make informed and prudent choices in these marketplaces could be a key obesity prevention strategy. Industry continuously develops new products and services in response to changing consumer demand, and its primary emphases—sales trends, marketing opportunities, product appeal, and expanding market share for specific product categories and product brands (Datamonitor, 2002; U.S. Market for Kids' Foods and Beverages, 2003)—could be profitably shifted toward healthier and more active lifestyles.

Although the private sector has not historically viewed its responsibility as changing consumers' preferences toward healthier choices, changes are under way that acknowledge the essential role that industry may play in related policy dialogues, public/private partnerships, and research (Crockett et al., 2002).

The increased media coverage of childhood obesity in recent years, and the consequent growth in public attention and potential for litigation have sensitized the food and beverage industries to examine the underlying causes of the problem and learn from the tobacco industry experiences (Daynard, 2003; Appendix D). Moreover, it provides an opportunity for many types of industries (e.g., food, beverage, entertainment, recreation) to explore new marketing opportunities (Datamonitor, 2002). To the extent that consumers want to purchase and consume a healthful diet, engage in physical activity, and maintain energy balance, private industry not only has a profit incentive but a public relations incentive to help them meet that goal and demonstrate that industry can be responsive to public concerns.

The committee recognizes that children, youth, and their adult care providers are immersed in a modern milieu, including a commercial environment that could be shaped to encourage behaviors relevant to preventing obesity (Peters et al., 2002). Consumers may initially be unsure about what to eat for good health. They often make immediate trade-offs in taste, cost, and convenience for longer term health (Wansink, 2004). But numerous opportunities for influencing consumers' purchase decisions present themselves as the food and beverage industries develop, package, label, promote, distribute, and price products and as retail food stores, full-service restaurants, and fast food establishments make similar sets of decisions. Each of these points offers opportunities for influencing consumers' purchase decisions.

Developing healthier food and beverage products or serving smaller portion sizes may be viewed by some private-sector businesses as risks rather than as opportunities; making changes in the absence of broad-based consumer demand, whatever the market, conceivably can be seen as a risk to the private sector. But in this case there is ample precedent. A variety of food-industry stakeholders have recently made positive changes by expanding healthier meal options for young consumers (Hurley and Liebman, 2004; Richwine, 2004), offering improved food products with reduced sugar content for children (PR Newswire, 2004), and reducing portion sizes at full-service and fast food restaurants (Hurley and Liebman, 2004). These changes can and should occur on a much larger scale. For that to happen, coordinated efforts among industry, government, and other sectors are needed to stimulate, support, and sustain consumer demand for healthful foods and beverages, appropriately portioned meals, and accurate and consistent nutritional information made readily available to the public.

Similarly, the leisure, entertainment, and recreation industries are faced with the challenge of maintaining profitability while portraying active living[1] as a desirable social norm for adults and children. These industries, which influence how leisure time is used, can create a wide range of new products and opportunities to increase energy expenditure through the incorporation of physical activity messages into sedentary pursuits (e.g., television commercials, video games and Internet websites that remind or prompt consumers to increase physical activity for a specified amount of time to balance screen time). This chapter presents a series of recommendations appropriate to the commercial environment in general and to various industries in particular.

Food and Beverage Industry

Product Development

The food and beverage industries' decisions are guided by key factors—including taste, palatability, cost, convenience, value, variety, availability, ethnic preferences, and safety—that drive consumer demand (FMI, 2003a,b; Wansink, 2004). The industry's decisions are also constrained by other conditions. For example, product and meal size are significant drivers of consumers' perceived value of the foods and beverages they purchase, whether for consumption at home or elsewhere (FMI, 2003a,b; Stewart et al., 2004; Wansink, 2004).

Similarly, modern retail food stores offer tens of thousands of food and beverage items from which to choose. While more than 14,000 new food and beverage products enter the U.S. marketplace annually, less than 6

---

[1]Active living is a way of life that integrates two types of physical activity—*recreational* or *leisure* activity (e.g., jogging, skateboarding, or playing basketball), and *utilitarian* or *occupational* activity (e.g., walking or bicycling to school or running errands)—into one's daily routine.

percent are innovative enough to be successful (Heasman and Mellentin, 2001). The majority of these new products fail for a variety of reasons including lack of consumer demand, cost, marketing strategies, or lack of positive reinforcement or support from other groups (such as the public health sector and health-care professionals) (Heasman and Mellentin, 2001).

But failure in the past, particularly with regard to healthier food and beverage offerings, does not necessarily mean failure in the future. The financial success of diet carbonated beverages and the greater availability of reduced-calorie food and beverage products—buttressed in part by the reduced fat or saturated fat processed food products created by industry in response to the *Healthy People 2000* objectives (NCHS, 2001)—are examples of how industry could be continually seeking new ways to meet consumer demand, earn a decent profit, and have its products positively affect public health.

Thus significant profit incentives now exist for industry to develop reduced-calorie and low-energy-dense foods, thereby helping consumers achieve their dietary and energy balance goals. Movement in that direction has already begun; food and beverage industries are currently seeking opportunities in product development and product reformulation, with an emphasis on eating for health (Datamonitor, 2002; FMI, 2003a). New products are also developed, packaged, and marketed to ethnically diverse children and youth with attention to cultural taste preferences and attractive packaging (Williams et al., 1993). **The committee recommends that as new products are developed or existing products are modified by the private sector, it should be imperative that energy balance, energy density, nutrient density, and standard serving sizes are primary considerations in the process. This can be assisted by government stakeholders providing general support, technical assistance, research expertise, and regulatory guidance.**

Energy Density of Foods

As discussed in Chapter 3, the energy density of a given food is the amount of energy it stores per unit volume or mass. At 9 kilocalories[2] stored per gram, fat has the highest energy density. Alcohol stores 7 kilocalories per gram, carbohydrates and protein both store 4, fiber stores 1.5-2.5, and water stores 0.0—i.e., it does not provide energy. Energy density is a determinant of the effects of foods and macronutrients on satiety (Rolls et

---

[2] In this report the term "kilocalories" is used synonymously with "calories."

al., 2004a), and it may have a significant influence on regulating food intake and body weight as well (Drewnowski, 2003; Prentice and Jebb, 2003).

High-energy-dense foods, such as potato chips and sweets, tend to be palatable but may not be satiating for consumers, calorie for calorie, thereby encouraging greater food consumption (Drewnowski, 1998; Prentice and Jebb, 2003). Humans may have a weak innate ability to recognize foods with a high energy density to down-regulate the amount of food consumed in order to maintain energy balance, thereby fostering a "passive overconsumption" of these types of foods (Prentice and Jebb, 2003). By contrast, low-energy-dense foods, such as fruits and vegetables, contain more fiber and water and less fat than high-energy-dense foods. As a result, they promote satiety and reduce energy intake but may be considered less palatable by some individuals (Drewnowski, 1998; Rolls et al., 2004b). Consumers typically ingest fewer calories when meals are low in energy density than high in energy density (Kral et al., 2002; Rolls et al., 2004b). There is a need for further research on the implications of dietary energy density on the short-term and long-term physiological regulation of satiety, and the role of energy density in total energy intake and achieving a healthy body weight.

An analysis of the 1999-2000 National Health and Nutrition Examination Survey (NHANES) and NHANES III data revealed that three food groups—sweets and desserts, soft drinks, and alcoholic beverages—comprised nearly 25 percent of all calories consumed by Americans between 1988 and 2000. Salty snacks and fruit-flavored beverages accounted for another 5 percent, bringing the total calories contributed by high-energy-dense/low-nutrient-dense foods to be at least 30 percent of Americans' total calorie intake during that period (Block, 2004). Nutrient composition data available from fast food company websites suggest that average menus are twice the energy density of recommended healthful diets (Prentice and Jebb, 2003).

Developing low-energy-dense but palatable food products, which will help consumers achieve and maintain energy balance by reducing the probability of excessive energy consumption, has been a significant challenge for the food industry (Drewnowski, 1998). While acknowledging this challenge, the committee emphasizes the need to identify specific incentives that will help the industry develop such new products. In the meantime, manufacturers can modify existing products—for example, by replacing fat with protein, fruit or vegetable purée, fiber, water, or even air—to reduce energy density but maintain palatability without substantially reducing the product size or volume.

Product Packaging and Portion Sizes

Packaging is the "interface" between food-industry products and the consumer—that is, it is the public's first point of contact—and food packages implicitly suggest portion sizes or food combinations (e.g., which foods are eaten together such as peanut butter and jelly). But a product package can be modified in three general ways—by size, visual appeal, and the type and amount of information it provides (such as the nutritional content according to the Nutrition Facts panel on food labels)—in order to assist consumers in making knowledgeable purchasing decisions and determining portion sizes for themselves.

Because energy requirements vary both by age and body size (IOM, 2002), parents need to be aware of the appropriate amount of food that will help meet but not exceed their child's own energy needs. In order to do so at present, however, they must overcome an established and unhealthy trend; research has revealed a progressive increase in portion sizes of many types of foods and beverages made available to Americans from 1977 to 1998 (Nielsen and Popkin, 2003; Smiciklas-Wright et al., 2003), the same period during which a rise in obesity prevalence has been observed (Nestle, 2003b; Rolls, 2003).

Some research on the effects of food portion size has shown that children 3 years old and younger seem to be relatively unresponsive to the size of the portions of food that they are served (Rolls et al., 2000; see also Chapter 8). By contrast, the food intake of older children and adults is strongly influenced by portion size, with larger portions often promoting excess energy intake (McConahy et al., 2002; Rolls et al., 2002; Orlet Fisher et al., 2003). Children 3 to 5 years of age consumed more of an entrée and 15 percent more total energy at lunch when presented with portion sizes that were double an age-appropriate standard size (Orlet Fisher et al., 2003). Portions that are currently served and consumed at home, and particularly away from home, may be several times the USDA-recommended serving size or recommended caloric level[3] (Orlet Fisher et al., 2003). In addition to food portion size, the frequency of eating and the types of foods consumed are important predictors of energy intake as children transition from being toddlers to preschoolers. One study that evaluated the relationship of food intake behaviors to total energy intake among

---

[3]A serving size is a standardized unit of measure used to describe the total amount of foods recommended daily from each of the food groups from the Food Guide Pyramid (FGP) or a specific amount of food that contains the quantity of nutrients listed on the Nutrition Facts panel. A portion size is the amount of food an individual is served at home or away from home and chooses to consume for a meal or snack. Portions can be larger or smaller than serving sizes listed on the food label or the FGP (USDA, 1999).

children aged 2 to 5 years who participated in the Continuing Survey of Food Intakes by Individuals (CSFII) 1994-1996, 1998 found that eating behaviors and body weight were positively related to energy intake (McConahy et al., 2004).

Research also suggests that individuals tend to overconsume high-energy-dense foods beyond physiological satiety (Kral et al., 2004), especially when they are unaware that the portion sizes served to them have been substantially increased (Rolls et al., 2004a). Satiety signals are not triggered as effectively with high-energy-dense foods (Drewnowski, 1998), and large portions of them consumed on a regular basis are particularly problematic for achieving energy balance and weight management in older children and adults.

A variety of physiological processes are involved in the regulation of dietary intake, satiety, energy metabolism, and weight. These include the neural pathways that regulate hunger and influence food intake, gastrointestinal mechanisms involved in providing signals to the brain about ingested food, and adipocyte-derived factors that provide information about energy stores, as well as the genetic and environmental factors that affect these physiological processes (see Chapters 3 and 8). There are a variety of external cues that may also influence dietary intake such as portion size and package size. For example, there is some evidence to support the hypothesis that larger food package sizes encourage greater consumption than smaller food package sizes (Wansink, 1996), and external cues such as packaging and container size may contribute to the volume of food consumed (Wansink and Park, 2000).

Thus, although the committee recognizes the difficulties faced by the food industry in developing new packaging options for consumers, industry should explore, through research and test-marketing, the best approaches for modifying product packages—multipackages with smaller individual servings or standard serving sizes, or resealable packages—so that products palatable to consumers may remain profitable while promoting consumption of smaller portions. Moreover, the food industry should investigate other approaches for promoting consumption of smaller portion sizes and standard serving sizes.

Leisure, Entertainment, and Recreation Industries

Americans now enjoy more leisure time than they did a few decades ago. As discussed in Chapter 1, trend data collected by the Americans' Use of Time Study through time use diaries indicated that adults' free time increased by 14 percent between 1965 and 1985 to an average total of nearly 40 hours per week (Robinson and Godbey, 1999). Data from other population-based surveys, including the National Health Interview Survey,

NHANES, Behavior Risk Factor Surveillance System (BRFSS), and the Family Interaction, Social Capital and Trends in Time Use Data (1998-1999), together with trend data on sports and recreational participation, suggest a significant increase in reported leisure-time physical activity in adults (Pratt et al., 1999; French et al., 2001a; Sturm, 2004).

Cross-sectional data from the National Human Activity Pattern Survey, based on the responses of 7,515 adults between 1992 and 1994, assessed time use and daily energy expenditure patterns of adults. Results suggested that sedentary and low-intensity activities dominated while leisure-time, high-intensity activities accounted for less than 3 percent of energy expenditure (Dong et al., 2004).

Americans are presented with trade-offs in how they allocate their time and money. Understanding how Americans in general, and children and youth in particular, use their leisure time will help to determine ways of promoting more physical activity into their lives. An analysis of time allocation and expenditure patterns for U.S. adults over the past several decades suggests that they are spending more time in leisure and travel or transportation and less time in productive home activities (e.g., meal preparation and cleanup) and occupational activities (Sturm, 2004). Leisure-time industries have exceeded gross domestic product growth for both active industries (e.g., bicycles, sporting goods, membership sports clubs) and sedentary industries (television, spectator sports). However, there has been a steeper growth in sedentary industries from 1987 to 2001—especially the growth of cable television and spectator sports (Sturm, 2004).

Trend data for children (spanning from 1981 to 1997) have shown that they now have less discretionary or free time—defined as time not spent eating, sleeping, attending to personal care, or at school—than they used to because more of their time is spent away from home in school, after-school programs, or daycare. There is also a noted increase in the amount of time children spend in organized sports (Hofferth and Sandberg, 2001; Sturm, 2005a), but active transportation (e.g., bicycling or walking) is not a significant source of physical activity for children and youth (Sturm, 2005b).

Modern technologies such as labor-saving home appliances have reduced the energy expended for home meal preparation and the amount of time needed to achieve the same task (Sturm, 2004). Other technological innovations such as home entertainment devices (including cable television, computers, video games) and automobiles have contributed to sedentary behaviors among Americans, causing them to expend less energy. This phenomenon of increased time spent in passive sedentary pursuits relative to active leisure activities has been associated with the rise in obesity (French et al., 2001a; Philipson and Posner, 2003). However, although the average American adult spends more than 20 hours per week watching television, videos, or digital video discs (DVDs), it is notable that the largest increase in television watching occurred prior to 1980, which preceded the obesity epidemic (Sturm, 2004). The leisure, entertainment, and recreation industries can help counter the physical inactivity trend by promoting active leisure-time pursuits, while at the same time developing new products and markets. The introduction of products that involve more physical activity by some industry leaders suggests that some already believe they can create a significant market for these types of products.

Some companies have used popular athletic figures, who are potential role models for active and healthful lifestyles, to promote sedentary lifestyles. Instead, the industries could leverage their existing relationships with celebrities to convey messages that encourage physical activity and healthful living and reduce sedentary behaviors.

Some potentially positive efforts are now under way. One athletic apparel manufacturer provides funding to build, upgrade, or refurbish sports courts and other athletic facilities throughout the United States; awards grants to nonprofit organizations and governmental partners; supports physical education classes in elementary schools; and is a partner in Shaping America's Youth, a national cross-sectoral initiative for promoting physical activity and healthful lifestyles during childhood (Nike, 2004). Activity-based games offer opportunities for the leisure industry to market a product that promotes physical activity in children and youth. The evaluation of private-sector programs is crucial in order to assess if they are effective in increasing physical activity, especially among high-risk populations, and determine if they may have unanticipated and adverse consequences.

Full-Service and Fast Food Restaurant Industry

Increased consumption of food outside of the home has been one of the most marked changes in the American diet over the past several decades. In 1970, household income allotted to away-from-home foods accounted for 25 percent of total food spending; by 1999, it had reached nearly one-half (47 percent) of total food spending (Lin et al., 1999c). Total consumer spending on food dispensed for immediate consumption outside the home amounted to $415 billion in 2002 (Stewart et al., 2004). Similarly, a greater proportion of consumers' nutrients is now derived from foods purchased outside the home.

Consumption of away-from-home foods comprised 20 percent of children's total calorie intake in 1977, rising to 32 percent in 1994-1996 (Lin et al., 1999b). For adults, such foods provided more than one-third (34 percent) of total calories in 1995 (Lin et al., 1999a).

The frequency of dining out rose by more than two-thirds over the past two decades, from 16 percent in 1977-1978 to 27 percent in 1995 (Lin et al., 1999a). Restaurant industry sales for commercial and noncommercial services were projected to exceed $426 billion in 2003 (National Restaurant Association, 2003) and are forecasted to reach $440 billion in 2004 (National Restaurant Association, 2004). Moreover, consumer spending at restaurants is projected to continue growing over the next decade (Stewart et al., 2004). Full-service and fast food restaurants alike have been enjoying this boom—in 2003, full-service restaurant sales reached $153.2 billion and fast food restaurant sales reached nearly $121 billion (National Restaurant Association, 2003)—and it appears likely to continue. Assuming modest growth in household income and demographic changes, consumer per-capita spending between 2000 and 2020 is expected to rise by 18 percent at full-service restaurants and by 6 percent at fast food outlets (Stewart et al., 2004).

Given the growing public concern about the rise in obesity, particularly childhood obesity, full service and fast food restaurants throughout the country have begun offering healthier food options. At present, however, most restaurants do not provide consumers with the calorie and selected nutrient content either of offered meals or individual food and beverage items[4]; this information would be useful for making more prudent menu decisions. While the culinary qualities of fast food meals tend to differ from those of full-service restaurants (Lin et al., 1999a), both of them are typically energy dense and served in large portions.

Fast food consumption is associated with a diet that is high in total energy and energy density but low in micronutrient density. For example, an analysis of the CSFII 1994-1996 data for adult men and women revealed that a typical fast food meal provided more than one-third of their daily energy, total fat, and saturated fat intake; and that energy density increased while micronutrient density concurrently decreased with frequency of fast food consumption (Bowman and Vinyard, 2004).

Published data are limited that compare the nutrient content of full-service restaurant meals for children. However, one review of the entrees offered to children at 20 table-service restaurants found fried chicken on every one of the children's menus, a hamburger or cheeseburger on 85 percent of the menus, and french fries on all but one of the menus (Hurley and Liebman, 2004). At nearly one-half of the restaurant chains, french fries were the only side dish on the children's menus, and while children could generally choose a beverage from among soft drinks, juice, or milk,

---

[4]Under the Nutrition Labeling and Education Act of 1990, food products exempted from calorie and nutrient labeling include foods served for immediate consumption, ready-to-eat food not for immediate consumption (i.e., take-out foods), and foods produced by small businesses with annual sales below $500,000 (IOM, 2004).

10 of the restaurants offered free refills only for soft drinks (Hurley and Liebman, 2004).

Children and youth aged 11 to 18 years visit fast food outlets an average of twice per week (Paeratakul et al., 2003), and this frequency is associated with increased intake of soft drinks, pizza, french fries, total fat, and total calories, as well as with reduced intake of vegetables, fruit, and milk (French et al., 2001b). In a study of 6,212 children and adolescents between the ages of 4 and 19 years of age participating in the CSFII, those who ate fast food consumed more total energy, more energy per gram of food (greater energy density), more total fat and carbohydrates, more added sugars, more sweetened beverages, less milk, and fewer fruits and non-starchy vegetables than those who did not consume fast food (Bowman et al., 2004). Adolescents aged 13 to 17 years were found to consume more fast food regardless of whether they were lean or obese. Moreover, obese adolescents were less likely to compensate for the extra energy consumed by adjusting their energy throughout the day than were their lean counterparts (Ebbeling et al., 2004).

Expanding Healthier Meals and Food Choices

Given these trends and data, full-service and fast food restaurants should continue to expand their healthier meal options and food choices—particularly for children and youth—through the inclusion of fruits, vegetables, low-fat milk, and calorie-free beverages among their offerings. It is also important for restaurants to expand options for healthier children's meals, encourage parents to help their children make smarter eating choices, and remind parents of their rights as customers to substitute side dishes and customize meals to their satisfaction. Research is needed to monitor consumers' and children's responses to these expanded options.

Restaurants should also initiate a voluntary, point-of-sale, nutrition-information campaign for consumers. Meanwhile, in accordance with the recommendations of the Food and Drug Administration (FDA) Obesity Working Group's recommendations (FDA, 2004), consumers at restaurants should be encouraged to request information about the nutritional content of complete meals, foods, and beverages offered and consequently be provided with accurate, standardized, and understandable details at the point of sale. This nutritional information should include total calories, fat, cholesterol, and fiber, together with instruction on meaningfully interpreting these values within the context of typical consumers' total energy and dietary needs.

Nutrition labeling of restaurant meals and individual foods should take varying sizes or options into account and should be located near the price of the selections; this will ensure that the consumer is made aware of the information and that increased demand for healthful items and appropriate portions is made more likely. Moreover, the restaurant industry should explore price incentives that encourage consumers to order smaller meal portions. Research initiatives are needed to identify the most effective types of information formats on menus for encouraging the selection of healthful options (Stubenitsky et al., 1999).

As these suggested actions are costly endeavors, consideration must be given to the practicality of implementing these actions in cost-effective ways, especially in expensive restaurants where there is great variability in meals requested by patrons, and small or individual restaurants with limited food volume sales. It is also unclear who will be expected to pay for the nutrient analyses as well as the menu labeling itself. One option would be to encourage local public health departments to contract with dietitians in conducting nutrition education for the public and analyzing the nutrient content of menus. This would represent a new role for local government, but it could be developed by adapting current food safety and sanitation inspection services. It could also generate fees, so that the activity would be self-supporting and sustainable in the long-term; and it could be a convenient way to give public recognition to restaurants in compliance.

Providing Nutrition Education at Restaurants

In addition to voluntary point-of-service menu labeling, the committee recognizes that parents currently have limited nutrition information to rely on in order to select portion sizes and foods that are appropriate for their child. Thus, the committee encourages the restaurant industry to provide nutrition education that is consistent with the Dietary Guidelines for Americans and the FGP in order to inform parents and older youth about appropriate energy intake for meals intended for children and adolescents of different ages.

The Dietary Guidelines for Americans is a federal summary, issued jointly by DHHS and USDA every 5 years, that provides sound guidance to the public about food choices based on the current scientific evidence. The first edition was released in 1980 and provided seven guidelines. The fifth edition was released in 2000 and provided 10 guidelines clustered into three categories: aim for a healthy weight, build a healthy base, and choose sensibly (Ballard-Barbash, 2001).

The FGP was released in 1992 by USDA to teach consumers how to put the Dietary Guidelines for Americans into action. The FGP serves as the official food guide for the United States (USDA, 1992; Achterberg et al., 1994). The FGP illustrates the concepts of variety, proportionality, and moderation emphasized in the Dietary Guidelines for Americans (Achterberg et al., 1994; Dixon et al., 2001). In 1999, USDA developed an

FGP for Young Children, based on the actual eating patterns of children aged 2 to 6 years, which aims to simplify educational messages and focus on young children's food preferences and nutritional requirements (USDA, 2003b; ADA, 2004).

These FGPs offer recommended daily serving sizes for each of the food groups, including bread, cereal, rice, and pasta; fruits; vegetables; milk, yogurt, and cheese; meat, beans, eggs, and nuts; and fats, oils, and sweets. Considerations used in determining serving sizes are the amount of a food that provides key nutrients, ease of use, and commonly recognized household measures of food and equivalents (USDA, 1999, 2000).

Unfortunately, despite the availability of the FGP and its adapted version specifically for younger children, most American children do not meet the recommended servings for fruit, dairy, and grain groups; and they do not meet the Dietary Guidelines' recommendations for total and saturated fat (ADA, 2004) (see Chapter 3).

The committee acknowledges that parents may have a difficult time understanding how portion sizes should be distributed for their children across an entire day, particularly when they are making selections at full-service and fast food restaurants. Another confounding factor is that younger children tend to eat smaller portions, compared to standardized serving sizes, more frequently throughout the day (McConahy et al., 2004). The current educational tools do not provide guidance pertinent to these considerations. **The committee therefore encourages enhancing or adapting the existing FGP model,[5] or developing a new food-guidance system and relevant educational materials, that will convey how portions should be distributed throughout the day for children of different age groups.** (For example, if a child is in a particular age group, he or she should eat a certain proportion of energy at each meal—for example, 20 percent at breakfast, 30 percent at lunch, 30 percent at dinner, and 20 percent for snacks, and the appropriate temporal distribution of snacks should account for the duration of fasting overnight and for variations in daytime energy demands due to age and activity.)

Because such an enhancement could be used by parents to determine a single restaurant meal's percentage of their child's daily required total energy intake, encouraging restaurants to adopt this educational tool may promote children's consumption of smaller food portions. **Additionally, the full-service and fast food restaurant industries should provide general nutri-**

---

[5]An example of an adapted FGP is the Radiant Pyramid, a daily food guide based on the concept of nutrient density. The most nutrient-dense food choices, at the bottom of the pyramid, should be consumed in appropriate serving sizes frequently, whereas the most energy-dense food choices at the (much smaller) top of the pyramid should be consumed only occasionally (Porter Novelli, 2003).

tion information that will facilitate consumers' informed decisions about food and meal selections and appropriate portion sizes (consistent with the energy balance principles of the Dietary Guidelines for Americans and illustrated by the FGP). Finally, consumer research is needed to identify the most effective types of information formats on menus for encouraging the selection of healthful options.

Recommendation 2: *Industry*
Industry should make obesity prevention in children and youth a priority by developing and promoting products, opportunities, and information that will encourage healthful eating behaviors and regular physical activity.

To implement this recommendation:

• Food and beverage industries should develop product and packaging innovations that consider energy density, nutrient density, and standard serving sizes to help consumers make healthful choices.
• Leisure, entertainment, and recreation industries should develop products and opportunities that promote regular physical activity and reduce sedentary behaviors.
• Full-service and fast food restaurants should expand healthier food options and provide calorie content and general nutrition information at point of purchase.

NUTRITION LABELING

The purpose of nutrition labeling is to provide consumers with useful information that will allow them to compare products and make informed food choices, thereby enhancing the likelihood of maintaining dietary practices and reducing the risk of chronic disease (IOM, 2004). In particular, the implementation of the regulations resulting from the 1990 Nutrition Labeling and Education Act (NLEA) was to be communicated in such a way that the public could "readily observe and comprehend such information and understand its relative significance in the context of a total daily diet" (FDA, 1993). The Nutrition Facts panel and nutrient and health claims that resulted from the NLEA are complementary approaches for providing guidance to consumers. They are discussed in turn below.

Nutrition Facts Panel

In 1993, the percent Daily Value (% DV) was added to the Nutrition Facts panel—a set of consistently formatted information items that are displayed on food product labels—to assist consumers in rapidly and efficiently understanding how various foods could fit into the context of a healthful diet. The Nutrition Facts panel's contents, regulated by the FDA, are specific to the food product or food-product category; they specify the number of servings per container and the key nutrients in a serving, according to the % DV for a 2,000-calorie-per-day diet (USDA, 2000; IOM, 2004). Serving sizes on the label are standardized so that consumers can compare nutritional information between products, even for packaged foods (such as frozen pizza) that contain ingredients from multiple food groups (USDA, 2000).

Data on consumers' actual use of the Nutrition Facts panel are limited since it was mandated by FDA in 1990. However, consumer research conducted by the FDA and the Food Marketing Institute (FMI) has found that one-half of U.S. adult consumers use food labels when purchasing a food item for the first time (FMI, 1993, 2001; Derby, 2002). The most common reason for using the label is to assess whether a product is high or low in a particular nutrient, especially fat, and the second most common use is to determine total calories (IOM, 2004).

Moreover, consumers often use the Nutrition Facts panel and the % DV to confirm a nutrient or health claim on the front of a product and to make product-specific judgments (Geiger et al., 1991; FDA, 1995). Consumer research indicates that the % DV in particular has been effective in helping consumers make judgments about different food products that are high or low in a particular nutrient and to put different food products in the context of a daily diet (IOM, 2004). Research shows that without the % DV, consumers could not accurately interpret metric values and distinguish between products (IOM, 2004).

Consumers generally report using the nutrition label more often to avoid rather than to purchase a specific food item (FMI, 1997). Research suggests that although food labels may influence some consumers under certain circumstances, particularly women, older consumers, and well-educated consumers (Kristal et al., 2001), many do not use the Nutrition Facts panel at all. This is attributed in part to lack of interest, lack of knowledge for using it appropriately, and difficulty of use (IOM, 2004). But even when consumers do have and understand the information, it may not change their behavior if their food purchases are primarily motivated by factors such as palatability, price, and convenience (Wansink, 2004).

The committee supports the FDA's current actions in exploring how best to revise the Nutrition Facts panel to prominently display products' standardized calorie serving and % DV (FDA, 2004). The committee endorses this as a step to assist consumers in making informed decisions to achieve energy balance. Energy requirements of children and adolescents differ by age, gender, and activity level. These differences are reflected in the Estimated Energy Requirements established in the Institute of Medicine's (IOM) report on Dietary Reference Intake values for macronutrients (IOM, 2002). However, the committee did not see a practical way in which the Nutrition Facts panel could incorporate all the % DV figures that would correspond to the energy needs of children at different ages (IOM, 2002; USDA, 2003a). Therefore, a recommendation to develop a specific % DV for children and youth based on age, gender, and three activity levels is currently not feasible.

FDA should establish mandatory guidelines for the display of total calorie content on the Nutrition Facts panel regarding products such as vending-machine items, single-serving snack foods, and ready-to-eat foods purchased at convenience stores—typically consumed in their entirety on one eating occasion. Although many prepackaged, ready-to-eat foods are provided in package sizes that may typically be consumed all at once, the nutrition label offers information only on one serving, as defined by the FDA standard serving size.

Thus, although the number of servings per package is also given, the purchaser must calculate the nutritional content of a multiple-serving portion that may be consumed at one sitting. For example, soft drinks are often sold in 20-ounce containers and are labeled as containing 2.5 servings. Because many consumers undoubtedly consume the entire 20 ounces and not precisely 8 ounces (one serving), which represents only 40 percent of the entire product, it would be easier for them to know the total nutritional value if this information was provided directly on the label.

Finally, the Nutrition Facts panel may be modified in other ways to enhance readability and consumer understanding (Kristal et al., 2001). Consideration should be given to the selection, organization, and display of nutrients to maximize the positive message and educational benefit conveyed by the label in order to assist consumers in making wise choices within a healthful diet while also serving to remind them to limit calories and other nutrients (e.g., cholesterol, fat) and thereby reduce their risk of chronic diseases related to obesity (IOM, 2004). In summary, the FDA, relevant industries, and other groups should conduct consumer research on the use of the nutrition label, on restaurant menu labeling, and on how to enhance or adapt the FGP or develop a new food-guidance system.

Nutrient Claims and Health Claims

A nutrient claim is a food-package statement consistent with FDA guidelines that characterizes the level of a nutrient in a food. Depending on the claim, the level is usually categorized as "free," "high," or "low." With a few exceptions, a nutrient-content claim may be made by manufacturers only if a DV has been identified for that nutrient and the FDA has established, by regulation, the criteria that a food must meet in order to list the claim (IOM, 2004). An estimated 33.7 percent of products sold in 2000-2001 had nutrient content claims related to energy, total fat, saturated fat, cholesterol, dietary fiber, sodium, or sugars (Legault et al., 2004).

A health claim[6] on a product package states that a scientifically demonstrated relationship exists between a food substance, legally defined as a specific food or food component, and a disease or health-related condition (IOM, 2004). Health claims (as well as nutrient claims) must be authorized by the FDA prior to their use in food labeling; the agency carefully assesses wording so that the claimed health-related relationship does not imply causation (IOM, 2004).

The FDA has approved 14 different health claims that may be used on food packages that emphasize both risks and benefits such as the relationship between heart disease and saturated fat; cancer and fruits and vegetables; and coronary heart disease risk and fruits, vegetables, grains, and soluble fiber (IOM, 2004). Approximately 4.4 percent of products sold in 2000-2001 had a health claim on their food package. The product groups with the highest percentage of health claims were hot cereal, refrigerated and frozen beverages, seafood, snacks (granola bars and trail mixes), eggs and egg substitutes, and meat and meat substitutes (Legault et al., 2004). These products provided a claim about the relationship between a diet low in saturated fat and cholesterol and a reduced risk of heart disease; high in soluble fiber and reduced risk of heart disease; and high in soy protein and reduced risk of heart disease (Legault et al., 2004).

Health claims advertising and labeling is product-specific so that the information imparted not only suggests a relationship between the food characteristics and health but also features a product that contains these characteristics (Mathios and Ippolito, 1999). Health claims, in conjunction with the Nutrition Facts panel, can help consumers make product-specific decisions and more informed food and beverage choices in the marketplace (Ippolito and Pappalardo, 2002).

The question has been raised as to whether the policy changes that occurred in the mid-1980s, which allowed food manufacturers to explicitly link diet to disease risks in advertising and labeling, assisted or confused consumers in making more healthful food choices to improve their diet (Mathios and Ippolito, 1999). An analysis that examined market share data in the ready-to-eat cereal market, consumer knowledge data, individual nutrient intake data, and per capita consumption data found that U.S. consumers' diets improved from 1985 to 1990 during the same time period that producers were permitted to use health claims in advertising and label-

---

[6]A "qualified" health claim uses appropriate qualifying language to describe the level of scientific evidence that the claim is truthful. The FDA offers guidance, including a method for systematically evaluating the evidence, on the review process for developing qualified health claims (IOM, 2004).

ing (Mathios and Ippolito, 1999), although it is not possible to determine the role that health claims played in these positive outcomes. Evidence from the ready-to-eat cereal market indicates that allowing producers to use health claims resulted in more healthful product innovations and motivated competition based on healthful products (Mathios and Ippolito, 1999).

Thus, health claims may serve to stimulate industry to develop new products, or modify existing ones, that encourage positive changes in consumers' eating habits. Food and beverage companies would benefit from being able to use simple and easily understood health claims in order to stimulate increased consumer selection of healthier food products, including their own.

New health claims may be added to products through a process whereby a food manufacturer notifies the FDA of its intent to use a health claim based on scientifically accurate and authoritative findings. No health claims currently exist for products that explicitly address preventing obesity. However, it will be essential to develop a standard nutrient claim or health claim definition for energy density and nutrient density. For example, by developing a health claim for food products that have an energy density below 1 calorie per gram, such foods might be considered supportive of maintaining a healthy body weight. However, this type of health claim could not apply to beverages.[7] A disclosure statement may be needed to accompany a health claim if consumer research reveals that a health claim on a food label would imply that a food is healthful in all respects (e.g., it has a low energy density but may not be nutrient dense) if this is not the case.

The regulatory environment in the early 1980s discouraged food and beverage manufacturers and advertisers from using health claims, but this policy was eased in 1993 when the FDA's health claim rules were revised (Ippolito and Pappalardo, 2002). The FTC has recently encouraged the FDA to consider giving manufacturers greater flexibility in making truthful, nonmisleading nutrient claims for foods,[8] allowing comparative claims[9]

---

[7]As discussed in Chapter 3 and Appendix B, beverages (such as soft drinks and fruit drinks), due to their high water content, are generally not energy dense. However, the energy density of soft drinks is disproportionately high for its nutrient content when compared to other nutrient-dense beverages such as low-fat milk. Therefore, comparisons of beverages should involve considerations of nutrient density.

[8]A nutrient content claim is an FDA-regulated statement on food packages that characterizes the level of a nutrient in a food such as "free," "high," "low," "more," and "reduced". The NLEA (1990) allows the use of nutrient-content claims that describe the amount of a nutrient according to the FDA's authorizing regulations (IOM, 2004).

[9]Comparative claims are a subset of nutrient content claims. Under NLEA rules, comparative claims are required to meet a number of specific restrictions and disclose the comparison product, the percentage that a nutrient is reduced, and the actual amount of the nutrient for both the product and the comparison food (Ippolito and Pappalardo, 2002).

between different types and portion sizes of food, and permitting health claims that specifically relate reduced calorie consumption to decreasing the risk of obesity-related diseases (FTC, 2003).

The committee encourages the FDA to examine ways to give the food and beverage industries greater flexibility in making nutrient content and health claims that help consumers including children achieve and maintain energy balance. The committee also recommends that consumer research be undertaken to determine the best formats for health claims that relate lowered calorie consumption with reductions in the risk of obesity and obesity-related disease. Finally, the committee suggests that the government, academia, and private sector work together to conduct the necessary research on which to base such health claims.

Recommendation 3: *Nutrition Labeling*
Nutrition labeling should be clear and useful so that parents and youth can make informed product comparisons and decisions to achieve and maintain energy balance at a healthy weight.

To implement this recommendation:

- The FDA should revise the Nutrition Facts panel to prominently display the total calorie content for items typically consumed at one eating occasion in addition to the standardized calorie serving and the percent Daily Value.
- The FDA should examine ways to allow greater flexibility in the use of evidence-based nutrient and health claims regarding the link between the nutritional properties or biological effects of foods and a reduced risk of obesity and related chronic diseases.
- Consumer research should be conducted to maximize use of the nutrition label and other food-guidance systems.

ADVERTISING, MARKETING, AND MEDIA

Children of all ages are spending a larger proportion of their leisure time using a combination of various forms of media, including broadcast television, cable networks, DVDs, video games, computers, the Internet, and cell phones (Roberts et al., 1999; Rideout et al., 2003). This trend has prompted concerns about the effects of these activities on their health (Kaiser Family Foundation, 2004). Children's exposure to advertising and marketing, particularly to the food, beverage, and sedentary-lifestyle messages delivered through the numerous media channels, may have a strong influence on their tendency toward increased obesity and chronic disease risk (Kaiser Family Foundation, 2004).

Advertising and promotion have long been intrinsic to the marketing of the American food supply (Gallo, 1999). Food and beverage companies and the restaurant industry together represent the second-largest advertising group in the American economy, after the automotive industry (Gallo, 1999), and young people are a major target. The annual sales of foods and beverages to young consumers exceeded $27 billion in 2002 (*U.S. Market for Kids Foods and Beverages*, 2003), and millions of dollars are spent annually by the food and beverage industry for specific product brands (Story and French, 2004). Food and beverage advertisers collectively spend $10 billion to $12 billion annually to reach children and youth (Nestle, 2003a; Brownell, 2004). Estimates are available for different categories of youth-focused marketing in the United States—more than $1 billion is spent on media advertising to children, primarily on television; more than $4.5 billion is spent on youth-targeted promotions such as premiums, coupons, sweepstakes, and contests; $2 billion is spent on youth-targeted public relations; and $3 billion is spent on packaging designed for children (McNeal, 1999).

Similarly, young people are major consumers of the products and services of the entertainment, leisure, and recreation industries. An accurate figure for children's and adolescents' comprehensive media and entertainment use is not readily available, though market research suggests there is great potential for the growth of this market; children are being raised in a technology-oriented culture that exposes them to modern media conveniences as noted above (Rideout et al., 2003; U.S. Kids Lifestyles Market Research, 2003). For example, it was projected that $4.2 billion would be spent on children's videos in 2001 (*Children's Video Market*, 1997) and on a typical day, children aged 4 to 6 years used computers (27 percent) and video games (16 percent) (Rideout et al., 2003).

The quantity and nature of advertisements to which children are exposed to daily, reinforced through multiple media channels, appear to contribute to food, beverage, and sedentary-pursuit choices that can adversely affect energy balance. It is estimated that the average child currently views more than 40,000 commercials on television each year, a sharp increase from 20,000 commercials in the 1970s (Kunkel, 2001). Studies of children's advertising content during that roughly 20-year period found that more than 80 percent of all advertising to children fell into four product categories: toys, cereal, candy, and fast food restaurants (Kunkel, 2001). Moreover, an accumulated body of research reveals that more than 50 percent of television advertisements directed at children promote foods and beverages such as candy, fast food, snack foods, soft drinks, and sweetened breakfast cereals that are high in calories and fat, low in fiber, and low in nutrient density (Kotz and Story, 1994; Gamble and Cotunga, 1999; Horgen et al., 2001; Hastings et al., 2003).

Dietary and other choices influenced by exposure to these advertisements may likely contribute to energy imbalance and weight gain, resulting in obesity (Kaiser Family Foundation, 2004). Based on children's commercial recall and product preferences, it is evident that advertising achieves its intended effects (Kunkel, 2001; CSPI, 2003; Hastings et al., 2003; Wilcox et al., 2004), and an extensive systematic literature review concludes that food advertisements promote food purchase requests by children to parents, have an impact on children's product and brand preferences, and affect consumption behavior (Hastings et al., 2003). Indeed, the *2003 Roper Youth Report*[10] suggests that an increased number of children aged 8 to 17 years are playing central roles in household purchasing decisions related to food, media, and entertainment (Roper ASW, 2003).

Industry has come to view children and adolescents as an important market force, given their spending power, purchase influence, and potential as future adult consumers (McNeal, 1998). Market research from the early 1990s suggests that children's purchase influence rises with age from $15 billion per year for 3- to 5-year-olds to $90 billion per year for 15- to 17-year-olds (Stipp, 1993). Marketers use a variety of techniques, styles, and channels to reach children and youth, including sales promotions, celebrity or cartoon-character endorsements, product placements, and the co-marketing of brands (Horgen et al., 2001; CSPI, 2003; Hastings et al., 2003; Wilcox et al., 2004).

Research suggests that long-term exposure to such advertisements may have adverse impacts due to a cumulative effect on children's eating and exercise habits (Horgen et al., 2001; CSPI, 2003; Hastings et al., 2003; Wilcox et al., 2004). Children learn behaviors and have their value systems shaped by the media (Villani, 2001). Just as portrayals in television and film shape viewers' perceptions of certain health-related behaviors, such as smoking cigarettes or drinking alcohol, the messages about consuming certain foods and beverages and engaging in sedentary activities may affect them as well (Hastings et al., 2003; Kaiser Family Foundation, 2004).

A recent report issued by the American Psychological Association (APA) Task Force on Advertising and Children concluded that young children (under the age of 8) are uniquely vulnerable to commercial promotion because they lack the cognitive skills to comprehend its persuasive intent; that is, they do not understand the difference between information and

---

[10]The *2003 Roper Youth Report*, based on a nationwide cross-sectional cohort of 544 children aged 8 to 17 years, was conducted by Roper ASW, a market-research firm. Face-to-face interviews were conducted in children's homes in 2003 (Roper ASW, 2003).

advertising (Wilcox et al., 2004). This finding is consistent with the policy statement of the American Academy of Pediatrics that "advertising directed toward children is inherently deceptive and exploits children under eight years of age" (AAP, 1995). A child is unable to critically evaluate these messages' content, intention, and credibility in order to assess their truthfulness, accuracy, and potential bias (Wilcox et al., 2004).

In general, children are exposed to up to one hour of advertising for every five hours of television watched (Horgen et al., 2001). This proportion complies with the Federal Communication Commission's enforcement of the Children's Television Act of 1990, which limits advertising to no more than 12 minutes per hour during the week, and fewer than 10.5 minutes per hour on the weekend, for television programs reaching children under 12 years old (FCC, 2002). However, this exposure to advertising may represent a conservative estimate given the growth in unregulated advertising reaching children through cable television and the Internet (Dale Kunkel, University of Arizona, personal communication, August 17, 2004).

After reviewing the evidence, the committee has concluded that the effects of advertising aimed at children are unlikely to be limited to brand choice. Wider impacts include the increased consumption of energy-dense foods and beverages and greater engagement in sedentary behaviors, both of which contribute to energy imbalance and obesity. The committee concurs with the APA Task Force's finding (Wilcox et al., 2004) that advertising targeted to children under the age of 8 is inherently unfair because it takes advantage of younger children's inability to attribute persuasive intent to advertising. There is presently insufficient causal evidence that links advertising directly with childhood obesity and that would support a ban on all food advertising directed to children. Additional research and public dialogue are needed regarding the potential benefits and consequences of instituting a food advertising ban for children. Recommending a ban may not be feasible due to concerns about infringement of First Amendment rights and the practicality of implementing such a ban (Engle, 2003).

There are historical insights that can be gained from the prior federal government efforts related to advertising food products to children. In 1978, the FTC proposed a rule that would ban or significantly restrict advertising to children, based on a long-standing and widespread concern about the possible adverse health effects from television advertising of food and beverage products to children. The FTC staff sought comment on the issues, including three proposed alternative actions (Engle, 2003).

During this process, the FTC presented a review of the scientific evidence with the conclusion that television advertising directed at young children is unfair and deceptive. The government rulemaking process found that the evidence of adverse effects of advertising on children was inconclusive, despite acknowledging some cause for concern; furthermore, it was found that it would be difficult to develop a workable rule that would address the concerns without infringing on First Amendment rights (Engle, 2003). Congress barred any rule based on unfairness, and the FTC terminated the rulemaking in 1981 (Engle, 2003; Story and French, 2004).

Protecting parents from children's requests for advertised products was not considered a sufficient basis for FTC action at that time. Furthermore, the process identified the complexities of designing implementable rules that restrict advertising directed at children (e.g., how to effectively place limits on the time of day when advertisements could appear and how to define the scope of advertisements directed at young children only) (Engle, 2003). Thus the committee feels that the immediate step is to strengthen industry self-regulation and corporate responsibility. Government agencies should also be empowered to be engaged with industry in these discussions and to monitor compliance.

The committee favors an approach to address advertising and marketing directed especially at young children under 8 years of age, but also for older children and youth, that would first charge industry with voluntary implementation of guidelines developed through diverse stakeholder input, followed by more stringent regulation if industry is unable to mount an effective self-regulating strategy. This approach is similar to that recommended for control of advertising of alcoholic beverages to youth (NRC and IOM, 2003).

It is not possible to determine whether industry self-regulation will lead to a favorable change in marketing and advertising of food and sedentary entertainment[11] products to children sooner than governmen- imposed regulation. However, it is desirable that industry is provided with an opportunity to implement voluntary changes to move toward marketing and advertising practices that do not increase the risk of obesity among children and youth, followed by government regulation if voluntary actions are determined to be unsuccessful.

DHHS should convene a national conference and invite the participation of a diverse group of stakeholders to develop standards for marketing of foods and beverages (e.g., portion sizes, calories, fat, sugar, and sodium) and sedentary entertainment (movies, videos and DVDs, and other electronic games). The group should include the food, beverage, and restaurant industries; the Children's Advertising Review Unit (CARU) of the Better Business Bureaus; media and entertainment industries; leisure and recre-

---

[11]Sedentary entertainment refers to activities and products that require minimal physical activity and encourage physical inactivity such as watching television, video rentals, and spectator sports.

ation industries; public health organizations; and consumer advocacy groups. This national conference should also establish appropriate objectives and methods for evaluating the ongoing effectiveness of the new guidelines.

In addition, further information should be collected about the impact of advertising on children's eating and physical activity behaviors and about how media literacy training may help children and parents make more informed choices.

Implementation of the guidelines will be the responsibility of the food and beverage industry and sedentary entertainment industry trade organizations, individual companies, advertising agencies, and the entertainment industry, with oversight from federal agencies. Appropriate advertising codes and monitoring mechanisms, including industry-sponsored and external review boards (e.g., CARU, National Advertising Review Board), should be implemented to enforce the guidelines. Moreover, industry should take actions to strengthen CARU guidelines and oversight in order to ensure compliance. Through these actions, it is expected that reasonable precautions will be put in place regarding the time, place, and manner of product placement and promotion (i.e., children's morning, afternoon, and weekend television programming and in-school educational programming) to limit children's exposure to products that are not consistent with the principle of energy balance and that do not promote healthful diets and regular physical activity.

Further, Congress should empower the FTC with the authority and resources to monitor compliance with the guidelines, scrutinize marketing practices of the relevant industries (including product promotion, placement, and content), and establish independent external review boards to investigate complaints and prohibit food and beverage and sedentary entertainment product advertisements that may be deceptive or have "particular appeal" to children that conflict with principles of healthful eating and physical activity. Potential guideline elements to consider might be:

- Restrict or otherwise constrain the content of food and beverage and sedentary entertainment advertising on programs with a substantial children's audience (i.e., children's morning, afternoon, and weekend television programming and in-school educational programming such as Channel One).
- Avoid implicit or explicit claims that high-energy-density and low-nutrient-density foods have nutritional value.
- Avoid linking such products to admired celebrities or sports figures, or to cartoon characters. This would include cross-promotion of food and sedentary entertainment products with branded children's programming or networks.

• Require inclusion of a disclaimer pointing to the need to limit consumption of food or participation in sedentary entertainment.

• Require a message recommending complementary consumption of healthier food or participation in more physically active entertainment.

Congress should also authorize and appropriate sufficient funding to support a study of the cumulative direct and indirect effects of advertising and marketing on the food and beverage and sedentary entertainment purchasing and health behaviors of children, adolescents, and parents; and investigate how approaches such as media literacy can provide children with the desirable skills to respond to marketing messages.

Recommendation 4: *Advertising and Marketing*
Industry should develop and strictly adhere to marketing and advertising guidelines that minimize the risk of obesity in children and youth.

To implement this recommendation:

• The Secretary of DHHS should convene a national conference to develop guidelines for the advertising and marketing of foods, beverages, and sedentary entertainment directed at children and youth with attention to product placement, promotion, and content.

• Industry should implement the advertising and marketing guidelines.

• The FTC should have the authority and resources to monitor compliance with the food and beverage and sedentary entertainment advertising practices.

MEDIA AND PUBLIC EDUCATION

Throughout this report there is discussion of the influence of media on childhood obesity. This section discusses use of the media as a positive strategy for addressing childhood obesity. The fundamental perspective of this report is that childhood obesity reflects numerous influences, and consequently that addressing the epidemic will require changes in the many ways in which American society interacts with its children. Deploying the media should be seen as part of a broader effort to change social norms— for youth about their own behavior, for parents about their actions on behalf of their children, and for society at large about the need to support policies that protect its most vulnerable members.

There is perhaps some irony in using the mass media to address the childhood obesity epidemic when the sedentary lifestyles associated with viewing television are noted to be contributing causes of that epidemic (see

Chapter 8). Nonetheless, the committee recognizes that the behaviors associated with the obesity epidemic are widespread, and few other mechanisms are available for stimulating the required changes. Use of the mass media is the best way to reach large segments of the population. At the same time, the committee recognizes that there have been very few efforts to address the problem of childhood and youth obesity through the mass media, thus actions in this domain should be accompanied by careful and continuous monitoring and evaluation to ensure that they are doing what they were meant to do.

Finally, the committee recognizes that if a campaign is not designed with sensitivity, there may be an unintentional consequence that could increase stigmatization of obese children. Stigmatization of smokers was thought to be an effective tool for the tobacco control campaigns; however, obesity may be different. Therefore, the possibility that a campaign could increase negative attitudes and behaviors directed at obese children and youth, such as teasing and discrimination, needs to be explicitly considered in the design and development of the campaign. This should include adequate formative evaluation during development as well as surveillance, concurrent with and following campaign implementation, to detect and minimize any potential adverse effects.

Media-centered efforts must be closely linked with complementary efforts elsewhere in pursuit of the same objectives. For example, a media campaign to recommend that children walk to school might need to be complemented by a public-relations campaign to ensure that there are safe routes for walking, a campaign for reaching parents with a message that they should encourage their children to walk, and a campaign for motivating children to be excited about and interested in walking to school. Thus, media-centered efforts include not only those directed at children and youth themselves, and those directed at parents, but also those directed at policy makers. Throughout this report the committee has emphasized the central role of policy change in obesity prevention, and media-based efforts can have an important role in achieving these changes.

Policy changes occur more quickly if there is a strong social consensus behind them (Economos et al., 2001; Kersh and Morone, 2002). For example, it is worth considering the policy changes that have been important in the success of the anti-tobacco movement (Kersh and Morone, 2002; Daynard, 2003; Yach et al., 2003; see Appendix D). Restrictions on advertising, increases in taxation, and controls over smoking-permissible locations were important components of the tobacco-use decline (Hopkins et al., 2001), but these changes could be readily implemented only because a new public-opinion climate around tobacco supported them and permitted legislators and regulators to act (Kersh and Morone, 2002; Yach et al., 2003). This public opinion transformation likely resulted both from the natural diffusion of information about the health consequences of tobacco use and the deliberate efforts by advocacy agencies to affect public opinion (Warner and Martin, 2003). Similarly, it will likely be easier to implement policies to prevent childhood obesity if the general public is informed about the issues and strongly supportive of the need to address them.

Lessons Learned from Other Media Campaigns on Public Health Issues

A number of media campaigns covering a range of public health issues have been targeted to adults or the general public. For example, media efforts were successfully used to encourage parents to put their infants to sleep on their backs to avoid Sudden Infant Death Syndrome (Moon et al., 2004) and to discourage the use of aspirin for children's fevers to avoid Reye's syndrome (Soumerai et al., 1992). The outcomes of the "Back to Sleep" and the Reye's syndrome campaigns were encouraging, but their objective may be simpler than the sorts of actions recommended for energy-balance campaigns. A major national effort to encourage parents to monitor their children so as to reduce their risk of drug use has not yet shown evidence of behavior change, although it is still ongoing (Hornik et al., 2003).

A broader range of campaigns addressing parents' own behaviors related to energy balance has shown mixed results. Evaluations of a series of mass-media-based interventions undertaken in the 1990s to promote adult physical activity provide a mixed picture of success, with most reporting fairly good levels of recall of messages and changes in knowledge about the benefits of exercise. Only sometimes, however, did results show evidence of actual increases in self-reported physical activity, even over the short term (Owen et al., 1995; Vuori et al., 1998; Wimbush et al., 1998; Bauman et al., 2001, 2003; Hillsdon et al., 2001; Miles et al., 2001; Reger et al., 2002; Renger et al., 2002).

In addition to these predominantly mass-media-focused efforts, there were other multicomponent campaigns for which mass media was but one (albeit important) channel that addressed not only physical activity but other outcomes as well (see Chapter 6). Initial success from the Stanford Three Community Study and the North Karelia Project demonstrated the promise of this approach, and were followed by three large National Heart, Lung, and Blood Institute-funded community trials in the 1980s—the Stanford Five-City Project, the Minnesota Heart Health Program, and the Pawtucket Heart Health Program (Farquhar et al., 1990; Luepker et al., 1994; Carleton et al., 1995). The multiyear Minnesota Heart Health Program reported greater adult physical activity in its experimental communities than in its control communities (Luepker et al., 1994); and the Stanford Five-City Project reported similar patterns (Young et al., 1996), as well as lower resting heart rate (a measure of cardiorespiratory fitness), lower blood pressure, and lower body mass index levels (Taylor et al., 1991; Farquhar et al., 1990) in the intervention communities. The Stanford and Minnesota projects included change in diet among their objectives, but these studies did not report notable successes in affecting dietary fat or dietary cholesterol, although an effect on plasma cholesterol was reported in the Stanford Five-City Project (Farquhar et al., 1990).

There were also a small number of evaluated mass-media interventions focused on diet. These included the "1% or Less" campaign in Wheeling, West Virginia, which showed that more adults in the state switched to low-fat milk than in a control community after a campaign in 1996 (Reger et al., 1999); and the Victoria, Australia's "2 Fruit 'n' 5 Veg Every Day" campaign that ran from 1992 to 1995, which showed some increase in reported consumption of these targeted foods (Dixon et al., 1998).

The National Cancer Institute-sponsored "5 A Day for Better Health" program, for which mass-media promotion of fruit and vegetable consumption was a component, showed varying degrees of success. California data for the initial "5 A Day for Better Health" program from 1989 to 1991, as well as the subsequent national program, revealed small increases in consumption of daily servings of fruit and vegetables, though evaluators suggested that these may well have reflected ongoing secular trends (Foerster et al., 1995) or demographic shifts (Stables et al., 2002).

The findings on diet interventions, like those regarding physical activity, clearly were mixed. The 5-A-Day evaluations represented efforts of a different magnitude than any of the described physical activity interventions, yet there were no clear associations between those efforts and dietary changes. These results are of concern when considering large-scale dietary interventions. At the same time, it is evident that substantial changes in the U.S. adult diet have occurred during the last few decades, most strikingly in the reduction of dietary cholesterol and resulting levels of plasma cholesterol (Frank et al., 1993). Although evaluations of deliberate campaigns may not show consistent evidence of influence on dietary intake and outcomes, there are some influences producing large shifts in dietary knowledge and behavior. The idea that such shifts reflect general media coverage of dietary issues, creating in turn a substantial demand for low-cholesterol, low-fat products, and more recently, low-carbohydrate products, is worth serious consideration.

Approaches that seek to affect the shape of media coverage of diet and/or physical activity might merit high priority. One of the most difficult barriers to successful public education programs is achieving high rates of exposure to persuasive messages. Even if a carefully mounted intensive education effort was effective for the audience it could reach, it may not be feasible to reach large audiences with those messages. Resources may not be available to pay for the outreach channels and prime time exposure for target groups needed on a continuing basis. In contrast, ordinary mass-media programs and news do reach large audiences with their messages. They can achieve high and continuing exposure to healthy messages.

Such heavy exposure may be effective for a variety of reasons: sheer repetition so that messages (1) may be more likely to be heard and paid attention to, particularly if the repetition occurs across a variety of channels; (2) may communicate social expectations for behavior, and (3) may produce a greater likelihood of community discussion of the message possibly producing personal reinforcement for behavior change.

Thus if the media cover an issue extensively, it may be possible to achieve changes in behavior not practicable with controlled educational interventions. However the problem for programs that take this route is the difficulty of convincing media to cover an issue in a way consistent with sponsors' goals. The solutions that people have used include buying or obtaining donated advertising time; engaging in media advocacy—a deliberate attempt to create controversy or to leverage a news event to stimulate media coverage of an issue (Wallack and Dorfman, 1996); undertaking public relations efforts to encourage media coverage; and working with producers and writers of entertainment programs or talk shows to encourage incorporation of messages in those programs. Different programs have used each of these strategies, with varying success (Wallack and Dorfman, 1996; Hornik et al., 2003; Wray et al., 2004).

In March 2004, DHHS announced an obesity-focused campaign called "Small Steps" that is comprised of a series of public service announcements recommending that Americans take small and achievable steps toward increasing physical activity and reducing calorie consumption to improve their health and reverse the obesity epidemic (DHHS, 2004). The initiative and advertisements provide suggestions such as choosing fruit for dessert and doing sit-ups in front of the television—easily accomplished actions that DHHS anticipates will appeal to Americans searching for achievable weight-management goals. The campaign, which is part of a larger DHHS effort, the Steps to a Healthier U.S. Initiative, is addressed both to adults and children and is implemented through awards to large urban communities, rural communities, and tribal consortiums. Because this program was launched as this report was being written, results on effectiveness are not yet available.

Over the past 10 years, government and private groups have undertaken major media campaign efforts to influence a variety of other youth behaviors, including tobacco use and drug use. Current evidence suggests that the anti-tobacco campaigns have been successful, while the anti-drug campaigns have had less success. Tobacco use among youth has been declining since 1997, and there is evidence linking some of that decline to state-level media campaigns (Siegel, 2002). In contrast, the National Youth Anti-Drug Media Campaign, sponsored by the White House Office of National Drug Control Policy, has not shown success thus far in influencing youth marijuana consumption, despite having spent more than $1 billion in advertising and other efforts (Hornik et al., 2003). The inconsistent results from these two areas do not lead to easy conclusions about whether media campaigns are promising for obesity-related behaviors. They do suggest that the success of such campaigns will depend on the outcome sought and the ways in which the campaigns are mounted and maintained.

Industry-sponsored efforts to encourage increased levels of physical activity are currently under way (Nike, 2004), though the committee does not have any information about their possible influence of these efforts on youth behavior. The advantage of such industry-sponsored programs is that they do not require explicit public investment; however, reasonably enough, they will reflect their sponsors' interests, which may not always coincide with the agendas of those primarily concerned with youth obesity. In circumstances where they might play a useful complementary role in a national effort, industry-sponsored efforts should certainly be encouraged. However, national authorities must understand that such campaigns are likely to be only one part of a broad effort, and should not be seen as an alternative to mounting an urgent public-sector campaign focused on behavioral objectives.

Within the past two years, the Centers for Disease Control and Prevention (CDC) has launched the VERB campaign, a multi-ethnic media campaign based on social marketing principles and behavioral change models (Huhman, et al., 2004) with the goal of increasing and maintaining physical activity in tweens—youth aged 9 to 13 years. Parents and other influential sources on tweens (e.g., teachers and youth program leaders) are the secondary audiences of the VERB campaign. The CDC has conducted extensive formative research to design this social marketing campaign (Wong et al., 2004), which currently involves multiple media venues that include television, radio spots, print advertising, posters, the Internet, and out-of-home outlets such as movie theaters, billboards, and city buses (Wong et al., 2004).

A recently released summary of the VERB campaign's first-year results of a prospective study suggests a high recall of messages and some evidence that youth who had better campaign recall engaged in more physical activity than those who did not (Potter et al., 2004). It should be noted, however, that the extent to which the association between campaign recall and greater physical activity can be attributed to the campaign's influence cannot be determined from these results. One cannot rule out the alternative explanation that youth who are more naturally oriented toward being more physically active are also more likely to recall the campaign messages.

Given these preliminary, albeit positive results, and no other available evaluations of media campaigns, it is not possible at present to state that media campaigns can effectively increase physical activity in children aged 9 to 13 years.

Next Steps

The committee recognizes that there is limited evaluated experience in mass-media-centered interventions that address obesity prevention. Nonetheless, there is substantial experience in other related areas, along with the initial findings of positive evidence from some very recent obesity-focused efforts. In addition, the committee recognizes that most of its recommendations throughout the report require reaching the population at large, on a continuing basis, to generate popular support for policy changes and provide needed information to parents and youth about behaviors likely to reduce the risks of obesity. Only the mass media offer the possibility of reaching that sizeable and wide-ranging audience.

Thus the committee recommends that DHHS, in coordination with other federal departments and agencies and with input from independent experts, develop, implement, and rigorously evaluate a broad-based, long-term, national multimedia and public relations campaign focused on obesity prevention in children and youth. This campaign would vary in its focus as the nature of the problem changes, including components focused on changing eating and physical activity behaviors among children, youth, and their parents as well as on raising support among the general public for policy actions. The outcome of this effort should be greater awareness of childhood obesity, increased public support for policy actions, and behavior change among parents and youth.

The three areas of focus for the recommended media campaign would involve:

• A continuing public relations or media advocacy effort designed to build a political constituency for addressing youth obesity, and for supporting specific policy changes on national, state, or local levels. This will include print and broadcast media press briefings and outreach, media support for other organizations focused on obesity issues, and efforts to encourage commercial media to incorporate obesity issues and positive role modeling in their programming.

• A systematic and continuing campaign to provide parents with the types of information described in Chapter 8, including the importance of serving as role models and of establishing household policies and priorities regarding healthful eating and physical activity.

- A systematic and continuing campaign to reach youth who are themselves making energy balance decisions that affect their risk of obesity.

The federal government's recently launched VERB campaign is one example of a youth-focused campaign and presents an opportunity to examine the long-term impact of a multimedia campaign focused on promoting physical activity in youth, one component of preventing obesity. As noted above, preliminary results are positive for an early phase of the campaign. CDC has made substantial investment in this program and, given the positive first results, further investments should follow over a longer term.

Regarding the systematic campaign to reach youth, the committee specifically endorses the continuation of VERB funding to ensure the possibility of fully realizing the social marketing campaign's potential and to evaluate its long-term impact. This proposal is costly. Thus, based on a rigorous evaluation over the long term, resources should be redirected if results are not promising in meeting the three components of the campaign. In addition, the committee notes that physical activity is but one side of the energy equation. Additional resources should be provided for a complementary campaign focusing on energy-intake behaviors.

Funding for the national multimedia and public relations campaign should include sufficient budgets to purchase media time for the campaign's advertising, rather than relying on donated time, as well as to support the professional implementation and careful evaluation of the campaign's effects. While DHHS's Small Steps program intends to depend on contributed airtime under the auspices of the Advertising Council (DHHS, 2004), the committee suggests that it is not a promising route for frequently reaching the public. A recent Kaiser Family Foundation study showed that the average television station rarely plays such public service announcements during periods when most adults are in the viewing audience (Kaiser Family Foundation, 2002). Some campaigns have had success in obtaining donated time on stations where they had also purchased time (Randolph and Viswanath, 2004), but that is merely a strategy for stretching resources more effectively. In general, a campaign that depends on contributed time is quite unlikely to satisfy its objectives.

Input should be sought from independent experts and representatives of other federal, state, and local agencies, nonprofit organizations, and, where appropriate, industry representatives to construct a broad and evolving strategy that includes all three of the areas of focus described above. These efforts, which need a long-term mandate from Congress, should be aimed at the general population and specific high-risk subgroups, and their staffs should be able to carefully assess targets of opportunity and rebalance their strategies as circumstances change.

The committee realizes that many nonprofit organizations and other nongovernmental groups are involved in obesity prevention efforts. It encourages these organizations to undertake their own extensive media campaigns (print, electronic, Web-based, and other media) for addressing the obesity problem.

Recommendation 5: *Multimedia and Public Relations Campaign*
DHHS should develop and evaluate a long-term national multimedia and public relations campaign focused on obesity prevention in children and youth.

To implement this recommendation:

- The campaign should be developed in coordination with other federal departments and agencies and with input from independent experts to focus on building support for policy changes, providing information to parents, and providing information to children and youth. Rigorous evaluation should be a critical component.
- Reinforcing messages should be provided in diverse media and effectively coordinated with other events and dissemination activities.
- The media should incorporate obesity issues into its content, including the promotion of positive role models.

REFERENCES

AAP (American Academy of Pediatrics). Committee on Communications. 1995. Children, adolescents, and advertising. *Pediatrics* 95(2):295-297.

Achterberg C, McDonnell E, Bagby R. 1994. How to put the Food Guide Pyramid into practice. *J Am Diet Assoc* 94(9):1030-1035.

ADA (American Dietetic Association). 2004. Position of the American Dietetic Association: Dietary guidance for healthy children ages 2 to 11 years. *J Am Diet Assoc* 104(4):660-677.

Ballard-Barbash R. 2001. Designing surveillance systems to address emerging issues in diet and health. *J Nutr* 131(2S-1):437S-439S.

Bauman AE, Bellew B, Owen N, Vita P. 2001. Impact of an Australian mass media campaign targeting physical activity in 1998. *Am J Prev Med* 21(1):41-47.

Bauman A, McLean G, Hurdle D, Walker S, Boyd J, van Aalst I, Carr H. 2003. Evaluation of the national 'Push Play' campaign in New Zealand—Creating population awareness of physical activity. *N Z Med J* 116(1179):U535.

Block G. 2004. Foods contributing to energy intake in the US: Data from NHANES III and NHANES 1999–2000. *J Food Comp Analysis* 17(3-4):439-447.

Bowman SA, Vinyard BT. 2004. Fast food consumption of U.S. adults: Impact on energy and nutrient intakes and overweight status. *J Am Coll Nutr* 23(2):163-168.

Bowman SA, Gortmaker SL, Ebbeling CB, Pereira MA, Ludwig DS. 2004. Effects of fast food consumption on energy intake and diet quality among children in a national household survey. *Pediatrics* 113(1):112-118.

Brownell K. 2004. *Food Fight: The Inside Story of the Food Industry, America's Obesity Crisis, and What We Can Do About It.* New York: McGraw-Hill.

Carleton RA, Lasater TM, Assaf AR, Feldman HA, McKinlay S. 1995. The Pawtucket Heart Health Program: Community changes in cardiovascular risk factors and projected disease risk. *Am J Public Health* 85(6):777-785.

Children's Video Market. 1997. [Online]. Available: http://www.academic.marketresearch.com/ [accessed June 4, 2004].

Crockett SJ, Kennedy E, Elam K. 2002. Food industry's role in national nutrition policy: Working for the common good. *J Am Diet Assoc* 102(4):478-479.

CSPI (Center for Science in the Public Interest). 2003. *Pestering Parents: How Food Companies Market Obesity to Children.* Washington, DC: CSPI. [Online]. Available: http://www.cspinet.org/new/200311101.html [accessed November 21, 2003].

Datamonitor. 2002. *Childhood Obesity 2002: How Obesity Is Shaping the U.S. Food and Beverage Markets. Executive Summary.* [Online]. Available: http://www.researchandmarkets.com/reports/c3990/ [accessed April 14, 2004].

Daynard RA. 2003. Lessons from tobacco control for the obesity movement. *J Public Health Policy* 24(3-4):291-295.

Derby B. 2002. *Consumer Understanding of Nutrition Labels and Use of Daily Values.* Presentation at the workshop on Use of Dietary Reference Intakes in Nutrition Labeling. Committee on Use of Dietary Reference Intakes in Nutrition Labeling, Institute of Medicine. Washington, DC, May 23.

DHHS. 2004. *Citing "Dangerous Increase" in Deaths, HHS Launches New Strategies Against Overweight Epidemic.* [Online]. Available: http://www.hhs.gov/news/press/2004pres/20040309.html [accessed March 29, 2004].

Dixon H, Borland R, Segan C, Stafford H, Sindall C. 1998. Public reaction to Victoria's '2 fruit 'n' 5 veg every day' campaign and reported consumption of fruit and vegetables. *Prev Med* 27(4):572-582.

Dixon LB, Cronin FJ, Krebs-Smith SM. 2001. Let the pyramid guide your food choices: Capturing total diet concept. *J Nutr* 131(2S-1):461S-472S.

Dong L, Block G, Mandel S. 2004. Activities contributing to total energy expenditure in the United States: Results from the NHAPS study. *Int J Behav Nutr Phys Act* 1(1):4.

Drewnowski A. 1998. Energy density, palatability, and satiety: Implications for weight control. *Nutr Rev* 56(12):347-353.

Drewnowski A. 2003. The role of energy density. *Lipids* 38(2):109-115.

Ebbeling CB, Sinclair KB, Pereira MA, Garcia-Lago E, Feldman HA, Ludwig DS. 2004. Compensation for energy intake from fast food among overweight and lean adolescents. *J Am Med Assoc* 291(23):2828-2833.

Economos CD, Brownson RC, DeAngelis MA, Novelli P, Foerster SB, Foreman CT, Gregson J, Kumanyika SK, Pate RR. 2001. What lessons have been learned from other attempts to guide social change? *Nutr Rev* 59(3 Pt 2):S40-S56.

Engle MK. 2003. *FTC Regulation of Marketing to Children.* Presentation at the workshop on The Prevention of Childhood Obesity: Understanding the Influences of Marketing, Media, and Family Dynamics. Committee on the Prevention of Obesity in Children and Youth, Institute of Medicine. Washington, DC, December 9.

Farquhar JW, Fortmann SP, Flora JA, Taylor CB, Haskell WL, Williams PT, Maccoby N, Wood PD. 1990. Effects of communitywide education on cardiovascular disease risk factors: The Stanford Five-City Project. *J Am Med Assoc* 264:359-365.

FCC (Federal Communications Commission). 2002. *Children's Educational Television.* [Online]. Available: http://www.fcc.gov/cgb/consumer facts/childtv.html [accessed November 21, 2003].

FDA (U.S. Food and Drug Administration). 1993. Food labeling: Mandatory status of nutrition labeling and nutrient content revisions: Format of nutrition label. Final rule. *Fed Regist* 58(3):2079-2205.

FDA. 1995. Food labeling: Reference Daily Intakes. Part II; Final rule. *Fed Regist* 60(249):67164–67175.

FDA. 2004. *Calories Count. Report of the Working Group on Obesity.* Center for Food Safety and Applied Nutrition. [Online]. Available: http://www.cfsan.fda.gov/~dms/owg-toc.html#action [accessed April 19, 2004].

FMI (Food Marketing Institute). 1993. *Shopping for Health: A Report on Diet, Nutrition and Ethnic Foods.* Washington, DC: FMI.

FMI. 1997. *Shopping for Health: Balancing Convenience, Nutrition, and Taste.* Washington, DC: FMI.

FMI. 2001. *Shopping for Health: Reaching Out to the Whole Health Consumer.* Washington, DC: FMI.

FMI. 2003a. *Shopping for Health 2003: Whole Health for the Whole Family.* Washington, DC: FMI.

FMI. 2003b. *Trends in the United States: Consumer Attitudes & the Supermarket 2003.* Washington, DC: FMI.

Foerster SB, Kizer KW, Disogra LK, Bal DG, Krieg BF, Bunch KL. 1995. California's "5 a Day for Better Health!" campaign: An innovative population-based effort to effect large-scale dietary change. *Am J Prev Med* 11(2):124-131.

Frank E, Winkleby M, Fortmann SP, Farquhar JW. 1993. Cardiovascular disease risk factors: Improvements in knowledge and behavior in the 1980s. *Am J Public Health* 83(4):590-593.

French SA, Story M, Jeffery RW. 2001a. Environmental influences on eating and physical activity. *Annu Rev Public Health* 22:309-335.

French SA, Story M, Neumark-Sztainer D, Fulkerson JA, Hannan P. 2001b. Fast food restaurant use among adolescents: Associations with nutrient intake, food choices and behavioral and psychosocial variables. *Int J Obes* 25(12):1823-1833.

FTC (Federal Trade Commission). 2003. *Public Workshop: Exploring the Link Between Weight Management and Food Labels and Packaging.* Docket No. 2003N-0038. Before the Department of Health and Human Services Food and Drug Administration. Comments of the Staff of the Bureau of Consumer Protection, the Bureau of Economics, and the Office of Policy Planning of the Federal Trade Commission. December 12.

Gallo AE. 1999. Food advertising in the United States. In: Frazao E, ed. *America's Eating Habits: Changes and Consequences.* Agriculture Information Bulletin Number 750. Washington, DC: USDA.

Gamble M, Cotunga N. 1999. A quarter century of television food advertising targeted at children. *Am J Health Behav* 23(4):261-267.

Geiger CJ, Wyse BW, Parent CR, Hansen RG. 1991. Review of nutrition labeling formats. *J Am Diet Assoc* 91(7):808-812, 815.

Hastings G, Stead M, McDermott L, Forsyth A, MacKintosh A, Rayner, M, Godfrey C, Caraher M, Angus K. 2003. *Review of Research on the Effects of Food Promotion to Children.* Glasgow, UK. Center for Social Marketing, University of Strathclyde, Glasgow, UK. Available: http://www.food.gov.uk/multimedia/pdfs/foodpromotiontochildren1.pdf [accessed November 22, 2003].

Heasman M, Mellentin J. 2001. *The Functional Foods Revolution: Healthy People, Healthy Profits?* London, UK: Earthscan Publications.

Hillsdon M, Cavill N, Nanchahal K, Diamond A, White IR. 2001. National level promotion of physical activity: Results from England's ACTIVE for LIFE campaign. *J Epidemiol Community Health* 55(10):755-761.

Hofferth SL, Sandberg JF. 2001. Changes in American children's time, 1981-1997. In: Owens T, Hofferth S, eds. *Children at the Millennium: Where Have We Come From, Where Are We Going?* Advances in Life Course Research. New York: Elsevier Science.

Hopkins DP, Husten CG, Fielding JE, Rosenquist JN, Westphal LL. 2001. Evidence reviews and recommendations on interventions to reduce tobacco use and exposure to environmental tobacco smoke: A summary of selected guidelines. *Am J Prev Med* 20(2S):67-87.

Horgen KB, Choate M, Brownell KD. 2001. Television food advertising: Targeting children in a toxic environment. In: Singer DG, Singer JL, eds. *Handbook of Children and the Media.* Thousand Oaks, CA: Sage Publications. Pp. 447-461.

Hornik R, Maklan D, Cadell D, Barmada C, Jacobsohn L, Henderson V, Romantan A, Niederdeppe J, Orwin R, Sridharan S, Baskin R, Chu A, Morin C, Taylor K, Steele D. 2003. *Evaluation of the National Youth Anti-Drug Media Campaign: 2003 Report of Findings.* Washington, DC: Westat.

Huhman M, Heitzler C, Wong F. 2004. The VERB™ campaign logic model: A tool for planning and evaluation. *Preventing Chronic Disease* [Online]. Available: http://www.cdc.gov/pcd/issues/2004/jul/pdf/04_0033.pdf [accessed August 17, 2004].

Hurley J, Liebman B. 2004. Kids' Cuisine: "What would you like with your fries?" *Nutrition Action Health Letter.* Washington, DC: CSPI.

IOM (Institute of Medicine). 2002. *Dietary Reference Intakes for Energy, Carbohydrate, Fiber, Fat, Fatty Acids, Cholesterol, Protein, and Amino Acids.* Washington, DC: The National Academies Press.

IOM. 2004. *Dietary Reference Intakes. Guiding Principles for Nutrition Labeling and Fortification.* Washington, DC: The National Academies Press.

Ippolito PM, Pappalardo JK. 2002. *Advertising Nutrition & Health. Evidence from Food Advertising 1977-1997.* Washington, DC: Federal Trade Commission.

Kaiser Family Foundation. 2002. *Shouting to be Heard: Public Service Advertising in a New Media Age.* Menlo Park, CA: Henry J. Kaiser Family Foundation. [Online]. Available: http://www.kff.org/entmedia/20020221a-index.cfm [accessed June 24, 2004].

Kaiser Family Foundation. 2004. *The Role of Media in Childhood Obesity.* Menlo Park, CA: Henry J. Kaiser Family Foundation.

Kersh R, Morone J. 2002. How the personal becomes political: Prohibitions, public health, and obesity. *Studies in American Political Development* 16(2):162-175.

Kotz K, Story M. 1994. Food advertisements during children's Saturday morning television programming: Are they consistent with dietary recommendations? *J Am Diet Assoc* 94(11):1296-1300.

Kral TV, Roe LS, Rolls BJ. 2002. Does nutrition information about the energy density of meals affect food intake in normal-weight women? *Appetite* 39(2):137-145.

Kral TVE, Roe LS, Rolls BJ. 2004. Combined effects of energy density and portion size on energy intake in women. *Am J Clin Nutr* 79(6):962-968.

Kristal AR, Hedderson MM, Patterson RE, Neuhouser M, Neuhauser ML. 2001. Predictors of self-initiated, healthful dietary change. *J Am Diet Assoc* 101(7):762-766.

Kunkel D. 2001. Children and television advertising. In: Singer DG, Singer JL, eds. *Handbook of Children and the Media.* Thousand Oaks, CA: Sage Publications. Pp. 375-394.

Legault L, Brandt MB, McCabe N, Adler C, Brown AM, Brecher S. 2004. 2000-2001 food label and package survey: An update on prevalence of nutrition labeling and claims on processed, packaged foods. *J Am Diet Assoc* 104(6):952-958.

Lin BH, Guthrie J, Frazao E. 1999a. *Away-from-Home Foods Increasingly Important to Quality of American Diet*. Washington, DC: Economic Research Service/U.S. Department of Agriculture. Agriculture Information Bulletin No. 749.

Lin BH, Guthrie J, Frazao E. 1999b. Quality of children's diets at and away from home: 1994-96. *Food Rev* 22(1):2-10.

Lin BH, Guthrie J, Frazao E. 1999c. Nutrient contribution of food away from home. In Frazao E, ed. *America's Eating Habits: Changes and Consequences*. Washington, DC: Economic Research Service/U.S. Department of Agriculture. Agriculture Information Bulletin No. 750. Pp. 213-242.

Luepker RV, Murray DM, Jacobs DR Jr, Mittelmark MB, Bracht N, Carlaw R, Crow R, Elmer P, Finnegan J, Folsom AR, Grimm R, Hannan PJ, Jeffrey R, Lando H, McGovern P, Mullis R, Perry CL, Pechacek T, Pirie P, Sprafka JM, Weisbrod R, Blackburn H. 1994. Community education for cardiovascular disease prevention: Risk factor changes in the Minnesota Heart Health Program. *Am J Public Health* 84(9):1383-1393.

Mathios AD, Ippolito P. 1999. Health claims in food advertising and labeling. In: Frazao E, ed. *America's Eating Habits: Changes and Consequences*. Washington, DC: Economic Research Service/U.S. Department of Agriculture. Agriculture Information Bulletin No. 750. Pp. 189-212.

McConahy KL, Smiciklas-Wright H, Birch LL, Mitchell DC, Picciano MF. 2002. Food portions are positively related to energy intake and body weight in early childhood. *J Pediatr* 140(3):340-347.

McConahy KL, Smiciklas-Wright H, Mitchell DC, Picciano MF. 2004. Portion size of common foods predicts energy intake among preschool-aged children. *J Am Diet Assoc* 104(6):975-979.

McNeal JU. 1998. Tapping the three kids' markets. *Am Demog* 20(4):37-41.

McNeal J. 1999. *The Kids Market: Myths and Realities*. Ithaca, NY: Paramount Marketing Publishing.

Miles A, Rapoport L, Wardle J, Afuape T, Duman M. 2001. Using the mass-media to target obesity: An analysis of the characteristics and reported behaviour change of participants in the BBC's 'Fighting Fat, Fighting Fit' campaign. *Health Educ Res* 16(3):357-372.

Moon RY, Oden RP, Grady KC. 2004. Back to Sleep: An educational intervention with women, infants, and children program clients. *Pediatrics* 113(3 Pt 1):542-547.

National Restaurant Association. 2003. *Restaurant Industry Forecast. Executive Summary*. [Online]. Available: http://www.restaurant.org/research/forecast.cfm [accessed April 19, 2004].

National Restaurant Association. 2004. *Restaurant Industry Forecast. Executive Summary*. [Online]. Available: http://www.restaurant.org/pdfs/research/2004_forecast_exec summary.pdf [accessed April 26, 2004].

NCHS (National Center for Health Statistics). 2001. *Healthy People 2000 Final Review*. Hyattsville, MD: Public Health Service.

Nestle M. 2003a. *Food Politics: How the Food Industry Influences Nutrition and Health*. Berkeley, CA: University of California Press.

Nestle M. 2003b. Increasing portion sizes in American diets: More calories, more obesity. *J Am Diet Assoc* 103(1):39-40.

Nielsen SJ, Popkin BM. 2003. Patterns and trends in food portion sizes, 1977-1998. *J Am Med Assoc* 289(4):450-453.

Nike. 2004. *NikeGo Programs: What Are You Going To Do About It?* [Online]. Available: http://www.nike.com/nikebiz/nikego/programs.html [accessed June 7, 2004].

NRC (National Research Council), IOM. 2003. *Reducing Underage Drinking: A Collective Responsibility*. Washington, DC: The National Academies Press.

Orlet Fisher J, Rolls BJ, Birch LL. 2003. Children's bite size and intake of an entree are greater with large portions than with age-appropriate or self-selected portions. *Am J Clin Nutr* 77(5):1164-1170.

Owen N, Bauman A, Booth M, Oldenburg B, Magnus P. 1995. Serial mass-media campaigns to promote physical activity: Reinforcing or redundant? *Am J Public Health* 85(2):244-248.

Paeratakul S, Ferdinand DP, Champagne CM, Ryan DH, Bray GA. 2003. Fast food consumption among US adults and children: Dietary and nutrient intake profile. *J Am Diet Assoc* 103(10):1332-1338.

Peters JC, Wyatt HR, Donahoo WT, Hill JO. 2002. From instinct to intellect: The challenge of maintaining healthy weight in the modern world. *Obes Rev* 3(2):69-74.

Philipson TJ, Posner RA. 2003. The long-run growth in obesity as a function of technological change. *Perspect Biol Med* 46(3S):S87-S107.

Porter Novelli, Inc. 2003. *The Radiant Pyramid Concept. A Daily Food Choice Guide.* Washington, DC: Porter Novelli.

Potter LD, Duke JC, Nolin MJ, Judkins D, Huhman M. 2004. *Evaluation of the CDC VERB Campaign: Findings from the Youth Media Campaign Longitudinal Survey, 2002-2003.* Atlanta, GA: CDC.

PR Newswire. 2004. Kellogg introduces reduced-sugar versions of leaping kids' brands, frosted flakes and fruit loops. *News Release.* April 21.

Pratt M, Macera CA, Blanton C. 1999. Levels of physical activity and inactivity in children and adults in the United States: Current evidence and research issues. *Med Sci Sports Exerc* 31(11 Suppl):S526-S533.

Prentice AM, Jebb SA. 2003. Fast foods, energy density and obesity: A possible mechanistic link. *Obes Rev* 4(4):187-194.

Randolph W, Viswanath K. 2004. Lessons learned from public health mass media campaigns: Marketing health in a crowded media world. *Annu Rev Health* 25:419-437.

Reger B, Wootan MG, Booth-Butterfield S. 1999. Using mass media to promote healthy eating: A community-based demonstration project. *Prev Med* 29(5):414-421.

Reger B, Cooper L, Booth-Butterfield S, Smith H, Bauman A, Wootan M, Middlestadt S, Marcus B, Greer F. 2002. Wheeling Walks: A community campaign using paid media to encourage walking among sedentary older adults. *Prev Med* 35(3):285-292.

Renger R, Steinfelt V, Lazarus S. 2002. Assessing the effectiveness of a community-based media campaign targeting physical inactivity. *Fam Community Health* 25(3):18-30.

Richwine L. 2004. McDonald's launches anti-obesity campaign. *Reuters. News Release.* April 15.

Rideout VJ, Vandewater EA, Wartella EA. 2003. *Zero to Six: Electronic Media in the Lives of Infants, Toddlers and Preschoolers.* Kaiser Family Foundation.

Roberts D, Foehr U, Rideout V, Brodie M. 1999. *Kids and Media @ the New Millennium.* Menlo Park, CA: The Henry J. Kaiser Family Foundation.

Robinson JP, Godbey G. 1999. *Time for Life. The Surprising Ways That Americans Use Their Time.* 2nd ed. University Park, PA: Pennsylvania State University Press.

Rolls BJ. 2003. The supersizing of America. Portion size and the obesity epidemic. *Nutrition Today* 38(2):42-53.

Rolls BJ, Engell D, Birch LL. 2000. Serving portion size influences 5-year-old but not 3-year-old children's food intakes. *J Am Diet Assoc* 100(2):232-234.

Rolls BJ, Morris EL, Roe LS. 2002. Portion size of food affects energy intake in normal-weight and overweight men and women. *Am J Clin Nutr* 76(6):1207-1213.

Rolls BJ, Roe LS, Kral TV, Meengs JS, Wall DE. 2004a. Increasing the portion size of a packaged snack increases energy intake in men and women. *Appetite* 42(1):63-69.

Rolls BJ, Ello-Martin JA, Carlton Tohill B. 2004b. What can intervention studies tell us about the relationship between fruit and vegetable consumption and weight management? *J Nutr* 62(1):1-17.

Roper ASW. *2003 Roper Youth Report.* New York, NY. [Online]. Available: http://www.roperasw.com/products/ryr.html [accessed May 3, 2004].

Siegel M. 2002. The effectiveness of state-level tobacco control interventions: A review of program implementation and behavioral outcomes. *Annu Rev Public Health* 23(1):45-71.

Smiciklas-Wright H, Mitchell D, Mickle S, Goldman J, Cook A. 2003. Foods commonly eaten in the United States, 1989-1991 and 1994-1996: Are portion sizes changing? *J Am Diet Assoc* 103(1):41-47.

Soumerai SB, Ross-Degnan D, Kahn JS. 1992. Effects of professional and media warnings about the association between aspirin use in children and Reye's syndrome. *Milbank Q* 70(1):155-182.

Stables GJ, Subar AF, Patterson BH, Dodd K, Heimendinger J, Van Duyn MA, Nebeling L. 2002. Changes in vegetable and fruit consumption and awareness among US adults: Results of the 1991 and 1997 5 a Day for Better Health Program surveys. *J Am Diet Assoc* 102(6):809-817.

Stewart H, Blisard N, Bhuyan S, Nayga RM Jr. 2004. *The Demand for Food Away from Home. Full Service or Fast Food?* Washington, DC: Economic Research Service/U.S. Department of Agriculture. Agricultural Economic Report No. 829. [Online]. Available: http://www.ers.usda.gov/publications/AER829/ [accessed June 3, 2004].

Stipp H. 1993. New ways to reach children. *Am Demog* 15(8):50-56.

Story M, French S. 2004. Food advertising and marketing directed at children and adolescents in the US. *Int J Behav Nutr Phys Act* 1(1):3-20. [Online]. Available: http://www.ijbnpa.org/content/1/1/3 [accessed August 9, 2004].

Stubenitsky K, Aaron JI, Catt SL, Mela DJ. 1999. The influence of recipe modification and nutritional information on restaurant food acceptance and macronutrient intakes. *Public Health Nutr* 3(2):201-209.

Sturm R. 2004. The economics of physical activity: Societal trends and rationales for interventions. *Am J Prev Med* 27(3S):126-135.

Sturm R. 2005a (in press). *Childhood Obesity—What Can We Learn from Existing Data on Societal Trends. Part 1. Preventing Chronic Disease* [Online]. Available: http://www.cdc.gov/pcd/issues/2005/jan/04_0038.htm [access after December 15, 2004].

Sturm R. 2005b (in press). *Childhood Obesity—What Can We Learn from Existing Data on Societal Trends. Part 2. Preventing Chronic Disease* [Online]. Available: http://www.cdc.gov/pcd/issues/2005/apr/04_0039.htm [access after March 15, 2005].

Taylor CB, Fortmann SP, Flora J, Kayman S, Barrett DC, Jatulis D, Farquhar JW. 1991. Effect of long-term community health education on body mass index. The Stanford Five-City Project. *Am J Epidemiol* 134(3):235-249.

USDA (U.S. Department of Agriculture). 1992. *The Food Guide Pyramid. A Guide to Daily Food Choice.* Home and Garden Bulletin 252. Washington, DC: USDA Human Nutrition Information Service.

USDA. 1999. *Food Portions and Servings: How Do They Differ?* Washington, DC: USDA Center for Nutrition Policy and Promotion. Nutrition Insights 11.

USDA. 2000. *Serving Sizes in the Food Guide Pyramid and the Nutrition Facts Panel: What's Different and Why?* Washington, DC: USDA Center for Nutrition Policy and Promotion. Nutrition Insights 22.

USDA. 2003a. *Federal Register Notice on Technical Revisions to the Food Guide Pyramid.* Table 2: Energy Levels for Proposed Food Intake Patterns. Center for Nutrition Policy and Promotion. [Online]. Available: http://www.cnpp.usda.gov/pyramid-update/FGP%20docs/TABLE%202.pdf [accessed August 25, 2004].

USDA. 2003b. *The Food Guide Pyramid for Young Children.* Center for Nutrition Policy and Promotion. [Online]. Available: http://www.usda.gov/cnpp/KidsPyra/LittlePyr.pdf [accessed April 21, 2004].

U.S. Kids' Lifestyles Market Research. 2003. *Kids' Lifestyles–US.* [Online]. Available: http://www.the-infoshop.com/study/mt16815_kids_lifestyles.html [accessed June 4, 2004].

U.S. Market for Kids Foods and Beverages. 2003. 5th edition. Report summary. [Online]. Available: http://www.marketresearch.com/researchindex/849192.html#pagetop [accessed April 17, 2004].

Villani S. 2001. Impact of media on children and adolescents: A 10-year review of the research. *J Am Acad Child Adolesc Psychiatry* 40(4):392-401.

Vuori I, Paronen O, Oja P. 1998. How to develop local physical activity promotion programmes with national support: The Finnish experience. *Patient Educ Couns* 33(S1):S111-S120.

Wallack L, Dorfman L. 1996. Media advocacy: A strategy for advancing policy and promoting health. *Health Education Quarterly* 23(3):293-317.

Wansink B. 1996. Can package size accelerate usage volume? *Journal of Marketing* 60(3):1-14.

Wansink B. 2004. The de-marketing of obesity. In: Wansink B, Smith AF, eds. *Marketing Nutrition: Soy, Functional Foods, Biotechnology and Obesity.* Champaign, IL: University of Illinois Press.

Wansink B, Park S. 2000. Accounting for taste: Prototypes that predict preference. *J Database Marketing* 7(4):308-320.

Warner KE, Martin EG. 2003. The US tobacco control community's view of the future of tobacco harm reduction. *Tob Control* 12(4):383-390.

Wilcox BL, Kunkel D, Cantor J, Dowrick P, Linn S, Palmer E. 2004. *Report of the APA Task Force on Advertising and Children.* Washington, DC: American Psychological Association.

Williams JD, Achterberg C, Sylvester GP. 1993. Target marketing of food products to ethnic minority youth. *Ann NY Acad Sci* 699:107-114.

Wimbush E, MacGregor A, Fraser E. 1998. Impacts of a national mass media campaign on walking in Scotland. *Health Promot Int* 13(1):45-53.

Wong F, Huhman M, Heitzler C, Asbury L, Bretthauer-Mueller R, McCarthy S, Londe P. 2004. VERB™ —A social marketing campaign to increase physical activity among youth. *Preventing Chronic Disease* 1(3). [Online]. Available: http://www.cdc.gov/pcd/issues/2004/jul/04_0043.htm [accessed June 17, 2004].

Wray R, Hornik R, Gandy O, Stryker J, Ghez M, Mitchell-Clark K. 2004. Preventing domestic violence in the African American community: Assessing the impact of a dramatic radio serial. *J Health Commun* 9(1):31-52.

Yach D, Hawkes C, Epping-Jordan JE, Galbraith S. 2003. The World Health Organization's framework convention on tobacco control: Implications for global epidemics of food-related deaths and disease. *J Public Health Policy* 24(3/4):274-290.

Young DR, Haskell WL, Taylor CB, Fortmann SP. 1996. Effect of community health education on physical activity knowledge, attitudes, and behavior. The Stanford Five-City Project. *Am J Epidemiol* 144(3):264-274.

6

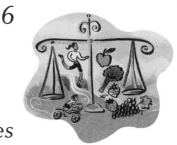

Local Communities

Prevention of obesity in children and youth is, ultimately, about *community*—extending beyond individuals and families and often beyond geographic boundaries to encompass groups of people who share values and institutions (Pate et al., 2000). In recent years, many public health professionals and community leaders have recognized the need for community involvement in preventing disease and promoting healthful lifestyles. Consequently, they have attempted to capitalize on the naturally occurring strengths, capacities, and social structures of local communities to institute health-promoting change.

Many factors in the community setting affect the health of children and youth. Does the design of the neighborhood encourage physical activity? Do community facilities for entertainment and recreation exist, are they affordable, and do they encourage healthful behaviors? Can children pursue sports and other active-leisure activities without excessive concerns about safety? Are there tempting-yet-healthful alternatives to staying-at-home sedentary pastimes such as watching television, playing video games, or browsing the Internet? Are sound food choices available in local stores and at reasonable prices?

Communities can consist of people living or working in particular local areas or residential districts; people with common ethnic, cultural, or religious backgrounds or beliefs; or people who simply share particular interests. But intrinsic to any definition of a community is that *it seeks to protect for its members what is shared and valued.* In the case of obesity prevention in children and youth, what is "shared and valued" is the ability of children to grow up with healthy and productive bodies and minds. But "to protect" is not necessarily a given. Achieving the vision of *Healthy People 2010*— "healthy people in healthy communities"—depends on the capacity of communities to foster social norms that support energy balance and a physically active lifestyle (DHHS, 2000b).

This report as a whole examines a variety of types of communities and the ways in which improvements can be made in order to foster and promote healthful food and physical activity choices and behaviors. This chapter focuses on the *local* community, using the term "community" to refer to the town, city, or other type of geographic entity where people share common institutions and, usually, a local government. Of course, within each local community there are many interdependent smaller networks of residential neighborhoods, faith-based communities, work communities, and social communities.

The intent of this chapter's recommendations is not only to make a case for raising the priority of childhood obesity prevention in our communities, but also to identify common interests that can spark collaborative community initiatives for addressing that goal. Many communities and organizations across the United States are actively working to address physical activity and nutrition-related issues; examples are highlighted throughout the chapter (Boxes 6-1 through 6-5).

MOBILIZING COMMUNITIES

By stepping outside the traditional view of obesity as a medical problem, we may more fundamentally focus on the many institutions, organizations, and groups in a community that have significant roles to play in making the local environment more conducive to healthful eating and physical activity. Table 6-1 illustrates categories of many of the stakeholder groups that could be involved in obesity prevention efforts. For community efforts, key stakeholders include youth organizations, social and civic organizations, faith-based groups, and child-care centers; businesses, restaurants, and grocery stores; recreation and fitness centers; public health agencies; city planners and private developers; safety organizations; and schools.

Community-based obesity prevention efforts differ from those of school and home settings (Pate et al., 2000), but potentially supplement and reinforce the messages received in those settings. Young people, particularly adolescents, often spend a large part of their free time in community locales (e.g., recreational or entertainment centers, shopping areas, parks, fast food restaurants). These informal settings, which do not have the stresses of grades or other school situations, may offer environments that are more conducive to trying new activities and foods. Additionally, community settings offer the potential for involving parents and other adult role models in

TABLE 6-1 Examples of Stakeholder Groups in the Prevention of Childhood Obesity

Children, Youth, Parents, Families

Child- and Youth-Centered Organizations
Program, service, and advocacy organizations (e.g., Boys and Girls Clubs, 4H, Girl Scouts, Boy Scouts, YMCA, YWCA, National Head Start Association, Children's Defense Fund, National Association for Family Child Care)

Community-Based Organizations
Community coalitions, civic organizations, faith-based organizations, ethnic and cultural organizations

Community Development and Planning
Architects, civil engineers, transportation and community planners, private developers, neighborhood associations

Employers and Work Sites
Employers and corporate policy makers, employee advisory committees

Food and Beverage Industries, Food Producers, Advertisers, Marketers, and Retailers
Corporate and local food producers and retailers (e.g., food and beverage industries, grocery stores, supermarkets, restaurants, fast food outlets, corner stores, farmers' markets, community gardens)

Foundations and Nonprofit Organizations
Government Agencies and Programs
Federal, state, county, and local elected or appointed decision-makers (e.g., education boards and agencies, public health agencies, parks and recreation commissions, planning and zoning commissions, law enforcement agencies)

Health-Care Providers
Pediatricians, family physicians, nurses and nurse practitioners, physician assistants, dietitians, occupational-health providers, dentists

Health- and Medical-Care Professional Societies
Disciplinary organizations and societies

Health-Care Delivery Systems
Hospitals, health clinics, school-based facilities, work-site health facilities

Health-Care Insurers, Health Plans, and Quality Improvement and Accrediting Organizations
Public and private health-care providers and insurance reimbursement institutions such as Medicaid and health maintenance organizations; quality improvement and accrediting organizations (e.g., National Committee for Quality Assurance)

Mass Media, Entertainment, Recreation, and Leisure Industries
Television, radio, movies, print, and electronic media; journalists; commercial sponsors and advertisers; Internet websites and advertisers; computer and video-entertainment industry representatives

Public Health Professionals

Recreation and Sports Enterprises
Local, collegiate, and professional sports organizations; recreation facilities; recreation and sport equipment manufacturers, advertisers, marketers, and retailers

Researchers
Biomedical, public health, and social scientists; universities; private industry

Schools, Child-Care Programs
Educators and school administrators, food service personnel, after-school program providers, coaches, school boards, school designers (siting and construction), child-care providers

promoting healthful behaviors (Pate et al., 2000). In enhancing local assets for promoting physical activity—that is, in designing and revamping community facilities and neighborhoods—communities should consider issues related to cultural and social acceptability, availability (proximity), affordability, and accessibility (ease of use).

Community Stakeholders and Coalitions

Community-Based Interventions: Framework and Evidence Base

"Ecological frameworks," which have been applied across a variety of settings and public health issues to change people or change the environment (Glanz, 1997), suggest that it is important to involve individuals, organizations, communities, and health policy makers in producing desired effects on health (Baker and Brownson, 1998). Given the interactive nature of virtually all elements of a community, most effective interventions act at multiple levels. Moreover, tapping a wide range of local community leaders, organizations, businesses, and residents can result in local ownership of the issue and effectively leverage limited resources (Pate et al., 2000).

Community-wide campaigns and interventions. The most relevant evidence for large-scale community-wide efforts comes from studies aimed at reducing cardiovascular risk factors through dietary change and increased physical activity. These interventions have often used multiple strategies, including media campaigns (see Chapter 5), community mobilizations, education programs for health professionals and the general public, modifications of physical environments, and health screenings and referrals; in some cases, home- and school-based interventions were also incorporated (Shea and Basch, 1990).

The Stanford Three Community Study, Stanford Five-City Project, Minnesota Heart Health Program (MHHP), Pawtucket Heart Health Program, and North Karelia Project (in Finland) have demonstrated the feasibility of community-based approaches in promoting physical activity and changes in dietary intake (Farquhar et al., 1977, 1990; Maccoby et al., 1977; Luepker et al., 1994; Young et al., 1996; Puska et al., 2002). The results of these studies for adults have been somewhat inconsistent, although modest positive changes in diet and physical activity have generally been seen when a community that received the intervention was compared with one that had not. The strongest positive results were obtained by the extensive North Karelia project, which examined the effects of multiple interventions on the high incidence of coronary artery disease (Pietinen et al., 2001; Puska et al., 2002). This study, being long-term and multifocal, may be the best model for childhood obesity prevention efforts.

MHHP's Class of 1989 Study provides some insights into the potential impact of community-based programs focused on children and youth (Kelder et al., 1993, 1995). This study examined changes in nutrition and aerobic activity among groups of students, starting when they were sixth-graders and extending through 12th grade. Interventions included a school-based curriculum and a number of other community-based approaches that were not designed specifically for children (including labeling of heart-healthful restaurant and grocery store items; media campaigns; and screening for heart disease risk factors). Positive changes were seen in the young people's levels of physical activity and their nutritional knowledge and decision-making.

Community campaigns aimed at preventing tobacco use by children and youth also provide evidence of the feasibility of using this approach for addressing major public health problems. The Midwestern Prevention Project, the North Karelia Youth Project, and MHHP's Class of 1989 Study each found reductions in youth smoking rates that were maintained over time (IOM, 1994). It should be stressed that each of these studies had a strong school-based prevention intervention that complemented a community-wide program, and isolating the effects of the community-wide program was not possible.

Community programs for children and youth. Programs involving specific community-based organizations have also been found to aid health promotion efforts. Studies with civic, faith-based, and social organizations have established the feasibility of developing programs in a variety of settings that can be effective in improving nutritional knowledge and choices, increasing physical activity, and in some cases in reducing body weight or

---

BOX 6-1
Girls on the Run

Girls on the Run is a nonprofit organization that works with local volunteers and community-level councils to encourage preteen girls to develop self-respect and healthful lifestyles through running (Girls on the Run, 2004). A 12-week, 24-lesson curriculum has been developed for use in after-school programs and at recreation centers and other locations. Evaluation of the program has found improvements in participants' self-esteem, body-size satisfaction, and eating attitudes and behaviors (DeBate, 2002).

maintaining healthy body weight (IOM, 2003). For example, Cullen and colleagues (1997) found that Girl Scouts who participated with their troop in nutrition classes including tasting sessions and materials sent home exhibited increased levels of fruit and vegetable consumption. Furthermore, community programs often are focused on high-risk populations and offer the opportunity to implement culturally appropriate interventions and evaluate their impact (Yancey et al., 2004).

Community coalitions. Building coalitions involves a range of public- and private sector organizations that, together with individual citizens, focus on a shared goal and leverage the resources of each group through joint actions (Table 6-2). It has been pointed out, however, that while the strength of

TABLE 6-2 Unique Characteristics of Effective Community Coalitions

Characteristic	Description
Holistic and comprehensive	Allows the coalition to address issues that it deems as priorities; well illustrated in the Ottawa Charter for Health Promotion
Flexible and responsive	Coalitions address emerging issues and modify their strategies to fit new community needs
Build a sense of community	Members frequently report that they value and receive professional and personal support for their participation in the social network of the coalition
Build and enhance resident engagement in community life	A structure is provided for renewed civic engagement; the coalition becomes a forum where multiple sectors can engage with each other
Provide a vehicle for community empowerment	As community coalitions solve local problems, they develop social capital, allowing residents to have an impact on multiple issues
Allow diversity to be valued and celebrated	As communities become increasingly diverse, coalitions provide a vehicle for bringing together diverse groups to solve common problems
Incubators for innovative solutions to large problems	Problem solving occurs not only at local levels, but at regional and national levels; local leaders can become national leaders

SOURCE: Adapted from Wolff, 2001.

coalitions is in mobilizing the community to work for change, they are not generally designed to develop or manage specific community services or activities (Chavis, 2001).

Community collaborative efforts focused on health are of growing interest across the United States. Models are being refined on ways to link community organizations, community leaders and interested individuals, health-care professionals, local and state public health agencies, and universities and research organizations (Lasker et al., 2001; Lasker and Weiss, 2003). Community coalitions have played significant roles in efforts to prevent or stop tobacco use. The American Stop Smoking Intervention Study (ASSIST), which was funded by the National Cancer Institute and featured the capacity building of community coalitions, targeted tobacco control efforts at the state and local levels. States with ASSIST programs had greater decreases in adult smoking prevalence than non-ASSIST states (Stillman et al., 2003); factors identified as contributing to participation and satisfaction with the ASSIST coalitions included skilled members and effective communication strategies (Kegler et al., 1998). Coalition building and community involvement also have been effective in community fluoridation efforts (Brumley et al., 2001).

Health Disparities

Although this report focuses primarily on population-wide approaches that have the potential to improve nutrition and increase physical activity among all children and youth, the committee recognizes the additional need for specific preventive efforts. Children and youth in certain ethnic groups including African-American, Mexican-American, American-Indian, and Pacific Islander populations, as well as those whose parents are obese and those who live in low-income households or neighborhoods, are disproportionately affected by the obesity epidemic (Chapter 2). Many issues—including safety, social isolation, lack of healthy role models, limited access to food supplies and services, income differentials, and the relative unavailability of physical activity opportunities—may be barriers to healthier lifestyles for these and other high-risk populations. Moreover, as discussed in Chapter 3, perceptions about body image and healthy weight can vary between cultures and ethnic groups, and these groups can manifest differing levels of comfort with having an elevated weight. Furthermore, there may be a "communication gap" in making information about the health concerns of childhood obesity widely available.

As a result, culturally appropriate and targeted intervention strategies are needed to reach high-risk populations. There are examples of these types of strategies having positive results. For example, a 10-county study of churches participating in the North Carolina Black Churches United for

Better Health project found that church-based interventions (including group activities, changes in food served at church events, and dissemination of educational materials) resulted in increased fruit and vegetable consumption by adults participating in the intervention (Campbell et al., 1999). Pilot studies from the Girls Health Enrichment Multi-site Study (GEMS), a research program designed to develop and test interventions for preventing overweight and obesity in African-American girls, have included a variety of community, after-school, and family-based components in a range of settings (Baranowski et al., 2003; Beech et al., 2003; Robinson et al., 2003; Story et al., 2003). For example, the Stanford GEMS pilot study in 61 families tested a model that combined after-school dance classes for girls with family-based efforts to reduce time spent watching television. Positive trends were observed regarding body mass index (BMI), waist circumference, physical activity, and television viewing in the treatment group when compared to the control group (Robinson et al., 2003). These studies demonstrate the feasibility of implementing relevant community programs; two of these studies have been expanded to evaluate programs with larger study populations over a 2-year period (Kumanyika et al., 2003).

However, much remains to be learned about interventions that can reduce or alleviate the risk factors for childhood obesity in high-risk populations. Prevention efforts must be considerate of culture, language, and inequities in social and physical environments (PolicyLink, 2002). Furthermore, because these populations traditionally have been disenfranchised, special efforts must be made to gain their trust, both among individuals and at the community level. The 39-community Partnership for the Public's Health project in California and other community-centered public health initiatives have demonstrated that the most progress is made when an intervention engages community members themselves in the program's assessment, planning, implementation, and evaluation (Partnership for the Public's Health, 2004).

Private and public efforts that work to eliminate health disparities should include obesity prevention as one of their primary areas of focus. Some of the many ongoing efforts span the public and private sectors as well as the local, regional, state, and national levels and focus on diabetes and other chronic diseases for which obesity is a risk factor. For example, the Centers for Disease Control and Prevention's (CDC's) REACH 2010 initiative has broad-based collaboration within the U.S. Department of Health and Human Services (DHHS) and the private sector (CDC, 2004b) to fund and support demonstration projects and community coalitions focused on eliminating health disparities. Each coalition includes community-based organizations and the local or state health department or a university or research organization. Efforts to date have included community and tribal efforts to address diabetes and cardiovascular disease risk factors.

These efforts should aim to increase access to culturally and linguistically appropriate nutritional and physical activity information and skills and should support community-based collaborative programs that address the inequities in obesity rates between populations.

The communities themselves, meanwhile, need to involve all segments of the local population in developing both community-wide interventions and those that focus on high-risk populations. Furthermore, local communities—with the assistance of state and federal governments, nonprofit organizations, and the private sector—need to grapple with the underlying and long-standing socioeconomic barriers that result in limited opportunities for physical activity (e.g., safe parks and playgrounds) and affordable healthful foods (e.g., produce markets or large grocery stores). Opportunities to foster such coalitions and to develop effective programs for high-risk populations will be widened if there is grassroots participation by the citizens most affected by the problem.

Next Steps for Community Stakeholders

Many community organizations are currently involved in efforts to improve the well-being of their children and youth regarding a number of health and safety concerns, such as tobacco and alcohol abuse, sexually transmitted diseases, pedestrian and bike safety, and prevention of motor

---

BOX 6-2
Kids Off the Couch

Kids Off the Couch is a community collaborative pilot project in Modesto, California, that works with parents and caregivers to prevent obesity in children up to 5 years of age. The project's goal is to influence behavioral changes in food selection and physical activity among parents and primary caregivers. The program provides parents and caregivers with:

- Information on the risks of childhood obesity
- Tools to assist their children in achieving normal growth and healthy development
- Hands-on demonstrations on how to prepare healthful and tasty foods that families will eat and enjoy
- Instruction on how to engage their families in physical activity.

This project is a collaborative effort of numerous partners including the local school system, health services agency, hospitals, and health clubs; the American Cancer Society; Blue Cross of California; and the University of California Cooperative Extension.

vehicle injuries. Increased media coverage and the voices of concerned individuals and groups should now be prompting these community groups and others, including the broad range of stakeholders they work with, to focus on childhood obesity prevention. In particular, there is a need to galvanize action and expand opportunities for healthful eating and physical activity at the community level.

Community youth organizations can have an impact not only by adapting their own programs to include emphasis on healthful eating and physical activity, but also by joining with other organizations to form coalitions to promote community-wide efforts. Additionally, innovative approaches to community recreational programs are needed. Traditional organized competitive sports programs are an important facet of the community and offer physical activity opportunities for many children and adolescents. However, competitive sports programs are not of interest to all individuals and it is important to expand the range of options to include not only team and individual sports but also other types of physical activity (e.g., dance, martial arts) (CDC, 1997b). It will also be important to help families overcome potential obstacles—including transportation, fees, or special equipment—to program participation (CDC, 1997b).

Community youth organizations (such as Boys and Girls Clubs, Girls Scouts, Boy Scouts, 4H, and YMCA) should expand existing programs and establish new ones that widen children's opportunities to be physically active and maintain a balanced diet. These programs should complement and seek linkages with similar efforts by schools, local health departments, and other community organizations. Furthermore, evaluation of these programs should be encouraged.

Employers and work sites are another important component of community coalitions. The work site affects children's health both indirectly, through its influence on employed parents' health habits, and directly, through programs that may engage the entire family. Workplaces should offer healthful food choices and encourage physical activity. In businesses where on-site child care is provided, attention should be paid to ensuring that children have a balanced diet and adequate levels of physical activity.

Local organizations, businesses, local public health agencies, and other stakeholders increasingly have been joining together to address health issues through community coalitions, wherein the sum is greater than the parts, and meaningful progress on an issue becomes more likely. Coalitions can make obesity prevention a local priority and can design and implement programs that best fit the local area. It is important for coalitions to be inclusive, promote broad involvement, and represent as many constituencies as possible (see Table 6-2). As coalitions become established, it is also important for them to periodically reassess their status to ensure they remain inclusive and do not outlive their usefulness. Because of their nature, coalitions exhibit wide variation in their structure and in the range of organizations, agencies, and individuals involved. However, to be sustained all require strong and ongoing leadership that is selected by coalition members.

Communities should establish and promote coalitions of key public and private stakeholders (including community youth organizations, local government, state and local public health agencies, civic and community groups, businesses, faith-based groups) to address the problem of childhood obesity by increasing the opportunities for physical activity and a balanced diet. Partnering with academic centers will be important for community-based research.

To have a long-term and significant impact on the public's health, community health initiatives should include programs that work towards initiating changes at many levels including changes in individual behaviors, family environments, schools, workplaces, the built environment, and public policy (Kaiser Permanente, 2004). This ecologic approach (see Chapter 3) is a critical part of a framework for community-level initiatives that support a health-promoting environment. Communities should seek to undertake a comprehensive, interrelated set of interventions operating at each ecological level and in multiple sectors and settings. Factors that have been found to be involved in sustaining successful community change efforts include a large number of environmental changes focused on a small number of categorical outcomes; intensity of behavior change strategy; duration of interventions; and use of appropriate channels of influence to reach appropriate targets (Fawcett et al., 2001).

Community-level approaches are among the most promising strategies for closing the disparities gap (PolicyLink, 2002; Prevention Institute, 2002). These strategies include improvements in the social and economic environment (e.g., through the creation of health-promoting social norms, economic stability, and social capital development), the physical environment (e.g., access to affordable healthful food and physical activity resources), and community services (e.g., after-school programs) (Prevention Institute, 2003). The goals of improving community health and addressing racial and ethnic health disparities are closely aligned.

The committee acknowledges the limited amount of empirical research that directly examines the effects of changes in community programs or formation of coalitions on obesity prevalence. However, interventions such as GEMS demonstrate the feasibility of these interventions, and the experience gained in other public health areas provides additional support for recommendations in these areas. As with other types of obesity prevention interventions (noted throughout this report), there is a critical need to ensure that community intervention programs are thoroughly evaluated. The impacts of coalitions have sometimes gone undetected because of inappropriate (or weak) evaluation plans. This is most likely to occur when (1) the evaluation timeline is too short, (2) the evaluation strategy focuses on unrealistic or distant health outcomes instead of intermediate indicators that can be influenced by coalition activity, (3) measures are incapable of detecting valid indicators of change, or (4) alternative explanations for effects are not taken into account (Kreuter and Lezin, 2002). In order to assess a community coalition's level of change, and to allow communities elsewhere to profit from its experience (good, bad, or in between), realistic evaluation plans must be set up and be incorporated into the initial planning and implementation of coalitions and interventions. Ongoing evaluation that relies on learning and feedback is also an integral component of the community change process. Community health initiatives by their nature are confronted with unpredictable variables; feedback should be used to adjust subsequent efforts.

The standard of practice in comprehensive community health improvement efforts is to fully engage community organizations and community residents, not just as subjects of research but as the drivers and owners of evaluation—"community-based participatory research" (Minkler and Wallerstein, 2003). Using this approach, community members are involved in identifying and framing of the problem or goals; developing a logic model or framework for achieving success; identifying research questions and appropriate research methods; documenting the intervention and its effects; understanding the data; and using the data to make midcourse adjustments (Fawcett et al., 2004).

To provide the impetus for community programs and efforts, a coordinated network of community-based demonstration projects should be established. These projects would be run by community organizations linked with public health departments and in partnership with academic institutions to provide support, training, and evaluation. Seed funding for the projects could come from an expansion of federal programs, particularly CDC's state-based Nutrition and Physical Activity Program to Prevent Obesity and Other Chronic Diseases (see Chapter 4) and the DHHS Steps to a Healthier U.S. initiative.

Built Environment

Designing Communities and Neighborhoods to Encourage Physical Activity

Communities should provide places where children can play outside, particularly within their residential neighborhoods, and where they can safely walk, bike, or travel by other self-propelled means to destinations such as the park, playground, or school. Hoefer and colleagues (2001) found that local neighborhood and parks were the most frequent settings for physical activity among middle school students. Three studies of young children found that the amount of time a child spent outside was the most powerful correlate of his or her physical activity level (Klesges et al., 1990; Baranowski et al., 1993; Sallis et al., 1993). However, pedestrian injuries that result from collisions with automobiles are a leading cause of injury death for children aged 5 years and older (Grossman, 2000), and traffic speed is a key determinant of their injury risk (Jacobsen et al., 2000). The challenge is thus to create places where children are safe to walk, bike, and play, so that the benefits of increased physical activity are not offset by increases in injuries.

Because changes to the built environment can enhance opportunities for children and youth to safely play outside and be more physically active, such changes are a critical component of any action plan to prevent childhood obesity. Interest in the role of the built environment in determining levels of physical activity has grown over the past decade, and renewed efforts are currently under way to reconnect the goals of urban planning and public health and to identify the factors that influence physical activity and travel behavior (Handy et al., 2002; Hoehner et al., 2003; Corburn, 2004). A concurrent study by the Transportation Research Board is examining issues regarding transportation, land use, and health in greater depth than this report, though for the population as a whole.

Encouraging children and youth to be physically active involves providing them with opportunities to walk, bike, run, skate, play games, or engage in other activities that expend energy. However, in many neighborhoods children do not have safe places—because of vehicular traffic, or high crime rates, or both—in which to play outside. In other locales, children may lack adequate sidewalks or paths on which to bike, skate, or simply walk to local destinations such as schools, parks, or grocery stores. This is a result of regulations and practices that guide the development of transportation systems and design of neighborhoods. The needs of the car have often been emphasized over the needs of pedestrians and bicyclists.

A recently published observational study examined the associations between community physical activity-related settings (e.g., sports areas, public pools and beaches, parks and green space, and bike paths) and race, ethnicity, and socioeconomic status in 409 communities throughout the United States (Powell et al., 2004). The researchers found that higher median household income and lower poverty rates were associated with increasing levels of available physical activity-related facilities and settings. Communities with higher proportions of ethnic minorities had fewer physical activity-related settings. There are many communities and neighborhoods where access to facilities for physical activity is an issue that needs to be addressed.

BOX 6-3
Discovering Public Spaces as Neighborhood Assets in Seattle

Feet First, a Seattle-area nonprofit organization, is using its Active Living by Design grant from the Robert Wood Johnson Foundation to help neighborhood residents take a closer look at their streets. As part of their project's activities, Feet First staff organize neighborhoods through monthly walking audits. On these walks, the staff train groups of up to 40 neighbors to see their streets as an untapped resource with potential for physical activity. At the end of the one-mile, two-hour inspections, participants receive notes with photos and maps documenting assets, possible improvements, and needed policy changes. The organization assists citizens in working with city agencies and departments to address the neighborhood concerns.

Evaluation has been built into the design and implementation of the Feet First program and is now in progress. Results will be used to assess next steps and inform the planning of future programs.

Correlational studies. Convenient access to recreational facilities emerges as a consistent correlate of physical activity, although most research has been conducted with adults (Sallis et al., 1998; Humpel et al., 2002). A 2002 review by Humpel and colleagues summarized the results of 16 cross-sectional studies, published between 1990 and 2001, on the link between physical activity and the physical environment. Access to facilities such as bicycle paths or parks showed significant positive associations with physical activity, while measures of a lack of facilities (or inadequate facilities) showed significant negative associations. Awareness of and satisfaction with facilities also showed significant associations with physical activity, as did measures of local aesthetics, such as attractive neighborhoods or enjoyable scenery.

Although there are fewer studies on the relationships between young people's access to recreational facilities and their levels of physical activity, they are nevertheless consistent with the findings for adults. A comprehensive review by Sallis and colleagues (2000a) on the correlates of physical activity among children found a significant positive association with access to recreational facilities and programs, and two out of three studies involving adolescents found a significant positive association as well. However, a study of the neighborhoods of low-income preschoolers in Cincinnati, Ohio, found that overweight was not associated with proximity to playgrounds (Burdette and Whitaker, 2004). These results suggest that access to recreational facilities may be more important for youth than for young children or that reported physical activity may not always translate into differences in weight.

Available evidence (limited to the behavior of all residents or of adults only) shows that the design of streets and neighborhoods is correlated with walking. A recent review of studies (Saelens et al., 2003) comparing "high-walkable" and "low-walkable" neighborhoods found that among persons aged 18 to 65 years, the frequency of walking trips was twice as high in the high-walkable locales. The high-walkable neighborhoods were characterized as those that had higher residential density, street connectivity (few cul-de-sacs), aesthetics, safety, and mixed land use (stores and services located within close proximity to residential areas).

Safety is often an important consideration in decisions by parents and children regarding outside activity. Safety concerns pertain to the speed and proximity of nearby traffic and to fears of crime; but other factors, such as unattended dogs and lack of street lighting, may also be pertinent. Research has shown that parents are more likely now than in the past to restrict their children's use of public spaces because of fear for their safety (Loukaitou-Sideris, 2003). Concerns about "traffic danger" and "stranger danger" have been reported as important influences on the decisions by parents to drive their children to school or not allow them to walk to the neighborhood park (Roberts, 1993; DiGuiseppi et al., 1998); furthermore, parents report that safety considerations are the most important factor in selecting play spaces for their young children (Sallis et al., 1997).

Among adults, data from five states (Maryland, Montana, Ohio, Pennsylvania, and Virginia) document a higher level of physical inactivity among persons who perceive their neighborhoods to be unsafe (CDC, 1999). There also appear to be large gaps in neighborhood safety across socioeconomic groups. For example, a national study found that perception of neighborhood crime was almost twice as great among lower income populations as in higher income populations (Brownson et al., 2001). Thus, the crime rate, or the perception of crime, is likely to affect the likelihood of people walking or bicycling in their neighborhoods.

Studies on the link between neighborhood crime and rates of physical activity among children and youth have shown inconsistent results. Gordon-Larsen and colleagues (2000) studied a large adolescent cohort and found that living in a high-crime neighborhood was associated with a decreased likelihood that teenagers would participate in moderate-to-vigorous physical activity at high levels. However, a study by Zakarian and colleagues (1994) looking at physical activity among minority adolescents or children, who were predominantly of low socioeconomic status, found no association with convenient facilities or neighborhood safety; another study found no association between these factors and overweight (Burdette and Whitaker, 2004). On the other hand, Romero and colleagues (2001) studied fourth-grade students of diverse economic backgrounds and found that children from families of lower socioeconomic status perceived more neighborhood hazards (including crime and traffic), but that this perception was significantly associated with *more* reported physical activity rather than less. This finding points to a problem documented by others (Doxey et al., 2003): children from families with lower socioeconomic status are more dependent on walking as a means of transportation than are children from families with higher socioeconomic status, but they also live in neighborhoods where walking is not as safe.

Intervention studies. Research that directly examines the impact of changes made in the built environment on physical activity has been limited simply because increasing physical activity is often not the primary goal of these interventions and "pre-/post-" studies are difficult to conduct. Instead, changes to the built environment are often made because of safety concerns and the need to reduce the likelihood of traffic-related injuries. For example, the primary goal of traffic-calming programs—such as speed humps, traffic diverters, and "bulb-outs" (pavement structures that extend from the sidewalk at an intersection to force cars to take slower turns around corners)—has been to reduce speeds and to lower the levels of traffic on residential streets. Studies have been conducted of traffic levels and speeds, pedestrian-vehicle crashes, and pedestrian behavior both before and after the installation of traffic-calming devices (Huang and Cynecki, 2000, 2001; Retting et al., 2003). One recent study, for example, showed that speed humps were associated with a lower probability of children being injured within their neighborhood (Tester et al., 2004). However, no studies of the impact of the installation of such devices on the physical activity of residents in the area are available.

A small group of studies has used a pretest/posttest design to test the impact of a specific change to the built environment in a relatively limited area (e.g., street-scale interventions). Painter (1996) examined the impact of improved lighting on the use of footpaths in London and found an intervention effect ranging from 34 percent to 101 percent increases in footpath use, depending on the location. Similarly, a 23 percent increase in bicycle use was found with the addition of bike lanes (Macbeth, 1999). Researchers examining the impact of the redesign of two residential streets in Hannover, Germany, into "Woonerven" (designed for shared use by cars and people) observed 11 percent to 100 percent more children on the street and 53 percent to 206 percent more incidents of street play after the changes in street design (Eubanks-Ahrens, 1987).

The research needs in this area are many. Most obviously, future studies should determine the specific elements of the built environment that influence physical activity in children and youth. DHHS and the Department of Transportation should fund community-based research to examine the impact of changes to the built environment on the levels of physical activity in the relevant communities; in addition, population-wide demonstration projects should be funded and carefully evaluated, as should studies of natural experiments.[1] In addition, carefully designed intervention studies together with studies using longitudinal designs are needed to improve our understanding of the relationships between changes to the built environment and resulting physical activity behavior in youth; such studies will require collaborations between researchers and the responsible public officials. Furthermore, better measures of physical activity collected through travel diary surveys (widely used in transportation planning) and ongoing surveillance systems such as the Youth Risk Behavior Surveillance System are needed, as are better measures of the built environment itself.

The *Guide to Community Preventive Services,* a systematic review of population-based interventions, strongly recommends the "creation of and enhanced access to places for physical activity combined with informational outreach activities" (p. 91) as an approach to promote physical activity, though the focus of this review was on adults (Kahn et al., 2002). But it is clear that improvements to many different elements of the built environment—parks, hike/bike trails, sidewalks, traffic-calming devices, pedestrian crossings, bicycle-route networks, street connections, and mixed land-use developments—will contribute to the solution.

Next steps. It is incumbent upon local governments to find ways to increase the opportunities for physical activity in local communities and neighborhoods. Achieving this goal may involve revising zoning and subdivision ordinances, where necessary, to ensure that new neighborhoods provide opportunities and facilities for physical activity. For example, a growing number of communities are revamping their local development codes to adhere to smart-growth principles (see Box 6-4) (Local Government Commission, 2003).

To enhance the quality and extent of opportunities for physical activity within existing neighborhoods, local governments will need to prioritize such projects in their capital improvement programs. Federal, state, and regional policies can also contribute to these efforts, primarily by providing the funding necessary to effect physical changes to the built environment. The Federal Transportation Enhancements Program, for example, funded $1.9 billion in pedestrian and bicycle projects throughout the United States between 1992 and 2002 (Federal Highway Administration, 2004). As a

---

[1]In this context, the term "demonstration projects" refers to interventions specifically designed to examine the effects of a change in the built environment on physical activity, whereas "natural experiments" are changes that occur or are put in place for other reasons (e.g., an urban policy or practice) but that can be evaluated to determine their effect on physical activity levels. The researcher or practitioner has a much higher level of control over a demonstration project compared with a natural experiment.

BOX 6-4
Trends in City Planning

- Communities throughout the United States are turning to the concept of "smart growth" as a way of fostering walkable and close-knit neighborhoods, providing a variety of transportation choices, taking advantage of community assets, and encouraging mixed land uses (Smart Growth America, 2004). Organizations such as Smart Growth America and the Smart Growth Network represent coalitions of nonprofit organizations and government agencies working toward these goals.

- The Congress for the New Urbanism has brought together architects, developers, planners, and others involved in the creation of cities and towns to promote the principles of coherent regional planning, walkable neighborhoods, and attractive and accommodating civic spaces (CNU, 2004). This nonprofit organization lists hundreds of recent development projects built according to these principles, on which the neighborhood-design ordinances of a number of cities are now based.

- Traditional approaches to street and street-network design are changing in response to concerns over the impact of increasing levels of traffic on communities. The Institute of Transportation Engineers has published recommended practices for street design that encourage narrower streets in residential areas to reduce traffic speeds (ITE, 1999). A growing number of the nation's communities have revised their land development codes to encourage greater connectivity in the street network and require improved access for pedestrians and bicycles (Handy et al., 2003).

---

result, many Metropolitan Planning Organizations, agencies responsible for implementing federal transportation programs in metropolitan areas, now put significant emphasis on bicycle and pedestrian planning (Chauncey and Wilkinson, 2003). Professional organizations such as the Institute of Traffic Engineers and the American Planning Association should also work to assist the efforts of local governments by developing and disseminating best practices for expanding opportunities for physical activity.

Citizens themselves have a responsibility to advocate for changes in policy so that the built environment may ultimately offer increased opportunities for physical activity among children and youth. The public may bring significant influence to bear over policy, particularly if a large and vocal constituency urges change and if prominent community groups, nonprofit organizations, and business organizations lend their support. In many communities, neighborhood associations play a formal role in the planning process and have successfully advocated for new or improved parks, additional side walks, traffic-calming programs, and other changes in the built environment. In addition, legal approaches may be useful (Perdue et al., 2003; Mensah et al., 2004).

Local governments, in partnership with private developers and community groups, should ensure that every neighborhood has safe and well-designed recreational facilities and other places for physical activity for children and youth. Communities can require such environmental characteristics in new developments and use creative approaches to retrofit existing neighborhoods. Furthermore, local governments should ensure that streets are designed to encourage safe walking, bicycling, and other physical activities within the neighborhood and the larger community. Child-safe street design includes well-maintained sidewalks, safe places for crossing, adequate bike lanes, and features that slow traffic.

Walking and Bicycling to School

Compared with 30 years ago, few students in the United States are walking or bicycling to school. In 1969, an average of 48 percent of all students walked or biked to that destination; among those living no more than a mile away, nearly 90 percent did so (EPA, 2003). In comparison, the 1999 HealthStyles Survey found that of the participating households, 19 percent reported that their children walked to or from school at least once a week in the preceding month and that 6 percent rode their bikes (CDC, 2002a). Similar results were seen in a study by the Georgia Division of Public Health, which found that fewer than 19 percent of the state's school-aged children who lived a mile or less from school commuted by foot most days of the week (CDC, 2002b).

The HealthStyles Survey households reported that barriers to their children's walking or bicycling to school included: long distances (noted by 55 percent of respondents), traffic-related safety concerns (40 percent), adverse weather conditions (24 percent), crime danger (18 percent), school policy (7 percent), or other reasons (26 percent) (CDC, 2002a). Sixteen percent acknowledged that there were *no* barriers to walking or bicycling to school.

Two other studies also identified distance as a determinant. In one small study of six school sites, respondents said that it was more likely that their children would walk or bike to school if their home was a mile or less away (McMillan, 2002), while the other found that the probability of walking or bicycling declined with travel time (EPA, 2003). The situation at present is that the majority of children arrive and leave school in automobiles, vans, trucks, and buses (Figure 6-1) (TRB, 2002). Research also suggests that parents, students, and school officials often select or encourage motorized travel because of convenience, flexibility, budget, or expectation rather than to maximize safety (TRB, 2002).

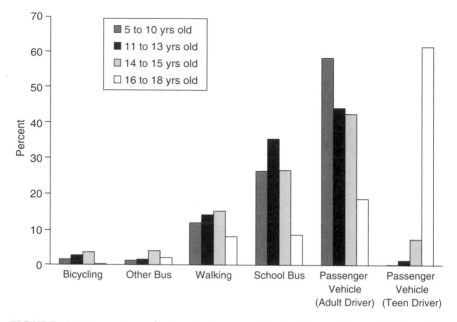

FIGURE 6-1 Percentage of trips during normal school travel hours, Nationwide Personal Transportation Survey, 1995.
SOURCE: *Special Report 269: The Relative Risks of School Travel.* Transportation Research Board, National Research Council, Washington, D.C., 2002, Figure 3-1(a), p. 88. Reproduced with permission.

Because the majority of children and youth attend school five days per week, throughout a large part of the year, trips to and from school offer a potential opportunity to substantially increase their daily physical activity and energy expenditure. Observational studies have in fact demonstrated that children can get some of their most vigorous school-day physical activity during the times they travel between home and school (Cooper et al., 2003; Tudor-Locke et al., 2003). Cooper and colleagues (2003) found, in a study of 114 British children aged 9 to 11 years, that the boys who walked to school were generally more active than those who were transported by car (although similar results were not seen for girls).

While the committee acknowledges that there is no direct evidence that walking or bicycling to school will reduce the prevalence of obesity in children, clear evidence does exist that increases in physical activity can have positive impacts on weight loss or on maintaining a healthy weight. Further, there are potential ancillary benefits, which include enhancing the neighborhood environment (e.g., so that families may walk or bike more often during after-school hours), lowering busing costs, and fostering social interaction within the community.

Interventions to promote safe walking and bicycling to schools have already become popular in some communities, thereby demonstrating a broader potential for feasibility and acceptability (Box 6-5). In Chicago, for example, 90 percent of the nearly 422,000 public school children walk to school and the city has encouraged a Walking School Bus program in which one or more adults walk to school with and supervise a small group of children from the neighborhood (Chicago Police Department, 2004). Since 1997,[2] National Walk Our Children to School Day and a similar international effort have attracted substantial interest.

Safe Routes to School programs have produced increases in the number of students walking or bicycling between home and school. Demonstration projects in 10 British towns showed an increase in walking and bicycling among children and reductions in car use (Sustrans, 2001). An evaluation of the Safe Routes to School programs in seven schools in Marin County, California, found that from fall 2000 to spring 2002, there was a 64 percent increase in the number of children walking to school and a 114 percent increase in the number of students bicycling (Staunton et al., 2003). Another evaluation of the California program, which focused on schools in Southern California, showed strong evidence of success in five schools, weak evidence in one school, and no evidence in three schools (success was defined as improvements in safety conditions as well as increases in the numbers of children walking or bicycling to school) (Boarnet et al., 2003). These data suggest that Safe Routes to School programs show promise in promoting physically active means for children traveling to and from school.

Locating schools in close proximity to the neighborhoods they serve is another opportunity for increasing the likelihood that children and youth will walk or bike between them (EPA, 2003). Annual school construction costs in the United States (including new school construction and school building rehabilitation) were estimated to have grown from about $18 billion in 1990 to $25 billion in 1997 (GAO, 2000) and continue to increase. Given the scale of this spending and the numerous projects involved, school construction projects provide a tremendous opportunity for locating at least some new schools within walking or biking distance of the residential areas from which they draw their students.

Local governments and school districts should ensure that children and youth have safe walking and bicycling routes between their homes and schools and that they are encouraged to use them. Realizing this objective

---

[2]The first National Walk Our Children to School Day was sponsored by the Partnership for a Walkable America in 1997.

BOX 6-5
Safe Routes to School

Safe Routes to Schools was initiated in Western Europe and the United Kingdom. As its name implies, the program promotes walking and bicycling to school, and it does so through education and incentives that show how much fun it can be. The program also addresses the safety concerns of parents by encouraging greater enforcement of traffic laws, educating the public, and exploring ways to create inherently safer streets.

In the United States, the California legislature established a Safe Routes to School program in 1999 and extended it for three more years in 2001. This program provides $25 million in state and federal transportation funds to projects that improve the safety of walking and bicycling to schools. Administered by the state Department of Transportation, Safe Routes to School funded 268 projects in its first 4 years (Caltrans, 2004).

Other programs are emerging across the United States to promote safe walking and bicycling to school, and the nonprofit organization Transportation Alternatives provides a toolkit to help communities in starting their own Safe Routes to School-type programs (Transportation Alternatives, 2004).

The U.S. programs incorporate one or more of the following four key elements:

- An *encouragement* approach, which uses events and contests to entice students to try walking and bicycling
- An *education* approach, which teaches students important safety skills and launches driver-safety campaigns
- An *engineering* approach, which focuses on making physical improvements to the infrastructure surrounding the school, reducing speeds and establishing safer crosswalks and pathways
- An *enforcement* approach, which uses local law enforcement to ensure that drivers obey traffic laws.

will involve the efforts of many groups in local communities. Schools and school districts, in collaboration with community partners, need to develop and implement policies and programs that promote walking and bicycling (Chapter 7). Local governments need to allocate the resources to make the necessary improvements to sidewalks, crosswalks, signals, signs, and other traffic control devices. Collaborations between law enforcement officials and schools are needed to deploy pedestrian safety measures at the beginning and end of each school day; crossing guards are an important part of this process. Additionally, decisions regarding the locations of new schools need to carefully consider the benefits of being close enough to the neighborhoods they serve to facilitate students' walking or bicycling from one site to the other.

When interventions that promote walking or bicycling to school are implemented, it is crucial that researchers evaluate their effects on total daily physical activity and energy expenditure, and on changes in weight over time. Programs promoting safe routes to school, as well as other efforts to increase students' walking and bicycling, should include funding for evaluation, and the organizations that implement these programs should work with researchers to develop rigorous evaluation designs. Because so much remains to be learned about the various approaches to increasing walking and bicycling to school, thorough evaluations of such initiatives are critical.

Community Food Environment

All members in a community need access[3] to affordable and healthful food on a regular basis. Food security is commonly defined as "access by all people at all times to enough food for an active, healthy life and includes at a minimum: a) the ready availability of nutritionally adequate and safe foods, and b) the assured ability to acquire acceptable foods in socially acceptable ways (p. 1560)" (LSRO, 1990). Food security is one of the necessary conditions to ensure the health of a population.

In 2002, 11.1 percent of U.S. households, representing more than 35 million people, experienced food *insecurity*—that is, their access to nutritious food on a regular basis was limited or uncertain (Nord et al., 2003). In general, households with children report food insecurity at more than twice the rate of households without children (16.5 percent versus 8.1 percent, respectively) (Nord et al., 2003). Children living in food-insecure households are more likely to have compromised well-being than children living in food-secure households (Alaimo et al., 2001); evidence has linked food insecurity to declines in children's health, mental and psychological functioning, and academic achievement (ADA, 2004). As discussed in Chapter 3, however, evidence linking childhood food insecurity to obesity is inconclusive.

In 2002, a food-secure household in the United States spent 35 percent more on food than the typical food-insecure household of the same size and composition (Nord et al., 2003), though food accounted for a greater proportion of the latter's budget (Lang and Caraher, 1998). Thus, it stands to reason that food cost is a significant predictor of dietary choices and health outcomes, particularly in low-income ethnic minority urban communities (Perry, 2001; Morland et al., 2002a; Pothukuchi et al., 2002; Sloane et al., 2003) and rural communities (Holben et al., 2004). At the same time, while

---

[3]Food access is defined broadly in this context to represent improved availability of adequate amounts of healthful foods that households and communities have the financial resources to afford on a regular basis.

it is acknowledged that consumer food choices are shaped by taste, cost, and convenience, it has been suggested that high-fat, energy-dense foods and diets are often less expensive on a cost-per-calorie basis and are more palatable than high-fiber low-energy-dense foods such as the lean meats, fish, fresh fruits, and vegetables that comprise a healthful diet (Drewnowski and Specter, 2004). However, based on the ACNielsen Homescan 1999 data for household food purchases from all types of retail outlets, a price analysis of 154 types of fruits and vegetables found that more than one-half of the produce items were estimated to cost less than 25 cents per serving. The study concludes that all consumers, including low-income households, can meet the recommendations of three servings of fruit and four servings of vegetables for 64 cents per day (Reed et al., 2004). However, it is difficult to predict or understand consumer behavior from these types of analyses, as discussed in Chapters 3 and 5.

The availability and affordability of energy-dense foods has increased in recent years in low-income neighborhoods (Morland et al., 2002a,b; Sloane et al., 2003). This situation is associated with several trends: fewer supermarkets being located within a reasonable walking distance, supermarket relocation to the suburbs (Cotterill and Franklin, 1995; Shaffer, 2002; Bolen and Hecht, 2003), the lack of transportation to supermarkets offering a variety of healthful choices at affordable prices (Urban and Environmental Policy Institute, 2002; Bolen and Hecht, 2003), and the local proliferation of gas stations and convenience stores that often have a limited selection of healthful foods and at higher prices (Alwitt and Donley, 1997; Perry, 2001; Morland et al., 2002a).

Community food-security assessment toolkits and other methods, such as community mapping, have been used to assist communities throughout the United States in undertaking community assessments and inventories to identify the type and range of locally available food resources, including supermarkets, corner grocery stores, full-service and fast food restaurants, food banks, food pantries, farmers' markets, and community gardens (Perry, 2001; Cohen, 2002; Pothukuchi et al., 2002; Sloane et al., 2003). Knowing the inventory and its gaps, communities may then take appropriate action, and in fact they are addressing their food insecurity problems in a variety of ways.

For example, local governments are offering financial incentives such as grants, loans, and tax benefits to stimulate the development of neighborhood groceries in underserved urban neighborhoods (Shaffer, 2002; Bolen and Hecht, 2003; Baltimore Healthy Stores Project, 2004; Clark, 2004). Some communities are initiating farmers' markets or enhancing the existing Farmers' Market Nutrition Programs offered to participants in Special Supplemental Nutrition Program for Women, Infants, and Children and the Food Stamp Program (Connecticut Food Policy Council, 1998; Fisher,

1999; Kantor, 2001; Conrey et al., 2003). Others are promoting community gardens (Kantor, 2001; Twiss et al., 2003), school gardens (Edible Schoolyard, 2004; see Chapter 7), and farm-to-school and farm-to-cafeteria programs (Kantor, 2001; Bellows et al., 2003; Center for Food and Justice, 2004; Sanger and Zenz, 2004; see Chapter 7).

Recent research has demonstrated that children who grow some of their own food in school gardens have an increased preference for certain vegetables (Morris and Zidenberg-Cherr, 2002). Recent federal legislation (Public Law 108-265) includes provisions designed to strengthen partnerships between local agriculture and schools to ensure that fresh local produce can go from farms directly to schools.

These initiatives to enhance the community food environment and promote household and community food security are promising to expand healthful food choices, especially for neighborhoods that are now limited in their ability to obtain healthful and affordable food on a regular basis. However, evaluations will be required to determine the programs' effectiveness in meeting these goals.

Local governments should work with community groups, nonprofit organizations, local farmers and food processors, and local businesses to support multisectoral partnerships and networks that expand the availability of healthful foods within walking distance, particularly in low-income and underserved neighborhoods. Such efforts will expand healthful food choices at local grocery stores, supermarkets, and fast food restaurants, and they will encourage a broad range of community food-security initiatives that improve access to highly nutritional foods.

Health Impact Assessments and Community Health Evaluations

Evaluation of community-wide efforts can be a challenge, given the typically wide age range among members of the population; their ethnic, racial, and social diversities; the differences in settings of various community interventions; and the numerous barriers involved.

Nevertheless, it is important to assess the potential impact of proposed programs and changes as well as to conduct evaluations of recent and ongoing efforts. A prospective approach to community evaluation efforts involves a "health impact assessment" that gauges the potential effects of a proposed policy or intervention on the health of the population (WHO, 1999). Much as environmental impact assessments examine the potential effects of a new construction project on such indicators as an area's air and water quality, health impact assessments are used to evaluate and then modify a proposed action—that is, to remove or minimize that action's negative public health impacts, and to help enhance its positive effects (Taylor and Quigley, 2002). The health impact assessment may also be particularly useful in bringing potential health impacts to the attention of policy makers.

A major value of this approach is its focus on considering the input of multiple stakeholders, including those who would be directly affected by the project under consideration. As changes are proposed to the built environment, communities should consider this tool for examining how proposed changes in the community would affect health issues such as access to and availability of healthful foods and opportunities for physical activity. It will be important to identify and examine natural experiments in which initiatives based on health-impact assessments could be compared to those undertaken without such an assessment.

For an overall assessment of a community's health improvement efforts that are already underway, community health "report cards" (also termed community health assessments or health profiles) are an excellent tool, both to assess and convey progress (CDC, 1997a). A variety of approaches have been used, all with the goal of providing a concise and consistent collection of data that can be formatted for dissemination to the community. For example, state, county, and community health profiles have been developed using CDC's *Healthy Days Measures* among other community performance indicators (CDC, 2004a). In addition, the Community Health Status Indicators Project (CHSI)—a collaborative effort of the Association of State and Territorial Health Officials, the National Association of County and City Health Officials (NACCHO), and the Public Health Foundation—has developed report indicators and formats for county-specific information that allows comparisons with similar "peer" counties throughout the country (NACCHO, 2004). A CHSI report contains information on behavioral risks, preventive services use, access, and summary health measures. To assist in obesity prevention efforts, community health report cards should use measures that assess the community's progress toward encouraging good nutrition and physical activity. These measures could rate the built and social environments, local school policies and practices (Chapter 7), the community food environment, and the degree of involvement of local businesses, organizations, and other groups in supporting and participating in obesity prevention efforts.

To streamline efforts and encourage communities to engage in these types of evaluation efforts, common evaluation tools should be developed and shared, while also ensuring that evaluation tools have the flexibility to be sensitive to the needs of local communities. This is an area where it will be important to build on tools (those discussed above and others) that have already been developed. Leadership for these efforts should involve CDC, NACCHO, the American Planning Association, and other relevant organizations, including foundations such as the Robert Wood Johnson Foundation, with interests in community-based obesity prevention efforts.

Communities should use evaluation tools (e.g., health impact assessments, audits, or report cards) to assess the availability and impact of local opportunities for physical activity (e.g., sidewalks, parks, recreational facilities) and for healthful eating (e.g., grocery store access, farmers' markets).

Recommendations

Mobilizing communities to address childhood obesity will involve changes in the social and built environment. Several large-scale community-based interventions—primarily focused on improving diet and physical activity levels to address cardiovascular outcomes—show the feasibility of such efforts, although much remains to be learned about how to increase their effectiveness, particularly with regard to obesity prevention in youth. Efforts to address other public health issues such as tobacco prevention and control provide models for community coalition efforts.

A relatively new field of research is merging urban planning, transportation, and public health research tools to examine the impact of the built environment on human health. Observational and correlational studies, primarily conducted in adult populations, have shown that features in the built environment such as the walkability of neighborhoods or availability of recreational facilities are associated with level of physical activity. A few small-scale intervention studies have examined the effects of changes to the built environment; however, research is needed to explore what specific changes to the built environment will be the most effective in preventing childhood obesity. The committee recommends the implementation and evaluation of a range of community changes to facilitate improved nutrition and increased physical activity. These efforts are an integral part of a comprehensive approach to create healthier environments for children and youth.

Recommendation 6: *Community Programs*
Local governments, public health agencies, schools, and community organizations should collaboratively develop and promote programs that encourage healthful eating behaviors and regular physical activity, particularly for populations at high risk of childhood obesity. Community coalitions should be formed to facilitate and promote cross-cutting programs and community-wide efforts.

To implement this recommendation:

• Private and public efforts to eliminate health disparities should include obesity prevention as one of their primary areas of focus and should support community-based collaborative programs to address social, economic, and environmental barriers that contribute to the increased obesity prevalence among certain populations.

• Community child- and youth-centered organizations should promote healthful eating behaviors and regular physical activity through new and existing programs that will be sustained over the long term.

• Community evaluation tools should incorporate measures of the availability of opportunities for physical activity and healthful eating.

• Communities should improve access to supermarkets, farmers' markets, and community gardens to expand healthful food options, particularly in low-income and underserved areas.

Recommendation 7: *Built Environment*
Local governments, private developers, and community groups should expand opportunities for physical activity including recreational facilities, parks, playgrounds, sidewalks, bike paths, routes for walking or bicycling to school, and safe streets and neighborhoods, especially for populations at high risk of childhood obesity.

To implement this recommendation:

Local governments, working with private developers and community groups, should:
• Revise comprehensive plans, zoning and subdivision ordinances, and other planning practices to increase availability and accessibility of opportunities for physical activity in new developments
• Prioritize capital improvement projects to increase opportunities for physical activity in existing areas
• Improve the street, sidewalk, and street-crossing safety of routes to school, develop programs to encourage walking and bicycling to school, and build schools within walking and bicycling distance of the neighborhoods they serve

Community groups should:
• Work with local governments to change their planning and capital improvement practices to give higher priority to opportunities for physical activity

DHHS and the Department of Transportation should:
• Fund community-based research to examine the impact of

changes to the built environment on the levels of physical activity in the relevant communities and populations.

HEALTH CARE

Because health care is usually provided at the local level, it is best addressed in a community context. Health-care professionals have frequent opportunities to encourage children and youth to engage in healthful lifestyles. Unfortunately, treatment of obesity per se is rarely considered a reimbursable interaction between patient and doctor, and our current health-care system is not yet focused on preventive measures for childhood obesity. But the health-care delivery system can still have a significant impact on this issue. It is now up to health-care professionals and their professional organizations, as well as health insurers and quality improvement and accrediting agencies, to make obesity prevention a part of routine preventive health care.

Health-Care Professionals

Health-care professionals—physicians, nurses, and other clinicians— have an influential role to play in preventing childhood obesity. As health-care advisors both to children and their parents, they have the access and the influence to make key suggestions and recommendations on dietary intake and physical activity throughout children's lives. They also have the authority to elevate concern about childhood obesity and advocate for preventive efforts.

The 2002 National Health Interview Survey found that 74.5 percent of children (aged 18 years or younger) had seen a health-care professional at some time during the past six months (Dey et al., 2004), thereby providing numerous opportunities for doctors and other clinicians to measure and track height, weight, and BMI and to counsel the children—as well as their parents or other caregivers—about proper nutrition and physical activity. Measuring height and weight and plotting these measures on growth charts is already a standard part of children's health care, and recent recommendations by the American Academy of Pediatrics have added BMI to this list (AAP, 2003). Although there is little direct evidence of the impact of height, weight, and BMI screening and tracking on preventing obesity in children, BMI measures for adults have been found to be both easy to measure and a highly reliable method for identifying patients at risk of morbidity and mortality due to obesity (McTigue et al., 2003). The U.S. Preventive Services Task Force (USPSTF) recommends that clinicians use BMI to screen all adult patients for obesity (USPSTF, 2003). A survey of 940 pediatric health-care providers, however, found that more used clinical impression and weight-for-age or weight-for-height measures than used BMI or BMI percentiles (Barlow et al., 2002).

Because there are standardized BMI charts for children, and given that BMI is a reasonably good surrogate for adiposity, it is sensible to include BMI calculations in all health supervision visits for children. By routinely measuring height and weight and calculating BMI, clinicians communicate that this is an important matter, just as important as routine immunizations or screening tests in protecting children's health (see Chapter 8). Furthermore, BMI measures on an annual or similarly regular basis allow assessment of the individual child's growth trajectory, which offers better insights, and on an earlier basis, than height or weight measurement alone (see Chapter 3).

After determining the child's weight status, health-care professionals have a responsibility to carefully communicate the results to parents and, in an age-appropriate manner, to the children themselves; provide the information that the families need to make informed decisions about physical activity and nutrition; and explain the risks associated with childhood overweight and obesity. Behaviors that can be targeted include those most closely associated with improved nutrition and increased physical activity: increased breastfeeding, limited consumption of sweetened beverages, reduced television viewing or other screen time, and a greater amount of outdoor play (Whitaker, 2003). Careful attention should be paid to minimizing the stigmatization of obesity (Schwartz and Puhl, 2003).

Studies of such counseling on obesity-related issues have shown positive results. In one trial, African-American families were randomized to receive primary-care-based counseling alone or counseling plus a behavioral intervention (including goal-setting and an electronic television-time manager) as part of their regular clinic visits (Ford et al., 2002). Both groups reported similar within-group decreases (from baseline) in children's television, videotape, and video game use. In the between-group comparison, the behavioral intervention group reported medium to large (and statistically significant) increases in organized physical activity and increases in playing outside. There was also a slight decrease for the intervention group in the number of meals eaten in front of the television, though the differences were not statistically significant (Ford et al., 2002). A four-month primary-care-based assessment and counseling intervention involving adolescents showed the feasibility of such efforts and found short-term improvements in dietary and physical activity outcome measures (Patrick et al., 2001).

More generally, studies of counseling for adults may provide insights into the potential effectiveness of counseling for children and their parents. The USPSTF review of dietary intake counseling for adults in primary-care settings found it to be effective in reducing dietary fat consumption and increasing fruit and vegetable consumption (Pignone et al., 2003). The best evidence was for patients with known risk factors for cardiovascular and other chronic diseases, but there was also fair evidence that brief counseling in primary care can produce some improvements in diet among unselected patients as well.

Similar reviews of studies that focused on physical activity counseling of adults in primary care found mixed results, although most of the studies showed a trend toward increased physical activity in the intervention groups (Sallis et al., 2000b; Eden et al., 2002). For example, a nonrandomized controlled trial in healthy sedentary adults found short-term increases in moderate physical activity, particularly walking, among those who had received three to five minutes of physical activity counseling by their physician (Calfas et al., 1996).

Although research on the effectiveness of counseling children and their caregivers about obesity prevention is limited to date, and much remains to be learned, the seriousness of the problem and the emergence of tested strategies argue for routine counseling. The evidence that routine smoking-cessation counseling is effective, at least in changing adult behaviors, is another precedent for this kind of guidance (DHHS, 2000a).

Additionally, as visible and influential members of their communities, health-care professionals can serve as role models for good nutrition, for being physically active, and for maintaining a healthy weight. Health-care professionals can also have influential voices in increasing community awareness and advocating for actions to prevent childhood obesity. By giving speeches or conducting workshops at schools, testifying before legislative bodies, working in community organizations, or speaking out in any number of other ways, health-care professionals can press for changes to make the community one that supports and facilitates healthful eating and physical activity. A notable precedent is that physicians and other health-care professionals have played crucial roles in changing tobacco-related behaviors; they have been advocates both at the local and national levels, and they have served as personal role models by quitting smoking or by not starting in the first place.

Pediatricians, family physicians, nurses, and other clinicians should take active roles in the prevention of obesity in children and youth. As discussed above, this includes routinely measuring height and weight; tracking BMI; and providing feedback, interpretation, counseling, and guidance on obesity prevention to children, parents, and other caregivers. This assumes that clinicians will have learned the appropriate skills to deliver these preventive services, which has implications for training at all levels (see below). They should also serve as role models for healthful eating and regular physical activity and take leadership roles in advocating for childhood obesity prevention in local schools and communities.

Similarly, health-care professional organizations and their members have important roles to play in advocating across the range of community institutions for obesity prevention activities and policies (AAP, 2003). Areas of possible involvement include health insurance coverage policies, school nutrition and physical education, and community recreation and zoning policies. Professional organizations can also be influential in encouraging their members to adopt a more healthful lifestyle and serve as role models to their patients as well as to become more active in their offices and communities in working to prevent obesity. For example, the leadership of the American Academy of Family Physicians (AAFP) has recently challenged all of its members to increase their personal physical activity levels in order to serve as role models for their patients (as well as improve their own health); additionally, AAFP has initiated a program called "Americans in Motion" to help patients, their families, and communities fight obesity (AAFP, 2004).

Furthermore, many professional organizations are providing information on topics relevant to obesity prevention. The American Academy of Pediatrics has issued position statements on children's television viewing and on physical fitness and activity in schools (AAP, 2000, 2001). The American Medical Association recently published a 10-part monograph on assessment and treatment of adult obesity (Kushner, 2003); similar materials on children should also be prepared. Collaboration between groups could broaden their effectiveness; if health-care professional organizations work together to implement obesity prevention programs and initiatives and develop clinical guidance, they would help ensure that consistent messages are reaching both health-care professionals and their patients.

Health- and medical-care professional organizations should make childhood obesity prevention a high-priority goal for their organizations. This includes creating and disseminating evidence-based clinical guidance and other materials on obesity prevention; establishing programs to encourage members to be role models for proper nutrition and physical activity; advocating for childhood obesity prevention initiatives; and coordinating their efforts, wherever possible, with other health-care professional organizations.

It is also critical to address current limitations in health-care training with regard to obesity prevention, nutrition, and physical activity. Medical and other health-care students have traditionally received little education in nutrition and physical activity; further, instruction on counseling about these topics generally has not been included either in medical school or primary-care residency training curricula (Taren et al., 2001). Such omissions should be corrected in curricula at all levels, from preclinical science through the clinical training years and into postgraduate training programs and continuing medical education for practicing clinicians. In addition, if certifying entities such as medical specialty boards included questions about these areas in their formal examinations, this would provide an incentive to students and residents to master the associated material. Programs such as the Nutrition Academic Award Program sponsored by the National Heart, Lung, and Blood Institute have begun to focus attention on improving nutrition education efforts in medical schools (Pearson et al., 2001), and further efforts are needed regarding other relevant areas. A recent Institute of Medicine report confirms the need for expanding behavioral and social-science content in medical schools' curricula (IOM, 2004). **Health-care professional schools, postgraduate training programs, continuing professional education programs, professional organizations, and certifying entities should require knowledge and skills related to obesity prevention (e.g., child and adolescent BMI interpretation, nutritional and physical activity counseling) in their curricula and examinations.**

Health-Care Insurers, Health Plans, and Quality Improvement and Accrediting Organizations

Until recently, health-care concerns had largely focused on the treatment—as opposed to the prevention—of obesity, particularly the severe forms of adult obesity. But epidemiologic data showing increases in the numbers of obese children and youth, along with a rise in the prevalence of type 2 diabetes (formerly termed "adult onset diabetes") and increased hypertension in children (Muntner et al., 2004), have raised awareness that childhood obesity might be best addressed from a prevention perspective. Furthermore, the high economic costs of obesity (Chapter 2) provide incentives to health-care insurers and health plans to encourage healthful lifestyles and thereby reduce their costs.

The health-care insurance industry in particular has several paths by which it may address obesity prevention. For individuals and their families, health insurance companies and health plans can develop innovative strategies for encouraging policy holders and their children to maintain a healthy weight, increase their levels of physical activity, and improve the quality of their diet. Creative options may include incentives for participating in and documenting regular physical activity, or programs that provide discounts or other incentives for wellness-related products. For example, one insurance company includes discounts on health and wellness magazines as well as lowered fees for health club memberships and weight-reduction programs for adults (CIGNA, 2004). Furthermore, health-care insurers can take an active role in community coalitions and other activities; one example is the Jump Up and Go Program in Massachusetts (Blue Cross Blue Shield of Massachusetts, 2004). It will be particularly important for health-care insurers and health plans to consider incentives that are useful to high-risk populations, who often live in areas where easy access to recreational facilities is lacking or where costs are prohibitive.

For the providers of health-care services, it is important that obesity prevention (including assessment of weight status as well as counseling on nutrition and physical activity) become a routine part of clinical care. Moreover, measures related to successful delivery of clinical preventive services, such as rates of screening tests, should be important components of health-care quality-improvement programs that are promoted by health plans. The National Committee for Quality Assurance (NCQA) and other national quality-improvement and accrediting organizations should add obesity prevention efforts—such as routine measurement and tracking of BMI, counseling of children and their parents on diet and exercise—to the measures they develop and assess.

There may also be opportunities for incorporating obesity prevention measures and counseling into ongoing federal, state, and local programs that provide disease prevention and health promotion services to children. For example, Medicaid's Early and Periodic Screening, Diagnostic, and Treatment program offers preventive screenings for eligible children (generally in underserved populations) and it includes a comprehensive health and developmental history. More than 8.7 million children participated in the screening program in 1998 (CMS, 2004), thus offering many potential opportunities for obesity prevention in children.

As with other sectors, those involved in delivering and paying for health care need to become more proactive, preferably through a multifocal, coordinated set of initiatives, in working with families to promote physical activity and healthful diets among children. Medicare has recently removed barriers to coverage for obesity-related services (DHHS, 2004). Although this, of course, does not relate directly to children, it is an action that may well be emulated by other insurers and for preventive services as well as for treatment.

Health insurers, health plans, and quality-improvement and accrediting organizations should designate childhood obesity prevention as a priority health promotion issue. Furthermore, health plans and health-care insurers should provide incentives to individuals and families to maintain healthy body weight and engage in routine physical activity. Health insurers, health plans, and quality improvement and accrediting organizations (such as NCQA) should include screening and obesity prevention services (e.g., routine assessment of BMI or other weight-status measures, counseling of children and their parents on nutrition and physical activity) in routine clinical practice and in quality assessment measures relating to health care.

Recommendation

The health-care community offers a range of opportunities for interactions with children and youth regarding obesity prevention. Several controlled trials of counseling by health-care providers have resulted in patient improvements in physical activity levels or diet, although these studies have generally been conducted with small numbers of patients and have focused on counseling of adult patients. Further research is needed on effective counseling or other types of obesity prevention interventions that could be provided in health-care settings. Improved professional education regarding obesity prevention is an important next step, as is the active involvement of health professional organizations, insurers, and accrediting organizations, in making childhood obesity prevention efforts a priority.

Recommendation 8: *Health Care*
Pediatricians, family physicians, nurses, and other clinicians should engage in the prevention of childhood obesity. Health-care professional organizations, insurers, and accrediting groups should support individual and population-based obesity prevention efforts.

To implement this recommendation:

• Health-care professionals should routinely track BMI, offer relevant evidence-based counseling and guidance, serve as role models, and provide leadership in their communities for obesity prevention efforts.

• Professional organizations should disseminate evidence-based clinical guidance and establish programs on obesity prevention.

• Training programs and certifying entities should require obesity prevention knowledge and skills in their curricula and examinations.

• Insurers and accrediting organizations should provide incentives for maintaining healthy body weight and include screening and obesity preventive services in routine clinical practice and quality assessment measures.

REFERENCES

AAFP (American Academy of Family Physicians). 2004. *Americans in Motion*. [Online]. Available: http://www.aafp.org/x22874.xml [accessed May 14, 2004].

AAP (American Academy of Pediatrics), Committee on Sports Medicine and Fitness and Committee on School Health. 2000. Physical fitness and activity in schools. *Pediatrics* 105(5):1156-1157.

AAP. 2001. Children, adolescents, and television. *Pediatrics* 107(2):423-426.

AAP, Committee on Nutrition. 2003. Prevention of pediatric overweight and obesity. *Pediatrics* 112(2):424-430.

ADA (American Dietetic Association). 2004. Position of the American Dietetic Association: Dietary guidance for healthy children ages 2 to 11 years. *J Am Diet Assoc* 104(4):660-677.

Alaimo K, Olson CM, Frongillo EA Jr, Briefel RR. 2001. Food insufficiency, family income, and health in US preschool and school-aged children. *Am J Public Health* 91(5):781-786.

Alwitt LF, Donley TD. 1997. Retail stores in poor urban neighborhoods. *J Consumer Affairs* 31(1):139-164.

Baker EA, Brownson CA. 1998. Defining characteristics of community-based health promotion programs. *J Public Health Manag Pract* 4(2):1-9.

Baltimore Healthy Stores Project. 2004. *Baltimore Healthy Stores Project.* [Online]. Available: http://www.healthystores.org/BHS.html [accessed June 8, 2004].

Baranowski T, Thompson WO, DuRant RH, Baranowski J, Puhl J. 1993. Observations on physical activity in physical locations: Age, gender, ethnicity, and month effects. *Res Q Exerc Sport* 64(2):127-133.

Baranowski T, Baranowski JC, Cullen KW, Thompson DI, Nicklas T, Zakeri IE, Rochon J. 2003. The Fun, Food, and Fitness Project (FFFP): The Baylor GEMS pilot study. *Ethn Dis* 13(1 Suppl 1):S30-S39.

Barlow SE, Dietz WH, Klish WJ, Trowbridge FL. 2002. Medical evaluation of overweight children and adolescents: Reports from pediatricians, pediatric nurse practitioners, and registered dietitians. *Pediatrics* 110(1):222-228.

Beech BM, Klesges RC, Kumanyika SK, Murray DM, Klesges L, McClanahan B, Slawson D, Nunnally C, Rochon J, McLain-Allen B, Pree-Cary J. 2003. Child- and parent-targeted interventions: The Memphis GEMS pilot study. *Ethn Dis* 13(1 Suppl 1):S40-S53.

Bellows BC, Dufour R, Bachmann J. 2003. *Bringing Local Food to Local Institutions. A Resource Guide for Farm-to-School and Farm-to-Institution Programs.* [Online]. Available: http://attra.ncat.org/attra-pub/PDF/farmtoschool.pdf [accessed June 8, 2004].

Blue Cross Blue Shield of Massachusetts. 2004. *Jump Up and Go!* [Online]. Available: http://www.bcbsma.com/common/en_US/myWellbeingIndex.jsp [accessed August 5, 2004].

Boarnet MG, Day K, Anderson C, McMillen T, Alfonzo M. 2003. *Urban Form and Physical Activity: Insights from a Quasi-Experiment.* [Online]. Available: http://www.activeliving research.org/downloads/boarnet_presentation.pdf [accessed June 3, 2004].

Bolen E, Hecht K. 2003. *Neighborhood Groceries: New Access to Healthy Food in Low-Income Communities. California Food Policy Advocates.* [Online]. Available: http://www.cfpa.net/Grocery.PDF [accessed January 8, 2004].

Brownson RC, Baker EA, Housemann RA, Brennan LK, Bacak SJ. 2001. Environmental and policy determinants of physical activity in the United States. *Am J Public Health* 91:1995-2003.

Brumley DE, Hawks RW, Gillcrist JA, Blackford JU, Wells WW. 2001. Successful implementation of community water fluoridation via the community diagnosis process. *J Public Health Dent* 61(1):28-33.

Burdette HL, Whitaker RC. 2004. Neighborhood playgrounds, fast food restaurants, and crime: Relationships to overweight in low-income preschool children. *Prev Med* 38(1):57-63.

Calfas KJ, Long BJ, Sallis JF, Wooten WJ, Pratt M, Patrick K. 1996. A controlled trial of physician counseling to promote the adoption of physical activity. *Prev Med* 25(3):225-233.

Caltrans. 2004. *Safe Routes to School Program.* [Online]. Available: http://www.dot.ca.gov/hq/LocalPrograms/saferoute2.htm [accessed April 22, 2004].

Campbell MK, Demark-Wahnefried W, Symons M, Kalsbeek WD, Dodds J, Cowan A, Jackson B, Motsinger B, Hoben K, Lashley J, Demissie S, McClelland JW. 1999. Fruit and vegetable consumption and prevention of cancer: The Black Churches United for Better Health project. *Am J Public Health* 89(9):1390-1396.

CDC (Centers for Disease Control and Prevention). 1997a. Characteristics of community report cards, United States, 1996. *MMWR* 46(28):647-648.

CDC. 1997b. Guidelines for school and community programs to promote lifelong physical activity among young people. *MMWR* 46(RR-6):1-36.

CDC. 1999. Neighborhood safety and prevalence of physical inactivity-selected states. *MMWR* 48(7):143-146.

CDC. 2002a. Barriers to children walking and bicycling to school—United States, 1999. *MMWR* 51(32):701-704.

CDC. 2002b. School transportation modes—Georgia, 2000. *MMWR* 51(32):704-705.

CDC. 2004a. *State and Community Health Profiles*. [Online]. Available: http://www.cdc.gov/hrqol/community.htm [accessed July 6, 2004].

CDC. 2004b. *REACH: Racial and Ethnic Approaches to Community Health*. [Online]. Available: http://www.cdc.gov/reach2010/ [accessed August 4, 2004].

Center for Food and Justice. 2004. *Farm to School Projects: Improving School Food While Helping Local Farmers*. Urban and Environmental Policy Institute. [Online]. Available: http://www.farmtoschool.org/ [accessed June 8, 2004].

Chauncey B, Wilkinson B. 2003. *An Assessment of MPO Support for Bicycling and Walking*. Washington DC: National Center for Bicycling and Walking.

Chavis DM. 2001. The paradoxes and promise of community coalitions. *Am J Community Psychol* 29(2):309-320.

Chicago Police Department. 2004. *Protecting Our Children—Working Together for a Safer Chicago*. [Online]. Available: http://www.cityofchicago.org/cp/Alerts/SafetyTips/ChildSafety/WalkingSchoolbus.html [accessed May 21, 2004].

CIGNA. 2004. *Member Discounts from Healthy Rewards*. [Online]. Available: http://www.cigna.com/health/consumer/medical/discount.html [accessed April 22, 2004].

Clark V. 2004. Plan would add supermarkets in city: The $100 million statewide proposal is intended to promote healthy eating in low-income areas. *Philadelphia Inquirer*. News release. May 5.

CMS (Centers for Medicare & Medicaid Services). 2004. *Annual EPSDT Participation Report, All States*. [Online]. Available: http://www.cms.hhs.gov/medicaid/epsdt/ep1998n.pdf [accessed May 14, 2004].

CNU (Congress for the New Urbanism). 2004. *About CNU*. [Online]. Available: http://www.cnu.org/aboutcnu [accessed April 22, 2004].

Cohen B. 2002. *Community Food Security Assessment Toolkit*. Washington, DC: USDA, Economic Research Service. E-FAN-02-013. [Online]. Available: http://www.ers.usda.gov/publications/efan02013/efan02013.pdf [accessed June 8, 2004].

Connecticut Food Policy Council. 1998. *Making Room at the Table: A Guide to Community Food Security in Connecticut*. Hartford, CT: CFPC.

Conrey EJ, Frongillo EA, Dollahite JS, Griffin MR. 2003. Integrated program enhancements increased utilization of a farmers' market nutrition program. *J Nutr* 133(6):1841-1844.

Cooper AR, Page AS, Foster LJ, Qahwaji D. 2003. Commuting to school: Are children who walk more physically active? *Am J Prev Med* 25(4):273-276.

Corburn J. 2004. Confronting the challenges in reconnecting urban planning and public health. *Am J Public Health* 94(4):541-546.

Cotterill RW, Franklin AW. 1995. *The Urban Grocery Store Gap*. Storrs, CT: Food Marketing Policy Center, University of Connecticut.

Cullen KW, Bartholomew LL, Parcel GS. 1997. Girl Scouting: An effective channel for nutrition education. *J Nutr Educ* 92(5):86-91.
DeBate RD. 2002. *Girls on the Run International. Evaluation Report, Spring 2002.* Charlotte, NC: University of North Carolina.
Dey AN, Schiller JS, Tai DA. 2004. Summary health statistics for U.S. children: National Health Interview Survey, 2002. *Vital Health Statistics* 10(221).
DHHS (U.S. Department of Health and Human Services), USPHS Guideline Panel. 2000a. *Treating Tobacco Use and Dependence.* Washington, DC: DHHS.
DHHS. 2000b. *Healthy People 2010: Understanding and Improving Health.* 2nd edition. Washington, DC: U.S. Government Printing Office. [Online]. Available: http://www.healthypeople.gov/document/tableofcontents.htm [accessed April 9, 2004].
DHHS. 2004. *HHS Announces Revised Medicare Obesity Coverage Policy.* [Online]. Available: http://www.hhs.gov/news/press/2004pres/20040715.html [accessed August 4, 2004].
DiGuiseppi C, Roberts I, Li L, Allen D. 1998. Determinants of car travel on daily journeys to school: Cross sectional survey of primary school children. *Br Med J* 316(7142):1426-1428.
Doxey J, Tran T, Kimball K, Corliss J, Mercer M. 2003. *Can't Get There from Here: The Declining Independent Mobility of California's Children and Youth.* A Joint Project of the Surface Transportation Policy Project, Transportation and Land Use Coalition, Latino Issues Forum. [Online]. Available: http://www.transcoalition.org/reports/kids/kids_report.pdf [accessed April 18, 2004].
Drewnowski A, Specter SE. 2004. Poverty and obesity: The role of energy density and energy costs. *Am J Clin Nutr* 79(1):6-16.
Eden KB, Orleans CT, Mulrow CD, Pender NJ, Teutsch SM. 2002. Does counseling by clinicians improve physical activity? A summary of the evidence for the U.S. Preventive Services Task Force. *Ann Intern Med* 137(3):208-215.
Edible Schoolyard. 2004. *The Edible Schoolyard.* [Online]. Available: http://www.edibleschool yard.org [accessed June 4, 2004].
EPA (U.S. Environmental Protection Agency). 2003. *Travel and Environmental Implications of School Siting.* EPA 231-R-03-004. Washington, DC: EPA.
Eubanks-Ahrens B. 1987. A closer look at the users of Woonerven. In: Moudon AV, ed. *Public Streets for Public Use.* New York: Van Nostrand Reinhold.
Farquhar JW, Maccoby N, Wood PD, Alexander JK, Breitrose H, Brown BW Jr, Haskell WL, McAlister AL, Meyer AJ, Nash JD, Stern MP. 1977. Community education for cardiovascular health. *Lancet* 1(8023):1192-1995.
Farquhar JW, Fortmann SP, Flora JA, Taylor CB, Haskell WL, Williams PT, Maccoby N, Wood PD. 1990. Effects of communitywide education on cardiovascular disease risk factors. The Stanford Five-City Project. *J Am Med Assoc* 264(3):359-365.
Fawcett SB, Paine-Andrews A, Francisco VT, Schultz J, Richter KP, Berkley-Patton J, Fisher JL, Lewis RK, Lopez CM, Russos S, Williams EL, Harris KJ, Evensen P. 2001. Evaluating community initiatives for health and development. *WHO Reg Publ Eur Ser* 92:241-270.
Fawcett SB, et al. 2004. *Understanding and Improving the Work of Community Health and Development.* Paper presented at the VIII Biannual Symposium on the Science of Behavior. As cited in: Kaiser Permanente. 2004. *Kaiser Permanente's Framework for Community Health Initiatives.* [Online]. Available: http://www.kpihp.org/publications/briefs/chi_Framework.pdf.
Federal Highway Administration. 2004. *Federal–Aid Highway Program Funding for Pedestrian and Bicycle Facilities and Programs.* [Online]. Available: http://www.fhwa.dot.gov/environment/bikeped/bikepedfund.htm [accessed July 15, 2004].

Fisher A. 1999. *Hot Peppers and Parking Lot Peaches: Evaluating Farmers' Markets in Low Income Communities*. Venice, CA: Community Food Security Coalition. [Online]. Available: http://www.foodsecurity.org/executive.html [accessed April 22, 2004].

Ford BS, McDonald TE, Owens AS, Robinson TN. 2002. Primary care interventions to reduce television viewing in African-American children. *Am J Prev Med* 22(2):106-109.

GAO (U.S. General Accounting Office). 2000. *School Facilities: Construction Expenditures Have Grown Significantly in Recent Years*. HEHS-00-41. Washington, DC: GAO.

Girls on the Run. 2004. *Girls on the Run International*. [Online]. Available: http://www.girlsontherun.org/ [accessed May 14, 2004].

Glanz K. 1997. Perspectives on using theory. In: Glanz K, Lewis FM, Rimer BK, eds. *Health Behavior and Health Education*. 2nd ed. San Francisco, CA: Jossey-Bass Publishers. Pp. 441-449.

Gordon-Larsen P, McMurray RG, Popkin BM. 2000. Determinants of adolescent physical activity and inactivity patterns. *Pediatrics* 105:E83.

Grossman DC. 2000. The history of injury control and the epidemiology of child and adolescent injuries. *Future Child* 10(1):23-52.

Handy S, Boarnet MG, Ewing R, Killingsworth RE. 2002. How the built environment affects physical activity: Views from urban planning. *Am J Prev Med* 23(2 Suppl):64-73.

Handy S, Paterson R, Butler K. 2003. *Planning for Street Connectivity: Getting from Here to There. Planning Advisory Service Report*. Chicago, IL: American Planning Association.

Hoefer WR, McKenzie TL, Sallis JF, Marshall SJ, Conway JL. 2001. Parental provision of transportation for adolescent physical activity. *Am J Prev Med* 21(1):48-51.

Hoehner CM, Brennan LK, Brownson RC, Handy SL, Killingsworth R. 2003. Opportunities for integrating public health and urban planning approaches to promote active community environments. *Am J Health Promot* 18(1):14-20.

Holben DH, McClincy MC, Holcomb JP Jr, Dean KL, Walker CE. 2004. Food security status of households in Appalachian Ohio with children in Head Start. *J Am Diet Assoc* 104(2):238-241.

Huang HF, Cynecki MJ. 2000. Effects of traffic calming measures on pedestrian and motorist behavior. *Transp Res Rec* 1705:26-31.

Huang HF, Cynecki MJ. 2001. *The Effects of Traffic Calming Measures on Pedestrian and Motorist Behavior*. McLean, VA: Federal Highway Administration.

Humpel N, Owen N, Leslie E. 2002. Environmental factors associated with adults' participation in physical activity: A review. *Am J Prev Med* 22(3):188-199.

IOM (Institute of Medicine). 1994. *Growing Up Tobacco Free: Preventing Nicotine Addiction in Children and Youth*. Washington, DC: National Academy Press.

IOM. 2003. *Fulfilling the Potential of Cancer Prevention and Early Detection*. Washington, DC: The National Academies Press.

IOM. 2004. *Improving Medical Education: Enhancing the Behavioral and Social Science Content of Medical School Curricula*. Washington, DC: The National Academies Press.

ITE (Institute of Transportation Engineers). 1999. *Traditional Neighborhood Development Street Design Guidelines: Recommended Practice*. Washington, DC: ITE.

Jacobsen P, Anderson CL, Winn DG, Moffat J, Agran PF, Sarkar S. 2000. Child pedestrian injuries on residential streets: Implications for traffic engineering. *Inst Traffic Eng J Web* 70:71-75.

Kahn EB, Ramsey LT, Brownson RC, Heath GW, Howze EH, Powell KE, Stone EJ, Rajab MW, Corso P. 2002. The effectiveness of interventions to increase physical activity. A systematic review. *Am J Prev Med* 22(4 Suppl):73-107.

Kaiser Permanente. 2004. *Kaiser Permanente's Framework for Community Health Initiatives*. [Online]. Available: http://www.kpihp.org/publications/briefs/chi_Framework.pdf.

Kantor LS. 2001. Community food security programs improve food access. *Food Rev* 24(1):20-26.

Kegler MC, Steckler A, McLeroy K, Malek SH. 1998. Factors that contribute to effective community health promotion coalitions: A study of 10 Project ASSIST coalitions in North Carolina. American Stop Smoking Intervention Study for Cancer Prevention. *Health Educ Behav* 25(3):338-353.

Kelder SH, Perry CL, Klepp KI. 1993. Community-wide youth exercise promotion: Long-term outcomes of the Minnesota Heart Health Program and the Class of 1989 Study. *J Sch Health* 63(5):218-223.

Kelder SH, Perry CL, Lytle LA, Klepp KI. 1995. Community-wide youth nutrition education: Long-term outcomes of the Minnesota Heart Health Program. *Health Educ Res* 10(2):119-131.

Klesges RC, Eck LH, Hanson CL, Haddock CK, Klesges LM. 1990. Effects of obesity, social interactions, and physical environment on physical activity in preschoolers. *Health Psychol* 9(4):435-449.

Kreuter M, Lezin N. 2002. Coalitions, consortia and partnerships. In: Last J, Breslow L, Green LW, eds. *Encyclopedia of Public Health*. London, UK: MacMillan Publishers.

Kumanyika SK, Obarzanek E, Robinson TN, Beech BM. 2003. Phase 1 of the Girls health Enrichment Multi-site Studies (GEMS): Conclusion. *Ethn Dis* 13(1 Suppl 1):S88-S91.

Kushner RF. 2003. *Assessment and Management of Adult Obesity: A Primer for Physicans*. Chicago, IL: American Medical Association.

Lang T, Caraher M. 1998. Food poverty and shopping deserts: What are the implications for health promotion policy and practice? *Health Educ J* 58(3):202-211.

Lasker RD, Weiss ES. 2003. Broadening participation in community-problem solving: A multidisciplinary model to support collaborative practice and research. *J Urban Health* 80(1):14-47.

Lasker RD, Weiss ES, Miller R, Community-Campus Parternerships for Health. 2001. Promoting collaborations that improve health. *Educ Health* 14(2):163-172.

Local Government Commission. 2003. *Overcoming Obstacles to Smart Growth Through Code Reform*. Sacramento, CA: Local Government Commission.

Loukaitou-Sideris A. 2003. *Transportation, Land Use, and Physical Activity: Safety and Security Considerations*. Draft paper presented at a workshop of the Transportation Research Board and the Institute of Medicine Committee on Physical Activity, Health, Transportation, and Land Use. Washington, DC.

LSRO (Life Sciences Research Organization). 1990. Core indicators of nutritional state for difficult to sample populations. *J Nutr* 120(Suppl 11):1559-1660.

Luepker RV, Murray DM, Jacobs DR Jr, Mittelmark MB, Bracht N, Carlaw R, Crow R, Elmer P, Finnegan J, Folsom AR, Grimm R, Hannan PJ, Jeffrey R, Lando H, McGovern P, Mullis R, Perry CL, Pechacek T, Pirie P, Sprafka JM, Weisbrod R, Blackburn H. 1994. Community education for cardiovascular disease prevention: Risk factor changes in the Minnesota Heart Health Program. *Am J Public Health* 84(9):1383-1393.

Macbeth AG. 1999. Bicycle lanes in Toronto. *ITE J* 69:38-40, 42, 44, 46.

Maccoby N, Farquhar JW, Wood PD, Alexander J. 1977. Reducing the risk of cardiovascular disease: Effects of a community-based campaign on knowledge and behavior. *J Community Health* 3(2):100-114.

McMillan TE. 2002. The influence of urban form on a child's trip to school. Presented at the Association of Collegiate Schools of Planning Annual Conference, Baltimore. Cited in: EPA. 2003. *Travel and Environmental Implications of School Siting*. EPA 231-R-03-004. Washington, DC: EPA.

McTigue KM, Harris R, Hemphill B, Lux T, Sutton S, Bunton AJ, Lohr KN. 2003. Screening and interventions for obesity in adults: Summary of the evidence for the U.S. Preventive Services Task Force. *Ann Intern Med* 139(11):933-949.

Mensah GA, Goodman RA, Zaza S, Moulton AD, Kocher PL, Dietz WH, Pechacek TF, Marks JS. 2004. Law as a tool for preventing chronic diseases: Expanding the spectrum of effective public health strategies [Part 2]. *Preventing Chronic Disease* [Online]. Available: http://www.cdc.gov/pcd/issues/2004/apr/04_0009.htm [accessed April 20, 2004].

Minkler M, Wallerstein N. 2003. *Community-Based Participatory Research for Health*. San Francisco, CA: Jossey-Bass.

Morland K, Wing S, Diez Roux A, Poole C. 2002a. Neighborhood characteristics associated with the location of food stores and food service places. *Am J Prev Med* 22(1):23-29.

Morland K, Wing S, Diez Roux A. 2002b. The contextual effect of the local food environment on residents' diets: The atherosclerosis risk in communities study. *Am J Public Health* 92(11):1761-1767.

Morris J, Zidenberg-Cherr S. 2002. Garden-enhanced nutrition curriculum improves fourth-grade school children's knowledge of nutrition and preferences for some vegetables. *J Am Diet Assoc* 102(1):91-93.

Muntner P, He J, Cutler JA, Wildman RP, Whelton PK. 2004. Trends in blood pressure among children and adults. *J Am Med Assoc* 291(17):2107-2113.

NACCHO (National Association of County and City Health Officials). 2004. *Community Health Status Indicators Project*. [Online]. Available: http://www.naccho.org/project2.cfm [accessed July 6, 2004].

Nord M, Andrews M, Carlson S. 2003. *Household Food Security in the United States, 2002*. Alexandria, VA: USDA, Economic Research Service. Food Assistance and Nutrition Research Report 35.

Painter K. 1996. The influence of street lighting improvements on crime, fear, and pedestrian street use, after dark. *Landsc Urban Plan* 35:193-201.

Partnership for the Public's Health. 2004. *The Power of Partnership: Improving the Health of California's Communities. 2003 Annual Report*. [Online]. Available: http://www.partnershipph.org/col4/ar/ar03.pdf [accessed July 6, 2004].

Pate RR, Trost SG, Mullis R, Sallis JF, Wechsler H, Brown DR. 2000. Community interventions to promote proper nutrition and physical activity among youth. *Prev Med* 31:S138-S148.

Patrick K, Sallis JF, Prochaska JJ, Lydston DD, Calfas KJ, Zabinski MF, Wilfley DE, Saelens BE, Brown DR. 2001. A multicomponent program for nutrition and physical activity change in primary care: PACE+ for adolescents. *Arch Pediatr Adolesc Med* 155(8):940-946.

Pearson TA, Stone EJ, Grundy SM, McBride PE, Van Horn L, Tobin BW, NAA Collaborative Group. 2001. Translation of nutritional sciences into medical education: The Nutrition Academic Award Program. *Am J Clin Nutr* 74(2):164-170.

Perdue WC, Stone LA, Gostin LO. 2003. The built environment and its relationship to the public's health: The legal framework. *Am J Public Health* 93(9):1390-1394.

Perry D. 2001. *The Need for More Supermarkets in Philadelphia*. Philadelphia, PA: The Food Trust.

Pietinen P, Lahti-Koski M, Vartiainen E, Puska P. 2001. Nutrition and cardiovascular disease in Finland since the early 1970s: A success story. *J Nutr Health Aging* 5(3):150-154.

Pignone MP, Ammerman A, Fernandez L, Orleans CT, Pender N, Woolf S, Lohr KN, Sutton S. 2003. Counseling to promote a healthy diet in adults: A summary of the evidence for the U.S. Preventive Services Task Force. *Am J Prev Med* 24(1):75-92.

PolicyLink. 2002. *Reducing Health Disparities Through a Focus on Communities.* Oakland, CA: PolicyLink. [Online]. Available: http://www.policylink.org/pdfs/HealthDisparities. pdf [accessed July 6, 2004].

Pothukuchi K, Joseph H, Burton H, Fisher A. 2002. *What's Cooking in Your Food System? A Guide to Community Food Assessment.* Venice, CA: Community Food Security Coalition.

Powell LM, Slater S, Chaloupka FJ. 2004. The relationship between community physical activity settings and race, ethnicity and socioeconomic status. *Evidence-Based Prev Med* 1(2):135-144.

Prevention Institute. 2002. *Eliminating Health Disparities: The Role of Primary Prevention.* [Online]. Available: http://www.preventioninstitute.org/pdf/Health Disparities.pdf [accessed August 23, 2004].

Prevention Institute. 2003. *Environmental and Policy Approaches to Promoting Healthy Eating and Activity Behaviors.* Oakland, CA: Prevention Institute.

Puska P, Pietinen P, Uusitalo U. 2002. Influencing public nutrition for non-communicable disease prevention: From community intervention to national programme—Experiences from Finland. *Public Health Nutr* 5(1A):245-251.

Reed J, Frazao E, Itskowitz R. 2004. *How Much Do Americans Pay for Fruits and Vegetables?* Agriculture Information Bulletin Number 790. Washington, DC: USDA, Economic Research Service. [Online]. Available: http://www.ers.usda.gov/publications/ aib790/aib790.pdf [accessed August 4, 2004].

Retting RA, Ferguson SA, McCartt AT. 2003. A review of evidence-based traffic engineering measures designed to reduce pedestrian-motor vehicle crashes. *Am J Public Health* 93(9):1456-1463.

Roberts I. 1993. Why have child pedestrian death rates fallen? *Br Med J* 306(6894):1737-1739.

Robinson TN, Killen JD, Kraemer HC, Wilson DM, Matheson DM, Haskell WL, Pruitt LA, Powell TM, Owens AS, Thompson NS, Flint-Moore NM, Davis GJ, Emig KA, Brown RT, Rochon J, Green S, Varady A. 2003. Dance and reducing television viewing to prevent weight gain in African-American girls: The Stanford GEMS pilot study. *Ethn Dis* 13(1 Suppl 1):S65-S77.

Romero AJ, Robinson TN, Kraemer HC, Erickson SJ, Haydel KF, Mendoza F, Killen JD. 2001. Are perceived neighborhood hazards a barrier to physical activity in children? *Arch Pediatr Adolesc Med* 155(10):1143-1148.

Saelens BE, Sallis JF, Black JB, Chen D. 2003. Neighborhood-based differences in physical activity: An environment scale evaluation. *Am J Public Health* 93(9):1552-1558.

Sallis JF, Nader PR, Broyles SL, Berry CC, Elder JP, McKenzie TL, Nelson JA. 1993. Correlates of physical activity at home in Mexican-American and Anglo-American preschool children. *Health Psychol* 12(5):390-398.

Sallis JF, McKenzie TL, Elder JP, Broyles SL, Nader PR. 1997. Factors parents use in selecting play spaces for young children. *Arch Pediatr Adolesc Med* 151(4):414-417.

Sallis JF, Bauman A, Pratt M. 1998. Environmental and policy interventions to promote physical activity. *Am J Prev Med* 15(4):379-397.

Sallis JF, Prochaska JJ, Taylor WC. 2000a. A review of correlates of physical activity of children and adolescents. *Med Sci Sports Exerc* 32(5):963-975.

Sallis JF, Patrick K, Frank E, Pratt M, Wechsler H, Galuska DA. 2000b. Interventions in health care settings to promote healthful eating and physical activity in children and adolescents. *Prev Med* 31(2):S112-S120.

Sanger K, Zenz L. 2004. *Farm-to-Cafeteria Connections. Marketing Opportunities for Small Farms in Washington State.* Washington State Department of Agriculture, Small Farm and Direct Marketing Program. [Online]. Available: http://agr.wa.gov/Marketing/SmallFarm/102-FarmToCafeteriaConnections-Web.pdf [accessed June 8, 2004].

Schwartz MB, Puhl R. 2003. Childhood obesity: A societal problem to solve. *Obes Rev* 4(1):57-71.

Shaffer A. 2002. *The Persistence of L.A.'s Grocery Gap: The Need for a New Food Policy and Approach to Market Development.* Los Angeles, CA: Center for Food and Justice, Urban and Environmental Policy Institute.

Shea S, Basch CE. 1990. A review of five major community-based cardiovascular disease prevention programs. Part II: Intervention strategies, evaluation methods, and results. *Am J Health Promot* 4(4):279-287.

Sloane DC, Diamant AL, Lewis LB, Yancey AK, Flynn G, Nascimento LM, McCarthy WJ, Guinyard JJ, Cousineau MR. 2003. Improving the nutritional resource environment for healthy living through community-based participatory research. *J Gen Intern Med* 18(7):568-575.

Smart Growth America. 2004. *Smart Growth America.* [Online]. Available: http://www.smartgrowthamerica.com/ [accessed April 22, 2004].

Staunton CE, Hubsmith D, Kallins W. 2003. Promoting safe walking and bicycling to school: The Marin County success story. *Am J Public Health* 93(9):1431-1434.

Stillman FA, Hartman AM, Graubard BI, Gilpin EA, Murray DM, Gibson JT. 2003. Evaluation of the American Stop Smoking Intervention Study (ASSIST): A report of outcomes. *J Natl Cancer Inst* 95(22):1681-1691.

Story M, Sherwood NE, Himes JH, Davis M, Jacobs DR Jr, Cartwright Y, Smyth M, Rochon J. 2003. An after-school obesity prevention program for African-American girls: The Minnesota GEMS pilot study. *Ethn Dis* 13(1 Suppl 1):S54-S64.

Sustrans. 2001. *Safe Route to Schools. Sustrans Information Sheet FS01.* [Online]. Available: http://www.saferoutestoschools.org.uk/imagprod/downloads/fs01.pdf [accessed August 4, 2004].

Taren DL, Thomson CA, Koff NA, Gordon PR, Marian MJ, Bassford TL, Fulginiti JV, Ritenbaugh CK. 2001. Effect of an integrated nutrition curriculum on medical education, student clinical performance, and student perception of medical-nutrition training. *Am J Clin Nutr* 73(6):1107-1112.

Taylor L, Quigley R. 2002. *Health Impact Assessment: A Review of Reviews.* London: Health Development Agency. [Online]. Available: http://www.hda-online.org.uk/evidence [accessed May 26, 2004].

Tester JM, Rutherford GW, Wald Z, Rutherford MW. 2004. A matched case-control study evaluating the effectiveness of speed humps in reducing child pedestrian injuries. *Am J Public Health* 94(4):646-650.

Transportation Alternatives. 2004. *Safe Routes to School.* [Online]. Available: http://www.saferoutestoschools.org [accessed April 20, 2004].

TRB (Transportation Research Board). 2002. *The Relative Risks of School Travel. A National Perspective and Guidance for Local Community Risk Assessment.* Washington, DC: TRB.

Tudor-Locke C, Ainsworth BE, Adair LS, Popkin BM. 2003. Objective physical activity of Filipino youth stratified for commuting mode to school. *Med Sci Sports Exerc* 35(3):465-471.

Twiss J, Dickinson J, Duma S, Kleinman T, Paulsen H, Rilveria L. 2003. Community gardens: Lessons learned from California healthy cities and communities. *Am J Public Health* 93(9):1435-1438.

Urban and Environmental Policy Institute. 2002. *Transportation and Food: The Importance of Access*. [Online]. Available: http://departments.oxy.edu/uepi/cfj/resources/TransportationAndFood.htm#_edn2 [accessed June 8, 2004].

USPSTF (U.S. Preventive Services Task Force). 2003. Screening for obesity in adults: Recommendations and rationale. *Ann Intern Med* 139(11):930-932.

Whitaker RC. 2003. Obesity prevention in pediatric primary care: Four behaviors to target. *Arch Pediatr Adolesc Med* 157(8):725-727.

WHO (World Health Organization). 1999. *Health Impact Assessment: Main Concepts and Suggested Approach*. Brussels, Belgium: European Centre for Health Policy.

Wolff T. 2001. Community coalition building—Contemporary practice and research: Introduction. *Am J Community Psychol* 29(2):165-172, 205-111.

Yancey AK, Kumanyika SK, Ponce NA, McCarthy WJ, Fielding JE, Leslie JP, Akbar J. 2004. Population-based interventions engaging communities of color in healthy eating and active living: A review. *Prev Chronic Dis* 1(1):1-18. [Online]. Available: http://www.cdc.gov/pcd [accessed August 26, 2004].

Young DR, Haskell WL, Taylor CB, Fortmann SP. 1996. Effect of community health education on physical activity knowledge, attitudes, and behavior. The Stanford Five-City Project. *Am J Epidemiol* 144(3):264-274.

Zakarian JM, Hovell MF, Hofstetter CR, Sallis JF, Keating KJ. 1994. Correlates of vigorous exercise in a predominantly low SES and minority high school population. *Prev Med* 23(3):314-321.

7

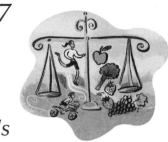

Schools

Schools are one of the primary locations for reaching the nation's children and youth. In 2000, 53.2 million students were enrolled in public and private elementary and secondary schools in the United States (U.S. Department of Education, 2002). Many of these schools are also locations for preschool, child-care, and after-school programs in which large numbers of children participate.

The school environment has the potential to affect national obesity prevention efforts both because of the population reach and the amount of time that students spend at school each day. Children obtain about one-third[1] of their total daily energy requirement from school lunch (USDA, 2004a), and should expend about 50 percent of their daily energy expenditure while at school, depending on the length of their school day. Given that schools offer numerous and diverse opportunities for young people to learn about energy balance and to make decisions about food and physical activity behaviors, it is critically important that the school environment be structured to promote healthful eating and physical activity behaviors. Further-

---

[1]These estimates are for a school day and do not take into account weekends, holidays, or school vacations. Students who eat breakfast at school could consume approximately 58 percent of their total daily energy requirement at school. This estimate is based on the federal School Breakfast Program's goal of providing one-fourth of the Recommended Dietary Allowances (RDAs) of certain nutrients through school breakfast and the National School Lunch Program's goal of providing one-third of the RDAs through school lunches (7CFR210.10; 7CFR220.8; USDA, 2004a).

more, consistency of the messages and opportunities across the school environment is vital—from the cafeteria, to the playground, to the classroom, to the gymnasium.

Increasingly, schools and school districts across the country are implementing innovative programs focused on improving student nutrition and increasing their physical activity levels. Parents, students, teachers, school administrators, and others play important roles in initiating these changes, and it is important to evaluate these efforts to determine whether they should be expanded, refined, or replaced and whether they should be further disseminated.

It is acknowledged that the school environment is complex, and schools face many economic and time constraints on their ability to address a broad array of student needs. Further, many food- and physical activity-related policies and practices are linked at multiple levels. A change in one practice may impact other areas of the school environment, either related directly to food or physical activity or indirectly to other areas (such as academic, extracurricular, financial, or administrative). The recommended actions, described below, therefore, were developed with the goal of being implemented concurrently and not as stand-alone strategies. Moreover, these actions should reinforce and support each other not only in the schools but in other settings, including the community and home environments (Chapters 6 and 8). Recommendations regarding schools also must acknowledge the diverse ways in which public schools are governed and funded throughout the United States. Although public school governance is primarily local (school boards that oversee school districts), there is variability in the additional role that states play (NRC, 1999).

The recommended actions in this chapter are intended to apply, as relevant, to all the settings where children and youth spend a majority of their organized time outside the home. For most children and youth over the age of 5 years, this will be a school setting (i.e., elementary school, middle school, or high school). For children below the age of 5 years, this may be kindergarten, formal preschool, early childhood education program, child development center, child-care center, or family or other informal child-care setting.

FOOD AND BEVERAGES IN SCHOOLS

The school food environment has undergone a rapid transition from a fairly simple to a highly complex environment, particularly in high schools. Traditionally, school cafeterias offered only the U.S. Department of Agriculture (USDA) federally subsidized school meal, which is required to meet defined nutritional standards. Recently there have been increases, however, in the amount of "à la carte" foods and beverages—items offered individually and not as part of a school meal—sold in or near the school cafeteria in tandem with the federally reimbursed school meal. Individual foods and beverages are also sold or served in vending machines, at school stores, or at school fundraisers.

Foods and Beverages Sold in Schools

Federal School Meal Programs

The National School Lunch Program (NSLP) was established in 1946 to "safeguard the health and well-being of the Nation's children and to encourage the domestic consumption of nutritious agricultural commodities and other food" (7CFR210.1). Each school day approximately 28 million school-aged children participate in the NSLP and some 8 million participate in the School Breakfast Program (SBP) (USDA, 2003).

Nutrition guidelines for the school meal programs have been revised periodically to maintain consistency with changes in nutritional recommendations. Current regulations for the programs require that the meals be consistent with the Dietary Guidelines for Americans and adhere to the RDAs for energy, protein, calcium, iron, vitamin A, and vitamin C. These guidelines are described in Box 7-1.

Several food-based menu-planning approaches are used in the NSLP to ensure that lunches and breakfasts are nutritionally balanced. The majority of schools use the "traditional" food-based menu-planning system, which

---

BOX 7-1
USDA Requirements for School Meal Programs

- Meet the applicable recommendations of the Dietary Guidelines for Americans, which recommend that no more than 30 percent of an individual's calories come from fat, and that less than 10 percent from saturated fat.
- Provide one-third of the RDAs of protein, vitamin A, vitamin C, iron, and calcium through school lunches and provide one-fourth of the RDA requirements through school breakfasts.
- "Foods of minimal nutritional value" (FMNV) as defined by federal regulations, cannot be sold in food service areas during the school meal periods. The four categories of foods defined as FMNV are soda water, water ices, chewing gum, and certain candies (including hard candy, jellies and gums, marshmallow candies, fondant, licorice, and spun candy).

SOURCES: 7CFR210.10; 7CFR220.8; 7CFR Appendix B to Part 210.

requires school lunches to offer five food items selected from four food types: fluid milk; meat or meat alternative; at least one serving of bread or grain products; and two or more servings of fruit, vegetables, or both. A second approach is the "nutrient-based" menu-planning approach used by about one-fourth of schools (USDA, 2004c). School food authorities prepare a nutrient analysis of meals for a one-week period to determine whether these meals meet the nutritional requirements outlined by the dietary guidelines (USDA, 2004b). Schools that use this approach must serve milk and offer at least one entrée and one side dish per meal. Requirements for fruit and vegetable servings are not specified under the current guidelines (USDA, 2004b), and it should be noted that high-calorie, energy-dense items (e.g., cookies, cake, and batter-fried foods) can be served to students as part of their school meals.

The target goals for the NSLP and SBP are that no more than 30 percent of calories should come from fat and less than 10 percent of calories from saturated fat (USDA, 2004b). Because milk with high saturated fat content has been a particular concern regarding the students' dietary intake, schools were required to offer both whole and low-fat milk (currently defined as having 1 percent fat content or less) beginning in 1994 (USDA, 2004b).

In response to research in the early 1990s indicating that school meals were generally not meeting key nutritional goals, USDA launched the School Meals Initiative for Healthy Children in 1995, which provides schools with educational and technical resources for meal planning and preparation (USDA, 2001b). According to data from the second School Nutrition Dietary Assessment Study (SNDAS-II), a nationally representative study of the NSLP and SBP conducted in the 1998-1999 school year, lunches in elementary schools provided an average of 33 percent of calories from fat (target goal is 30 percent or less) and 12 percent of calories from saturated fat (target goal is less than 10 percent). The average lunch in secondary schools provided about 35 percent of calories from fat and 12 percent of calories from saturated fat, also failing to meet the targets (USDA, 2001b). However, compared with the first SNDAS survey in the 1991-1992 school year, there were significant increases in the percentages of schools that served meals consistent with the Dietary Guidelines regarding fat and saturated fat content. In the second survey, approximately two-thirds of NSLP menus offered two fruit and vegetable choices, and more than 25 percent included five or more fruit and vegetable choices (USDA, 2001b).

All students are eligible to take advantage of the NSLP and SBP. The 1998-1999 SNDAS-II survey found that approximately 60 percent of students at participating schools did so, either through full-price or reduced-cost purchase or by being eligible to receive free meals. Participation was highest in elementary schools (67 percent) and lowest in high schools (39 percent) (USDA, 2001b). Participation was highest among students approved to receive free meals (80 percent) as compared with students receiving reduced-price meals (69 percent) or students paying full price (48 percent).

Only a few studies have compared dietary quality of NSLP participants and nonparticipants. Cullen and colleagues (2000) found that fifth-grade students who selected only the NSLP meal reported consuming up to twice as many servings of fruit, juice, and vegetables than students who ate from the snack bar or brought their lunch from home. In a two-year follow-up study, diets of students as fourth-graders (when they had access to NSLP lunches only) were compared with their diets during the subsequent year, when as fifth-graders they had access to the snack bar in middle school (Cullen and Zakeri, 2004). During that second year the students consumed fewer fruits, fewer nonfried vegetables, less milk, and more sweetened beverages.

Competitive Foods

The term "competitive foods" is used to describe all foods and beverages served or sold in schools that are not part of the federal school meal programs. This includes "à la carte" foods and beverages offered by the school food service; items sold from vending machines located inside or outside the school cafeteria; foods and beverages sold anywhere in the school as part of fundraising efforts by student, faculty, or parent groups; items served in the classroom for snacks and rewards; and foods and beverages made available during after-school activities. As discussed below, competitive foods from these various sources are typically lower in nutritional quality than those offered as part of the school meal programs.

Current federal nutritional guidelines for competitive foods are limited. Foods of "minimal nutritional value"—narrowly defined primarily as soft drinks and certain types of candy (Box 7-1) (7 CFR Appendix B to Part 210)—are prohibited from sale in the school cafeteria while meals are being served. However, no other national standards currently exist to screen competitive foods for nutritional quality within the school setting. Thus items of low nutrient density or high energy density, including cookies, candy bars, potato chips, and other salty or high-fat snack foods, are often allowed for sale in direct competition with the school meals. Furthermore, federal guidelines do not prohibit foods of minimal nutritional value from being sold in vending machines near the cafeteria or at other school locations.

States and school districts, however, may implement their own more-restrictive policies regarding competitive foods, and many states have passed legislation that limits the types of foods allowed for sale in the schools and the hours during which they are available. A recent report by the General Accounting Office (GAO) found that 21 states had policies that restrict competitive foods beyond USDA regulations (GAO, 2004). For example, California has mandated guidelines for foods and beverages offered in schools. This 2001 legislation includes a provision for funding pilot programs that would, among other things, require fruits and vegetables to be offered for sale in any school location where food or beverages are sold. Additionally, the board of the Los Angeles Unified School District in 2001 voted to implement standards for beverages, which led to a ban on the sale of carbonated beverages on all school campuses (Los Angeles Unified School District, 2004). West Virginia prohibits schools from serving or selling candy bars, foods, or drinks consisting of 40 percent or more added sugar or other sweeteners; juice or juice products containing less than 20 percent real juice; and foods with more than 8 grams of fat per 1-ounce serving. In addition, all soft drinks are prohibited in West Virginia elementary and middle schools (Stuhldreher et al., 1998; Wechsler et al., 2000). Local schools and school districts are also implementing their own restrictions on competitive foods (GAO, 2004). The issues surrounding competitive foods are currently being discussed in many other states and school districts.

Specific policies and nutritional standards are still needed, however, in most school districts. Data from the 2000 School Health Policies and Programs Study (SHPPS) found that only about 40 percent of school districts, but almost no state governments, required schools to offer a choice of two or more fruits or two or more vegetables at lunch time (Wechsler et al., 2001). With the exception of California, the 2000 SHPPS found that no states require schools to offer fruits and vegetables in school stores, snack bars, or vending machines. At the district level, 3.7 percent of school districts require fruits and vegetables to be available in school stores and snack bars, and 1.7 percent require fruits and vegetables to be available in vending machines (Wechsler et al., 2001). A recent statewide survey of Minnesota secondary school principals found that only 32 percent of their schools had policies of any kind about nutrition and food and that 18 percent had policies regarding items sold from school vending machines (French et al., 2002). Seventy-seven percent of these school principals reported having vending machine contracts with soft drink companies.

Competitive foods represent a significant share of the foods that students purchase and consume at school, particularly in high schools (Wechsler et al., 2001). National survey data from the 2000 SHPPS show that competitive foods are widely available in many elementary schools, most middle schools, and almost all secondary schools (Wechsler et al., 2001). In 2000, food and beverage items were sold to students from vending machines, school stores, or snack bars in 98 percent of secondary schools, 74 percent of middle schools, and 43 percent of elementary schools.

Data from a recent study of 20 high schools in Minnesota found a median of 11 vending machines in each school—typically four soft drink machines, five machines dispensing other beverages (e.g., fruit juice, sports drinks, or water), and two snack machines (French et al., 2003).

Available data show that competitive foods are often high in energy density (often high fat or high sugar) and low in nutrient density (Story et al., 1996; Harnack et al., 2000; Wechsler et al., 2001; Zive et al., 2002; French et al., 2003). National data from the SHPPS survey show that 80 percent of the à la carte areas in high schools sell high-fat cookies and baked goods, and 24 percent sell chocolate candy (Wechsler et al., 2001). Although fruits and vegetables are generally available—they are sold in the à la carte areas of 68 percent of elementary schools, 74 percent of middle schools, and 90 percent of secondary schools—energy-dense foods tend to comprise the majority of competitive foods offered for sale. For example, at the 20 Minnesota high schools noted above, chips, cookies, pastry, candy, and ice cream accounted for 51.1 percent of all à la carte foods offered, while fruits and vegetables were at 4.5 percent, and salads 0.2 percent (French et al., 2003).

Because students' food choices are influenced by the total food environment, the simple availability of healthful foods such as fruits and vegetables may not be sufficient to prompt the choice of these targeted items when other food items of high palatability (often high-fat or high-sugar items) are easily accessible, especially those that are heavily marketed to children and youth. Data from two recent studies conducted in middle schools provide empirical evidence for this hypothesis (Cullen et al., 2000; Kubik et al., 2003). Fruit and vegetable intake was lower among students at schools where à la carte foods were available, in comparison with schools where à la carte foods were not available. Not surprisingly, when given the choice many students select the higher fat and higher sugar items. However, data from a recent randomized trial involving 20 high schools indicate that offering a wider range of healthful foods can be an effective way to promote better food choices among high school students (French et al., 2004). In combination with student-led schoolwide promotions, increases in the availability of healthier à la carte foods led to significant increases in sales of the targeted foods to students over a 2-year period. Taken together, such findings suggest that restricting the availability of high-calorie, energy-dense foods in schools while increasing the availability of healthful foods might be an effective strategy for promoting more healthful food choices among students in schools.

The present reality, however, falls short of this situation. The rapid growth in the availability and marketing of à la carte foods and beverages, of soft drinks and other high-sugar beverages in school vending machines, and of other sources of competitive foods throughout the school environment has become an important issue. Bearing significantly as it does on student nutrition and obesity prevention efforts, this issue urgently needs attention from leaders at national, state, and local levels. New policies are needed, both to ensure that the foods available at schools are consistent with current nutritional guidelines and to support the goal of preventing excess energy intake among students and helping students achieve energy balance at a healthy weight.

School-Based Dietary Intervention Studies

School-based interventions to improve food choices and dietary quality among students have been designed primarily as multifaceted interventions that include one or more of the following components:

- Changes in food service and the food environment (e.g., food availability, preparation methods, price)
- Promotional activities (cafeteria-based or schoolwide)
- Classroom curricula on nutrition education and behavioral skills
- Parental involvement (e.g., informational newsletters or parent-child home activities).

Most often these interventions have targeted total fat, saturated fat, or fruit and vegetable intake. In addition, they may have addressed other weight-related behaviors such as physical activity or television viewing (reviewed later in this chapter). This section focuses on the large-scale controlled intervention studies that have examined weight status or body mass index (BMI) changes as an outcome measure. A much larger literature exists on school-based interventions to change the dietary behaviors of students, including the 5-A-Day and Know Your Body studies (Walter et al., 1985; Hearn et al., 1998).

Evaluation of the literature on such interventions is complicated because of their variety and the multicomponent nature of their designs, making comparisons of results difficult. In addition, differences exist across studies in the number and types of food-related behaviors and age groups targeted. Studies based in elementary, middle, and high schools differ not only in the developmental stage of the students, but in the corresponding physical and social environments, which contrast dramatically, for example, in the availability of à la carte foods, fast foods, snack bars, and vending machines. High school students are also more likely than elementary or middle school students to leave campus during the lunch period. These variables may moderate the effects of interventions designed to influence food choices in the school setting.

The Child and Adolescent Trial for Cardiovascular Health (CATCH), the largest and most comprehensive school-based intervention yet undertaken, targeted diet and physical activity behaviors as secondary outcome variables (Box 7-2). This randomized trial involving 96 elementary schools did not result in significant changes in body weight; however, significant changes did occur in the school food environment and in reported dietary intakes by students (Luepker et al., 1996). Compared to control schools, the fat content of meals at the intervention school meals was substantially lowered, and intervention students' reported dietary fat intake was significantly reduced relative to that of control students. Also, as noted below in the discussion on physical activity, the percentage of physical education classroom time with moderate to vigorous physical activity increased in the intervention schools. The researchers speculated that the reasons for the lack of changes in physiologic risk factors may be related to the growth and development stage of the students or to the relatively low magnitude of the changes in food intake and physical activity levels (Luepker et al., 1996).

Pathways, a large, multicomponent school-based intervention designed as an obesity prevention study, was conducted among third- to fifth-grade American-Indian children in reservation schools over a 3-year period (Caballero et al., 1998). Pathways did not significantly affect body-weight change, but significant intervention-related changes were observed for some dietary and physical activity behaviors, including lower fat intake and higher self-reported physical activity levels in the students in the intervention schools (Caballero et al., 2003). The goal of the food service intervention—to reduce the fat content of the school meals—was achieved. Both the CATCH and Pathways interventions show the feasibility of making positive changes in the school food environment, but also the challenges still to be faced in designing primary obesity prevention interventions in schools. As pointed out by the researchers in the Pathways study, restriction of energy intake is not an option in schools because there are students who are below the fifth BMI percentile, additionally, the school meals programs have to meet minimum mandatory levels for calorie content (Caballero et al., 2003).

Several other school-based intervention studies have shown significant effects on body-weight outcomes; these studies tested multicomponent interventions not limited only to targeting dietary change. Planet Health reported reductions in the prevalence of obesity among girls only (Gortmaker et al., 1999), and the Stanford Adolescent Heart Health Program observed reductions in BMI, triceps skinfold thickness, and subscapular skinfold thickness among boys and girls (Killen et al., 1988).

Overall, school-based interventions, both multicomponent and single component, have produced healthful food choices among students. Envi-

---

BOX 7-2
Selected School-Based Interventions

Child and Adolescent Trial for Cardiovascular Health (CATCH)—Designed as a health behavior intervention for the primary prevention of cardiovascular disease, CATCH was evaluated in a randomized field trial in 96 elementary schools in California, Louisiana, Minnesota, and Texas (Luepker et al., 1996). CATCH schools received school food service modifications and food service personnel training, physical education (PE) interventions and teacher training, and classroom curricula that addressed eating behaviors, physical activity, and smoking (Luepker et al., 1996). The primary individual outcome examined was change in serum cholesterol concentration; school-based outcomes were also examined.

Pathways—Designed to reduce obesity in American-Indian children in grades three through five, a randomized trial was conducted in 41 schools serving American-Indian communities in Arizona, New Mexico, and South Dakota (Caballero et al., 1998; Davis et al., 1999). This multicomponent program involved incorporation of high-energy activities in PE classes and recess; food service training and nutritional educational materials; classroom curricula enhancements; and family efforts including family fun nights, take-home action- and snack-packs, and family advisory councils. The primary outcome measure was the mean difference between intervention and control schools in percentage of body fat at the end of the fifth grade.

Planet Health—A curriculum-based health intervention, Planet Health lessons were integrated into the math, language arts, social studies, science, and PE curricula of grades six through eight. The lessons focus on teaching better dietary

---

ronmental interventions, which target reduced consumption of high-fat foods and greater intake of fruits and vegetables through variations in availability, pricing, and promotion in the school environment (Whitaker et al., 1993, 1994; Luepker et al., 1996; Caballero et al., 1998; Perry et al., 1998, 2004; Reynolds et al., 2000; French et al., 2001, 2004; French and Stables, 2003) may have a particularly significant independent effect on food choices (French et al., 2001; French and Stables, 2003). But their impacts are perhaps smaller in magnitude than when deployed as part of a multicomponent intervention program (Perry et al., 1998, 2004; French et al., 2001; French and Stables, 2003).

Because classroom education/behavioral skills curricula, for example, have typically been embedded in a multicomponent program, the effectiveness of this intervention component is difficult to evaluate as an isolated strategy. Furthermore, caution is needed in interpreting studies of self-reports of dietary intakes, which may be subject to reporting errors and bias.

habits, promoting physical activity, and reducing television viewing (Gortmaker et al., 1999). Evaluation of the intervention involved comparing obesity prevalence and behavioral changes among students in five intervention and five control schools in the Boston area.

Sports, Play and Active Recreation for Kids (SPARK)—A school-based intervention designed to improve the quantity and quality of physical education, the evaluation involved seven elementary schools in southern California in a 3-year study (McKenzie et al., 1997). The SPARK program involves enhancements to the PE curriculum, implementation of a self-management curriculum, and teacher in-service training programs. Outcomes assessed included changes in student BMI and physical activity levels.

Stanford Adolescent Heart Health Program—Designed to reduce cardiovascular disease risk factors in high school students, the intervention consisted of 20 50-minute classroom sessions on physical activity, nutrition, smoking, and stress (Killen et al., 1988). The evaluation of the intervention compared the results of 10th-grade students in four high schools in northern California on behavioral changes and physiological variables including BMI.

Stanford S.M.A.R.T. (Student Media Awareness to Reduce Television)—Designed to motivate children to reduce their television watching and video game usage, the intervention was evaluated in two elementary schools in California (Robinson, 1999). Students in the intervention third- and fourth-grade classrooms participated in an 18-lesson, six-month curriculum and families could use an electronic television time manager. The primary outcome measure was BMI; other physiologic variables and behavioral changes were also assessed.

Recent and Ongoing Pilot Program

Several pilot programs have been developed at the school, district, state, and federal levels to explore strategies to increase fruit and vegetable consumption among students in school. The committee is not aware of any published outcome evaluation of these studies but the programs are described here to illustrate current approaches that may warrant continued funding and more systematic analysis. The most recent and perhaps largest effort to increase the availability and consumption of fresh fruits and vegetables was implemented by USDA during the 2002-2003 school year (Buzby et al., 2003). One hundred schools in four states (Indiana, Iowa, Michigan, and Ohio) and seven schools in New Mexico's Zuni Indian Tribal Organization participated in the pilot program, which distributed fruit and vegetables free to participating schools. Schools could choose when and how to distribute the produce to students. The program requested, however, that the fruits and vegetables be made available to students outside the regular school meal periods. Due to limited funding, no quantitative data were collected on the effects of the program on students' fruit and vegetable consumption or on any other dietary outcomes. However, schools and school food-service staff reported that the program was positively received (Buzby et al., 2003), and there are plans to expand the program. A similar program was developed and pilot-tested on a national basis in the United Kingdom beginning in 2000. As far as the committee is aware, no quantitative evaluation data are available (United Kingdom Department of Health, 2002).

The Department of Defense's Fresh Produce Program has been working with schools in several states to provide fresh produce for the school meal programs. Schools have also begun to incorporate produce from school gardens (Morris and Zidenberg-Cherr, 2002; Stone, 2002), school salad bars (USDA, 2002), and farmers' markets (Misako and Fisher, 2002) into the school meal program in an effort to increase student participation and specifically to increase their fruit and vegetable consumption (Box 7-3). Evaluation of these and other similar programs is important in determining the effects of these changes on student dietary behaviors.

Next Steps

As discussed above, several large-scale school-based intervention studies demonstrate that changes in the school food environment can impact students' dietary choices and improve the nutrient quality of their diets while at school.

Schools, school districts, and state educational agencies need to ensure that all meals served or sold in schools are in compliance with the Dietary Guidelines for Americans. Additionally, schools should focus on improving

---

BOX 7-3
Edible Schoolyard

The Edible Schoolyard is a nonprofit program conducted at the Martin Luther King Junior Middle School in Berkeley, California, a public school for sixth- through eighth-graders. Students participate in all phases of the Seed to Table approach—planting vegetables, grains, and fruits; tending and harvesting the crops; preparing meals with the produce they have grown; and recycling the vegetable scraps back to the garden. This cooking and gardening program involves classroom lessons and hands-on experience in the garden and in the kitchen. The program's goals include an enhanced understanding of the cycle of food production; the focus of evaluation efforts to date has been on ecoliteracy.

SOURCE: Edible Schoolyard, 2004.

food quality in the school meal programs. Increasing the availability of whole-grain foods, low-fat milk, and fresh local produce will not only be more healthful for participating students, but has the potential to attract greater participation.

Current nutritional standards are extremely limited for regulating competitive foods sold in schools, and many schools are selling high-calorie, energy-dense food and beverage items, often in competition with school meal programs. To ensure that foods and beverages sold or served to students in school are healthful, **USDA, with independent scientific advice, should establish nutritional standards for all food and beverage items served or sold in schools.** Such standards need to be applied to *all* meals and *all* foods and beverages served or sold within the school environment.[2] Among the many nutritional issues, consideration should be given to setting standards for the fat and sugar content of school foods, because they are often high in calories and in energy density. **State education agencies and local school boards should adopt and implement these standards or develop stricter standards for their local schools.** Without such schoolwide standards, different sources compete for student sales under unequal conditions. Such competitive practices often give unfair advantage to those selling less healthful food and beverage items to students. Providing and enforcing uniform standards for meals, foods, and beverages on a schoolwide basis also establishes a social norm for healthful eating behaviors. The standards ensure that the school environment is one in which healthful eating is promoted and modeled, consistent with nutrition education messages taught in the classroom.

It is important that evaluations be conducted to assess the impact of changes on competitive foods' nutritional value and availability, on student dietary quality, and on revenues generated by food and beverage sales. Evaluations of the school food environment may benefit from point-of-service purchase information available from automated systems in school cafeterias. Additionally, evaluations of the efficacy and effectiveness of school-based multicomponent interventions are needed to determine whether these programs should be continued, replicated, expanded, or replaced.

In efforts to make changes in school foods, the school food industry should be an important partner in developing innovative approaches to preparing and serving healthful foods and beverages. Training of school

---

[2]Such changes in federal regulations may require changes in USDA's authority, as USDA's current authority extends only to foods sold in the cafeteria and other school food-service areas during school meal periods (GAO, 2004).

nutrition and food-service personnel should include a focus on obesity prevention efforts. Furthermore, as schools are built or renovated, school districts should take into consideration plans for school kitchens that have adequate preparation and serving space as well as plans for school cafeterias that are of adequate size and layout so that students will not be rushed, uncomfortable, or scheduled to eat lunch too early or too late in the school day.

Funding and Sales of School Meals and Competitive Foods

School Meal Funding

School nutrition programs are financially self-supporting and must generate sufficient revenues to pay for food-service staff, food purchases, and equipment. Schools that participate in the NSLP receive a fixed amount of reimbursement for each school meal served. Federal reimbursement rates are typically 9 to 10 times higher for free meals than for reduced-price or paid meals (FNS/USDA, 2003). Although some states contribute a supplemental amount and most schools also receive donated commodity foods through USDA, federal reimbursements at their present levels are insufficient to cover the remainder of the meals' actual costs.

To generate funds needed to function, school food services often sell additional foods and beverages that are not part of the school meals program (GAO, 2003). As noted earlier, these items are called "competitive foods" because they compete with the meal programs for students' spending on foods and beverages while in school. Thus, the federal funding structure places a school food service in the paradoxical situation of competing with itself as well as with other sources that sell food or beverages in school—such as student groups or the school administration (through vending machine contracts)—for student patronage.

In fact, the nationwide SNDAS-II school survey found that sales of à la carte items were inversely related to sales of NSLP meals (USDA, 2001b). Not surprisingly, states that restricted competitive food sales, such as Georgia, Louisiana, Mississippi, and West Virginia, had school meal program participation rates that were higher than the national average (USDA, 2001a).

Full funding for the school meal programs could relieve the pressure on schools' food services to generate extra funding through the sales of competitive foods. Such a policy may enhance food services by focusing on providing high-quality nutritious meals to encourage maximum participation and may also help alleviate any perceptions among students that only low-income individuals eat the school meals.

Sales of Competitive Foods

Local schools and school education agencies should consider examining policies and practices on the sale of competitive foods and beverages, including those sold in vending machines and as fundraisers. As discussed above, these foods and beverages are often calorie-laden and low in nutrient density. If nutritional standards are developed and implemented for competitive foods and beverages, as recommended in this report, the standards would apply to all food and beverage items sold in the schools, including those sold through vending machines and in fundraising. As seen in states and districts that have already implemented nutritional standards, the result of these standards and policies is that soft drinks and energy-dense foods are often precluded from being sold. The goal is, of course, a "win-win" situation where sales of healthful foods and beverages in vending machines and other venues would be more healthful for students as well as profitable to schools and school groups.

Current policies vary widely between schools and school districts about how funds are used from the different types of food and beverage sales. Vending machine revenues are often used by school administrators for discretionary budget purposes (Wechsler et al., 2000); examples include purchases of computers, sports equipment, and funding of other school programs and activities that are not funded in the school budget (Nestle, 2000). One of the issues that has been raised is the exclusivity of some schools' marketing contracts with specific soft drink companies that may include financial and in-kind incentives for the volume of beverages sold (Nestle, 2000; Wechsler et al., 2000).

Food and beverage sales have been used at special events to generate funds needed by student groups, school administrators, and booster clubs to support worthwhile activities such as field trips or the acquisition of uniforms, equipment, or other supplies that are not covered by existing budgets. Schools and school districts should consider adopting policies to discourage the sale of foods and beverages and instead encourage other types of fundraising activities, such as walkathons or fun runs.

Pricing strategies may also be an effective means of promoting the sales of healthful foods, while discouraging sales of high-fat or energy-dense foods and beverages. In an initial pilot study, purchase of fresh fruit and vegetables from à la carte areas in two high schools increased two- to fourfold when prices were reduced by 50 percent (French et al., 1997). In a second study over a 2-year period at 12 high schools and 12 worksites, purchases of more healthful vending machine snacks successively increased when prices of lower fat foods were reduced by 10 percent, 25 percent, and 50 percent compared to prices of the higher fat snacks that were also available (French et al., 2001). Importantly, no significant reduction in vending machine profits were observed during the price reduction intervention. More generally, reducing the prices of targeted foods has consistently produced increases in their purchase among adolescents in school settings, regardless of whether the target foods were vending machine snacks or fresh fruits and vegetables sold in food-service areas.

These pilot studies point to the need for further research and evaluation of pricing strategies. If competitive food sales to students continue, school food services should consider the strategy of price increases on higher fat, low-nutrient-dense foods in tandem with lower prices on more healthful foods (Hannan et al., 2002). This strategy could achieve the dual goals of promoting healthful food choices among students and maintaining needed school food-service revenues.

Next Steps

Innovative approaches are needed to encourage students to consume nutritious foods and beverages. Pilot programs offer the potential to implement and carefully evaluate a variety of strategies related to pricing and funding issues.

The committee proposes that USDA conduct pilot studies to examine the benefits and costs of providing full funding for school breakfast, lunch, and snack programs in a targeted subset of schools that include a large percentage of children at high risk for obesity. Outcomes to be examined would include the impact on student nutritional status and on obesity prevalence. It may also be valuable to examine whether the cost of providing free meals is less expensive than the cost to monitor and track free and reduced-price eligibility for school meals.

Pilot programs could also be used to develop, implement, and evaluate alternative models to financially support school and student programs without relying significantly on food and beverage sales.

Experimental research is needed to examine the effects of school-based interventions and policy changes on students' dietary intake and eating behaviors. For example, changes in food availability and access to both healthful and less healthful foods, pricing of foods and beverages sold through competitive food sources and pricing of the school meals, promotional programs to support healthful food choices, and corporate-sponsored in-school food and beverage marketing activities need to be evaluated to determine their effects on students' diet and eating behaviors. Experimental and quasi-experimental studies are needed to evaluate the effects of school- and district-level policies regarding school food and beverage availability and marketing on student dietary intake and on school revenues. Academic performance and classroom and social behavior are secondary outcomes of interest.

It is important to note that research should also focus on food service at child-care centers, preschools, and other sites that serve meals to young children. More needs to be known about improving nutrition for young children.

PHYSICAL ACTIVITY

At a time when many children and youth need to increase their physical activity levels, schools offer the environment, the facilities, and the teachers not only for meeting students' current physical activity needs, but for helping them form the lifelong habits of incorporating physical activity into their daily lives. As discussed in Chapter 3, current recommendations are for children to accumulate a minimum of 60 minutes of moderate to vigorous physical activity each day (Biddle et al., 1998; USDA and DHHS, 2000; Cavill et al., 2001; IOM, 2002; NASPE, 2004). Because children spend over half of their day in school, the committee felt it reasonable to recommend that at least 30 minutes, or half of the recommended daily physical activity time, be accrued during the school day. In addition to its contribution to preventing obesity, regular physical activity has numerous ancillary health and well-being benefits (Chapter 3).

Researchers are examining the extent and nature of the relationship between increased physical activity and enhanced academic performance, but the results to date are inconclusive. In a study involving 7,961 Australian children, Dwyer and colleagues (2001) found that higher academic performance was positively associated with physical fitness and physical activity. Other cross-sectional studies and a few limited longitudinal studies have found similar results, although correlations are often weak (reviewed by Shephard, 1997). Explanations for a positive association include improved motor development, increased self-esteem, and improved behavior due to physical activity; however, there are numerous confounders, including genetic factors, family environment, and changes in teacher and student attitudes.

Physical Education Classes and Recess During School Hours

Daily physical education (PE) for all students is a goal supported by several national health- and education-related organizations, including the National Association for Sport and Physical Education, the American Academy of Pediatrics, and the U.S. Department of Health and Human Services (CDC, 1997; AAP, 2000; DHHS, 2000; NASPE, 2004). But although more than three-fourths of the states and school districts responding to the SHPPS survey required that PE be taught, the nature and duration of the classes varied widely in practice (Burgeson et al., 2001) and the percentages requir-

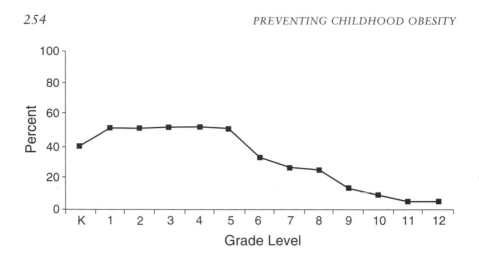

FIGURE 7-1 Percentage of schools that require physical education, by grade. SHPPS 2000.
SOURCE: Burgeson et al., 2001.

ing PE for all students were low. Only 8.0 percent of elementary schools, 6.4 percent of middle/junior high schools and 5.8 percent of senior high schools provided daily PE[3] for the entire school year for all of the students in each grade. Higher percentages of schools (though generally less than one-third) provided PE three days a week or for part of the school year for all students (Burgeson et al., 2001), but for the grades after elementary school the percentages steadily decreased (Figure 7-1 and Figure 7-2).

There have also been concerns about the nature and duration of physical activity levels during PE classes. The 2000 SHPPS survey found that in a typical PE class (lasting an average of 45 minutes), students at all levels spent an average of 15.3 minutes participating in games, sports, or dance and 9.6 minutes doing skill drills (Burgeson et al., 2001). Of the 55.7 percent of high school students who reported participating in PE class in the 2003 YRBSS survey, 80.3 percent reported that they exercised or played sports for more than 20 minutes in the average PE class (CDC, 2004b). Simons-Morton and colleagues (1993) found that in a typical 30-minute elementary school PE class, the average child was vigorously active for only two to three minutes (approximately 9 percent of the class time).

Traditionally PE teachers have been trained to conduct classes around

---

[3]Daily PE was defined as 150 minutes per week of PE class for elementary school students and 225 minutes for both middle/junior high and senior high school students (Burgeson et al., 2001).

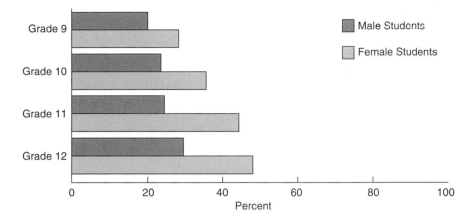

FIGURE 7-2 High school students not engaging in recommended amounts of physical activity (neither moderate nor vigorous) by grade and sex, United States, 2001. SOURCE: CDC, 2003.

a motor skill instruction paradigm. There are opportunities for exploring a variety of teaching methods that both optimize physical activity and that make PE classes more fun. Including a range of physical activity interests including dance and nontraditional activities such as Tai Chi and kick boxing is also important.

Recess is generally defined as unstructured time for physical activity during the school day. The Centers for Disease Control and Prevention's (CDC's) Guidelines for School and Community Programs to Promote Lifelong Physical Activity Among Young People recommend that schools provide ample time for unstructured physical activity and that this time should complement, not substitute for, PE classes (CDC, 1997). Elementary schools differ greatly in their recess policies. While only a small minority of states actually require elementary schools to provide students with regularly scheduled recess, many more (22.4 percent) recommend this practice (Burgeson et al., 2001). Among elementary schools surveyed in the 2000 SHPPS, 71.4 percent provided recess for all grades, and 96.9 percent offered regularly scheduled recess during the school day for students in at least one grade. (Burgeson et al., 2001). Among these schools, students were scheduled to have recess an average of 4.9 days per week for an average of 30.4 minutes per day.

Alternative approaches for incorporating physical activity into the school day continue to be explored and include integrating brief episodes of physical activity into the classroom curriculum.

School-Based Interventions

There have been few studies examining the possible correlations between PE enrollments and physical activity levels. Using the 1990 YRBSS data, Pate and colleagues (1996) found that 59 percent of high-active students were enrolled in PE as compared to 29 percent of low-active students. As described below, several large-scale school-based intervention studies have demonstrated increases in physical activity in PE classes, but only in isolated smaller scale studies have school interventions increased physical fitness, reduced obesity, or increased physical activity outside of PE classes.

To date, interventions focused on elementary school children have been the most successful at increasing activity levels, with interventions such as Go For Health (Simons-Morton et al., 1997) and SPARK (Sallis et al., 1997) reporting significant increases in the amount of moderate to vigorous physical activity performed during PE classes. In the SPARK intervention, students in the classes taught by physical education specialists spent more time being physically active (40 minutes) than those in the teacher-led classes (33 minutes) or those in control classes (18 minutes) (Sallis et al., 1997).

The largest elementary-school-based intervention to date has been CATCH, a multicenter trial (described above) that tested the effectiveness of a cardiovascular health promotion program in 96 elementary schools. Students in CATCH intervention schools participated in significantly more moderate-to-vigorous physical activity during PE classes than did students in control schools, but significant improvements in physical fitness levels or body weight were not observed (Luepker et al., 1996). An assessment of CATCH 5 years later found that the proportion of PE time spent in moderate to vigorous physical activity had been maintained in intervention schools, but vigorous activity levels declined (McKenzie et al., 2003). School-based programs are less likely to increase physical activity outside of PE classes, although students in the CATCH intervention schools did report participating in more vigorous physical activity during out-of-school hours, an effect that a 3-year follow-up study noted was still being maintained (Nader et al., 1999).

Although some elementary-school-based interventions have shown increased physical activity in PE classes, few have shown significant effects on physiological health risk variables such as body weight or composition. One notable exception was the South Australian Daily Physical Activity Program (Dwyer et al., 1983), which observed the effects of two interventions that markedly increased the exposure of elementary school children to PE. The first intervention emphasized participation in vigorous physical activity through endurance training for 75 minutes every day for 14 weeks, while the second maintained a traditional emphasis on motor-skill instruction but increased the duration and frequency to 75 minutes every day. Both of these interventions were compared to traditional PE classes for 30 minutes three days per week. Only the intervention that emphasized vigorous physical activity produced a significant reduction in skinfold thickness and an increase in objectively measured physical fitness, while traditional PE, even at increased frequency and duration, did not. The findings of this study suggest that physical education has the potential to improve body composition in children, but only if activity is at high intensity, with increases in frequency and duration. Physical education classes of 75 or more minutes are not feasible within most current school days; however, the impact of this intervention on students' BMI encourages the development of approaches for increasing physical activity that can realistically be implemented.

The other PE intervention that has demonstrated significant effects on body weight was the Stanford Dance for Health intervention, which substituted popular and aerobic dance classes (40 to 50 minutes, three times per week, over 12 weeks) for the standard physical activity class (Flores, 1995). In a randomized controlled trial among mostly low-income African-American and Latino middle-school students, girls who were randomized to the dance intervention significantly improved their physical fitness and reduced their BMI gain compared to girls in the standard class. There were no significant differences among boys. As in the South Australian study, changes in fitness and body weight/fatness were seen when the content of PE was made more vigorous.

A small number of school-based studies have focused on increasing physical activity in older students. The Lifestyle Education for Activity Program was a group randomized trial that examined the effects of a comprehensive school-based intervention on high school girls' physical activity levels. Girls in the intervention schools were significantly more likely to participate in vigorous physical activity, both in PE classes and in other settings, than girls in the control schools (Dishman et al., 2004). The Middle-School Physical Activity and Nutrition study tested the effects of an environmental and policy intervention on physical activity and fat intake in 24 middle schools. Boys in the intervention schools participated in significantly more physical activity than boys in the control schools, both in and out of PE classes. The same across-the-board effect was not observed for girls, although girls in the intervention schools did participate in more physical activity during PE classes (Sallis et al., 2003). The study found significant reductions in the BMIs of boys in the intervention schools as compared to boys in the control schools, based on self-reports of height and weight; however, similar results were not seen for girls. Issues regarding gender differences had been considered (e.g., the outside-of-PE component of the intervention was staffed primarily by female volunteers and the study involved physical activities of interest to middle-school girls), but much remains to be learned about how to design interventions that impact physical activity levels in both boys and girls. A recent comprehensive review of school-based physical activity programs (Kahn et al., 2002) identified 12 well-designed programs that met the CDC's *Guide to Community Preventive Services* criteria (Dwyer et al., 1983; Simons-Morton et al., 1991; Hopper et al., 1992, 1996; Vandongen et al., 1995; Donnelly et al., 1996; Fardy et al., 1996; Luepker et al., 1996; McKenzie et al., 1996; Sallis et al., 1997; Ewart et al., 1998; Manios et al., 1999; Harrell et al., 1999). These studies reported consistent increases in reported or observed time spent in physical activity in school, primarily through increases in moderate to vigorous physical activity in PE classes. Some of the studies also reported increases in energy expenditure and aerobic capacity. The effects on BMI and body fat, however, were minimal or inconsistent. Positive effects on physical activity were observed in both elementary school and high school studies, although the number of high school studies included in this review was small.

Inexpensive ways to enhance school breaks and recess periods to increase opportunities for physical activity have also been examined, including providing game equipment such as balls and painting school playground areas with markings for games (Jago and Baranowski, 2004).

Extracurricular Programs to Increase Physical Activity

One initiative that has shown a positive effect on physical activity is the Title IX legislation, which in recent decades increased the extent of interscholastic sports programs and participation, particularly for high school girls (Lopiano, 2000). However, these programs tend to serve only youth at the high school level, and only those who are attracted to competitive sports. The 2003 YRBSS nationwide survey found that 57.6 percent of students (grades 9 to 12) played on one or more sports teams during the previous year (CDC, 2004b). The 2000 SHPPS survey found that most middle and high schools had interscholastic sports teams, while only 49 percent offered intramural activities or PE clubs (Burgeson et al., 2001).

Research has shown that physical activity levels often decrease for middle- and high school students, especially among girls (Sallis, 1993; Pate et al., 1994; Trost et al., 2002). In those grades, there are fewer options for students who are not advanced athletes to be involved in physical activity. To fill that void, intramural sports and other physical activity opportunities—through clubs, programs, and lessons—can be tailored to meet the needs and interests of all students, with a wide range of abilities, who may lack the time, skills, or confidence to play interscholastic sports. Encouraging such a range of physical activity options in local schools and communities, through the development of programs and provision of support, may involve not only schools, but also the private sector and nonprofit foundations and organizations. It is critically important that a focused effort be made to enhance funding and opportunities so that intramural sports teams, as well as nonteam sports and activities, become staples of school and after-school programs.

Next Steps

There are opportunities for schools to improve the extent and nature of the physical activity opportunities that are offered so that students can attain at least 50 percent of their daily recommended physical activity (or approximately 30 minutes) while in school. Few studies of physical activity during school have examined weight status or body composition measures; most studies have focused on changes in the intensity or duration of physical activity during PE classes. School-based interventions that have involved teacher training, PE curriculum changes, increases in duration or intensity of physical activity, and other changes have resulted in increased levels of activity and in some cases reported increases in energy expenditure and aerobic capacity. An expansion of physical activity opportunities available through the school may result in benefits not only for students' health and well-being but also may potentially foster the formation of a lifelong practice of daily physical activity.

Schools should ensure that all children and youth participate in a minimum of 30 minutes of moderate to vigorous physical activity during the school day. This includes time spent being active during PE classes. This objective is equally important for young children in child development centers and other preschool and child-care settings, including Head Start programs—the benefits to young children include the nurturing and refinement of their gross motor development skills.

Furthermore, **schools should expand the physical activity opportunities available through the school, including intramural and interscholastic sports programs, and other physical activity clubs, programs, and lessons that meet the needs and interests of all students.** This includes physical activity programs both during the school day and after school.

Additionally, **schools should promote walking and bicycling to school.** As more thoroughly discussed in Chapter 6, schools should develop policies and promote programs that encourage these active ways of getting between school and home. Changes that are needed may include more support for crossing guards, bike racks, and education on pedestrian and biking safety.

Strategies and recommendations to achieve these goals include:

- Schools should provide PE classes of 30 to 60 minutes' duration on a daily basis. While attending these classes, children and youth should be engaged in moderate to vigorous physical activity for at least 50 percent of class time. Schools should examine innovative approaches that include an array of diverse and fun activities to appeal to the broad range of student interests.

- Child development centers, elementary schools, and middle schools should provide recess that includes a total of at least 30 to 60 minutes daily of physical activity.

- Schools should offer a broad array of after-school programs, such as interscholastic sports, intramural sports, clubs, and lessons, that together meet the physical activity needs and interests of all students.

- Schools and child development centers should support and encourage physical activity opportunities for teachers and staff for their own well-being and because they are important role models for their students.

- Schools should be encouraged to extend the school day as a means of providing expanded instructional and extracurricular physical activity programs.

- Regulations for managing Head Start and other publicly funded or licensed early-childhood-education programs should ensure that children engage in appropriate physical activity as part of the programs.

- Congress, state legislatures, state education agencies, local governments, school boards, and parents should hold schools and child development centers responsible for providing students with recommended amounts of physical activity. Concurrently, these authorities should ensure that schools and child development centers have the resources needed to meet the applicable standards.

- Schools should regularly evaluate the quantity and quality of their physical activity programs, and the results of these evaluations should be reported to the public.

The committee acknowledges the constraints and pressures on school boards and administrators, particularly limited resources and the focus on academic programs and homework to improve standardized test scores. Nevertheless, it urges schools and child-development centers to increase opportunities for students to participate in physical activity and to implement evidence-based programs. These institutions will need the help of federal, state, and local authorities, who should initiate and implement the necessary regulatory and curriculum changes. Such actions could well have influence beyond their nominal purposes. Programmatic requirements imposed by the state or district—which likely will be evaluated systematically, with results reported to the public—could provide the impetus for significant changes and innovative programs.

Much research is needed to identify effective school-based interventions for promoting and providing physical activity to children and youth. Specifically, large-scale studies are needed to identify ways in which modifications of physical education, school sports, intramural programs, and recess—singly and in combination—contribute to physical activity goals. It is important, moreover, to learn the effects of such interventions not only on physical activity during the school day, but also after school. Studies should also determine the influence of district or school-level policies on school practices and student physical activity. Furthermore, research is needed to determine the effects of school-based physical activity interventions on student academic performance, dietary and nutritional outcomes, classroom behavior, and social outcomes.

Research specific to preschool and child-care settings should emphasize feasible and generalizable interventions designed to increase physical activity (e.g., manipulations of outdoor play time), decrease sedentary behaviors (e.g., parenting skills interventions to reduce children's screen time), and improve dietary behaviors (e.g., systematic exposure to fruits and vegetables in a positive context to enhance taste preferences).

CLASSROOM CURRICULA

Health Education Requirements and Practices

National education and health organizations recognize the important role that schools can play in fostering healthful behaviors among children and youth (Kann et al., 2001). Priorities for health education include behavioral skills development, a set amount of time devoted to energy balance in the classroom curricula, adequately trained teachers, and periodic curriculum evaluation (NASBE, 1990; Kann et al., 2001). A comprehensive set of guidelines and recommendations for school health programs has been developed by CDC (1997). In practice, health education standards of the Joint Committee on National Health Education Standards (1995), which are followed by most states and school districts, also emphasize the importance of teaching students behavioral skills—such as effective decision-making and goal-setting—thereby making healthful behaviors more likely.

National data show that 69 percent of states require health education curricula to include instruction on nutrition and dietary behaviors, and 62 percent require the inclusion of physical activity and fitness (Kann et al., 2001). In 69 percent of districts, schools are required to follow national, state, or district-level standards or guidelines; 77.8 percent of the schools use the National Health Education Standards (Joint Committee on National Health Education Standards, 1995; Kann et al., 2001). Assessment of students' acquired skills is weak, however; only 16 percent of states require that they be tested on health education topics (Kann et al., 2001).

Numerous topics—including safety, first aid, alcohol and tobacco use prevention, growth and development, and personal hygiene—need to be covered in health education classes varying by the ages of the students. In the 2000 survey, 75 percent of health courses and 51 percent of other courses included content on nutritional and dietary behavior, and 69 percent and 29 percent, respectively, addressed physical activity and fitness (Kann et al., 2001). An average total of about five hours per year is spent on topics related to nutritional and dietary behavior, and about four hours per year on physical activity and fitness (Kann et al., 2001).

Behavioral Nutrition and Physical Activity Curricula

As described below, research findings support the effectiveness of behavior-oriented curricula—based on self-monitoring, goal-setting, feedback about behavior change efforts, incentives, and reinforcement methods—in promoting healthful food choices and physical activity. Skill-building activities, in which students engage in the desired behaviors and have a chance to practice new behaviors and receive feedback, are effective learning strategies.

However, there is still much to learn about the elements of nutrition and physical activity education programs that are key to changing behaviors and, subsequently, body weight. The most commonly used theoretical framework for developing behavior-based school interventions is social cognitive theory (SCT) (Bandura, 1986). "Self-efficacy," in particular, or the confidence in one's ability to perform a specific behavior, is a central concept in SCT. Self-efficacy is enhanced through skills building, practicing and mastering the behavior with feedback and reinforcement, and observing modeled behavior.

A recent review of 16 school-based cardiovascular risk factor prevention intervention studies found that interventions were most effective in changing cognitive variables, such as self-efficacy and outcome expectations, and were least effective in changing physiological variables such as body fatness (Resnicow and Robinson, 1997). However, these studies are difficult to compare because of the diversity of their intervention components and the primary outcomes targeted. Some interventions were only based on classroom curricula, while others include changes in the school food environment or PE classes.

Two of the most ambitious health behavior change interventions have been CATCH and Pathways, described above (Box 7-2). But despite tremendous commitments of resources and expertise, intervention effects were significant for some of the reported behavioral changes but not for the objectively measured physiological changes, including BMI or body fatness (Luepker et al., 1996; Caballero et al., 1998; Davis et al., 1999). The specific effects of the classroom curricula could not be evaluated because the studies were implemented as multicomponent interventions, including individual-level intervention targets (e.g., student knowledge and behavior) and environmental intervention targets (e.g., school meals, PE classes).

An interesting contrast is provided by the results of the Planet Health intervention (Gortmaker et al., 1999), which aimed to reduce the prevalence of obesity among students in grades six through eight. Ten schools were randomized to intervention or control for a 2-year period, and the interventions were classroom-based only; they did not include school food service, physical activity, or other environmental-change components. Classroom intervention sessions, which featured behavioral skills development and strategies (e.g., self-assessment and goal-setting) were incorporated into different curriculum content areas; behaviors targeted for change included increases in fruit and vegetable intake, increases in physical activity, and decreases in television viewing time. At the end of the study, obesity prevalence among girls in the five intervention schools was significantly lower than among girls in the five control schools. Differences in obesity prevalence were not significant among boys. Analysis of changes in behavioral variables showed that decreases in television viewing were significantly associated with decreases in obesity prevalence among the girls. The reason for the lack of an intervention effect in boys is not clear. There are few controlled studies in this area and further research is needed.

Curriculum-only interventions have also resulted in significant reductions in BMI or skinfolds among both boys and girls. The Stanford Adolescent Heart Health Program targeted tenth-graders in a four school randomized controlled trial (Killen et al., 1988). In addition to changes in body composition, the 20-session classroom curriculum also produced significant improvements in fitness.

Reducing Sedentary Behaviors

Television viewing time reduction has been examined in several school-based studies as a strategy for preventing obesity (Gortmaker et al., 1999; Robinson, 1999). In contrast to most other curriculum efforts, these intervention studies have shown positive effects on reducing the prevalence of obesity or weight gain. For example, Robinson (1999) examined the effects of the Stanford SMART (Student Media Awareness to Reduce Television) curriculum on changes in BMI among third- and fourth-grade children in two public elementary schools. Students in the intervention school received an 18-lesson, six-month curriculum designed solely to help children and families reduce television viewing time and videotape and video game use.

No other behaviors were targeted in the study in order to "isolate" the specific effects of reduced television viewing on changes in BMI. In addition to the classroom curriculum, parents also received newsletters and a television time-management monitor that allowed them to set time limits on the home television; 42 percent of parents reported that they actually installed the device. Results revealed significant reductions in BMI, triceps skinfold thickness, waist circumference, and waist-to-hip ratios among children in the intervention school compared with children in the control school, over a single school year.

The Planet Health intervention—a curriculum-based intervention for sixth- and seventh-grade students using behavioral choice and social cognitive approaches (discussed earlier)—also focused on reducing television viewing (Gortmaker et al., 1999). Other lessons included an emphasis on dietary and physical activity change. Teacher training sessions were held prior to implementation. Obesity prevalence decreased in girls in the intervention schools (from 23.6 percent to 20.3 percent) and increased in girls in the control schools (from 21.5 percent to 23.7 percent). For boys, obesity prevalence decreased in both groups, with no significant differences between groups. Number of television hours declined for both genders in the intervention schools as compared with controls and for girls in the intervention schools there was an increase in fruit and vegetable consumption.

The positive results of Stanford SMART and Planet Health suggest that obesity prevention efforts should involve reductions in sedentary television viewing time (see Chapter 8) and that school curricula should include television viewing reduction components.

Next Steps

Evidence from school intervention studies demonstrates some effectiveness of behavior-based nutrition and physical activity curricula. Evidence is most compelling from curricula for reducing television viewing, from vigorous PE interventions, and from large-scale, multicomponent intervention studies.

The extent to which schools are currently implementing such curricula, however, is unclear. Constraints include the limited availability of health educators who are trained in behavior-change methods, and the lack of sufficient time in the school day for specifically focusing on eating and physical activity behaviors. More staff training and the allocation of more time are two priorities. The impact of health education material can also be expanded by incorporating nutrition and physical activity information into science, math, history, social studies, and other courses.

Schools should ensure that nutrition, physical activity, and wellness concepts are taught throughout the curriculum from kindergarten through

high school. Schools should implement as part of the health curriculum an evidence-based program that includes a behavioral skills focus on promoting physical activity, healthful food choices, and energy balance and decreasing sedentary behaviors.

Given the limited resources in many schools and their varied priorities regarding the nature and duration of nutrition, health, and physical education classes and curricula, it is critically important for innovative approaches to be developed and evaluated to address obesity prevention in the schools. These approaches should involve evidence-based curricula that teach effective decision-making skills in the areas of diet and physical activity. Teacher training in health education and behavioral-change teaching methods is needed. **The departments of education and health at the state and federal levels, with input from relevant professional organizations, should develop and evaluate pilot programs to explore innovative approaches to both staffing and teaching about wellness, healthful choices, nutrition, physical activity, and sedentary behaviors.** Furthermore, it is hoped that health educators, school psychologists, and professional organizations (e.g., American Federation of School Teachers, American Psychological Association) will be brought into the discussions on how best to develop innovative curricula in this area.

ADVERTISING IN SCHOOLS

There have been growing concerns in recent years about the extent of commercial advertising in public schools and the influence that it may have on children's decision-making both for foods and other goods (Consumers Union, 1990, 1995; Greenberg and Brand, 1993; Bachen, 1998; Levine, 1999). Branded products are often advertised to students in a variety of school venues. Examples of these venues include required in-school television viewing such as Channel One, school textbooks, corporate-sponsored classroom materials, sports equipment, school cafeteria foods, signage and equipment (refrigerated display cases), vending machine signage, uniform logos, advertising on school buses, product giveaways, coupons, incentive contests, book covers, mouse pads, and book clubs.

Commercial activities involving schools have been categorized as follows (GAO, 2000; Wechsler et al., 2001):

- Product sales: short-term fundraising activities benefiting a specific student activity; cash or credit rebate programs; and commerce in products that benefit a district, school, or student activity (e.g., vending machine contracts; class ring contracts)
- Direct advertising on school property: billboards, signs, and product displays; signs on school buses; corporate logos or brand names on

school supplies or equipment; ads in school publications; media-based advertising (e.g., Channel One News); and free samples and coupons

• Indirect advertising: corporate-sponsored educational materials; teacher training; contests; incentive programs; and, in a small percentage of schools (<2 percent), lesson plans or curricula sponsored by companies (Wechsler et al., 2001)

• Market research conducted through or at schools: questionnaires, taste tests, and Internet surveys.

Only limited data are available on the extent of advertising in schools. The 2000 SHPPS nationwide survey found that the majority of high schools (71.9 percent) have contracts with one or more companies to sell soft drinks at the school (Wechsler et al., 2001). The percentages at middle schools (50.4 percent) and elementary schools (38.2 percent) are lower but still significant (Wechsler et al., 2001). Of those schools with soft drink contracts, most (91.7 percent) receive a proportion of the sales; some of the contracts include incentives for increased sales such as equipment, supplies, or cash awards. Advertising by soft drink companies is allowed in the school building at 37.6 percent of the schools with contracts; advertising is allowed on school grounds at 27.7 percent; and advertising on school buses is allowed by only 2.2 percent (Wechsler et al., 2001).

Data from the SHPPS survey (Table 7-1) give an overview of some of the commercial involvement of schools. In the 19 schools visited for the GAO report, most of the advertising was seen in high schools; examples included advertising on scoreboards, vending machines, posters, and on promotional materials such as free book covers and product samples (GAO, 2000). In many schools television programming is provided through Channel One News[4]—10 minutes of news, music, contests, and public service announcements interspersed with 2 minutes of commercials, including advertisements for candy, food, and beverages.

Although there is little published research on school commercialism, there are some indications of increases in the extent of commercialism in schools. In a survey of high school principals in North Carolina, 51.1 percent of the 174 respondents believed that corporate involvement in their school had increased over the past 5 years (Di Bona et al., 2003), the largest involvement being in the form of incentive programs (41.4 percent). Such changes have been noted by the press. An analysis of media references to school commercialism has found significant increases over the past 6 years (Molnar, 2003).

---

[4]Launched in 1990, Channel One News is viewed in approximately 12,000 U.S. schools representing an audience of 8 million teenagers (Di Bona et al., 2003).

TABLE 7-1 Schools That Allow Food Promotion or Advertising

		Total Schools (%)
Soft drink contracts:		
Have contract with company to sell soft drinks	Elementary schools:	38.2
	Middle/junior high schools:	50.4
	Senior high schools:	71.9
Of schools with soft drink contracts:		
Receive a specific percentage of soft drink sale receipts		91.7
Receive sales incentives from company[a]	Elementary schools:	24.0
	Middle/junior high schools:	40.9
	Senior high schools:	56.7
Allow advertising by the company in the school building		37.6
Allow advertising by the company on school grounds		27.7
Allow advertising by the company on school buses		2.2
Promotion of candy, meals from fast food restaurants, and soft drinks:		
Allow promotion of these products through coupons		23.3
Allow promotion of these products through sponsorship of school events		14.3
Allow promotion of these products through school publications		7.7
Prohibit or discourage faculty and staff from using these items as rewards		24.8

[a]Schools receive incentives such as cash awards or donations of equipment or supplies once receipts reach specified amounts.
SOURCE: Wechsler et al., 2001.

As discussed in Chapter 5, a number of studies have shown that advertising influences children's food and beverage choices. An extensive literature review by Hastings and colleagues (2003) concluded that food advertisements trigger food purchase requests by children to parents; have effects on children's product and brand preferences; and have an effect on consumption behavior. Furthermore, a recent analysis of the cognitive developmental literature (Wilcox et al., 2004) found that young children (generally under the age of 7 to 8 years) do not generally understand that difference between information and advertising.

Because public schools are institutions supported by taxpayer dollars, there are issues regarding whether it is appropriate for public schools to be a site for corporate or commercial advertising and marketing of products to children. Further, schools act in place of parents and advertising in school can be viewed as circumventing parental control over the types of advertising to which children are exposed. Additionally, children may interpret school-based advertising to mean that teachers or other adults at school endorse the use of the advertised product.

The problem of in-school advertising is complex and warrants a thorough and complete separate examination. Part of the difficulty in addressing issues regarding food and beverage advertising in schools is the issue of distinguishing advertising and promotion of healthful foods and beverages themselves from the companies or brands that may be associated with several different food or beverage products, some of which may be healthful and some less so. In addition, many foods and beverages currently sold in schools are packaged with branded corporate logos and labels. The extent to which such packaging is considered to be advertising is unclear.

The committee acknowledges that there are significant barriers to removing advertising completely from the school environment. Foremost is the anticipated loss of funding from corporate sponsors and what is perceived to be substantial revenue from the sale of soft drinks and other branded items (although this revenue often comes primarily from students and their families). Additionally, there is the potential for loss of free curriculum materials, incentives, sports equipment, food-service equipment, computers, televisions, and other items. However, as discussed earlier in the chapter, options need to be explored so that schools can provide the healthiest possible environment for children. It is important to note that some corporations donate goods, services, or money to schools without seeking advertising or marketing rights in return.

Nineteen states have state laws or regulations that are relevant to this issue, but in most cases they are not comprehensive (GAO, 2000). Throughout most of the United States, the local school districts make the decisions regarding school commercialism and advertising, and some schools and school districts appear to be more ready than others to eliminate such advertising. This presents an important opportunity to systematically study the potential benefits of different policies on obesity and other health and psychological parameters.

Research is needed to examine the impact of such advertising on youth dietary, physical activity, and sedentary behaviors within the school. As a first step, the Department of Education and USDA should fund quasi-experimental research comparing schools that introduce and/or eliminate such advertising, with respect to food and physical activity choices and behaviors at school and outside of school.

To date, the evidence on the impact of advertising in general, particularly on young children, favors removal of advertising and marketing from schools. Furthermore, the school environment needs to reinforce nutrition and physical activity messages taught in the classroom, and advertising may present conflicting messages. **Schools and school districts are urged to de-**

velop, implement, and enforce school policies to create schools that are advertising-free to the greatest possible extent.

SCHOOL HEALTH SERVICES

School health services should play a prominent role in addressing obesity-related issues among students and throughout the school environment. School health clinics and other school-based health services offer an often untapped resource because they have the opportunity to reach large numbers of students and the expertise to provide nutrition and health information as well as referrals to counseling and other health services. However, an emphasis on dietary behaviors and physical activity is not meant to be competitive with the other vital issues that school health services and health education curricula address, including prevention of tobacco and alcohol use and sexual education.

Although the 2000 SHPPS survey found that more than 75 percent of schools had at least a part-time school nurse, the extent and nature of health services at schools vary widely (Brener et al., 2001). Nearly all schools have provisions for administrating medications and first aid, but many lack the resources to deliver prevention services. The 2000 SHPPS survey found that 55.3 percent of schools reported offering nutrition and dietary behavior counseling and 37.2 percent offered physical activity and fitness counseling (Brener et al., 2001). Twenty-six percent of states required height and weight to be measured, or BMI to be assessed, in schools; of those, about 61.5 percent required parent notification (Table 7-2). Similarly, the survey found that physical fitness tests were required by approximately 20 percent of states or school districts.[5] Some states have developed their own fitness test, while others use the President's Challenge or the Fitnessgram (Burgeson et al., 2001). In most schools (91.1 percent) teachers provided students with explanations of what their fitness scores meant; in 59.8 percent of the schools, teachers informed the students' parents as well.

In Chapter 8, the committee recommends that parents make their child's weight status a priority for discussion with their medical-care provider, and in Chapter 6 the committee offers recommendations on the high priority that this issue should be given by health-care professionals themselves. However, there are an estimated 9.2 million children and youth[6] in the

---

[5]Physical fitness tests are required in elementary schools by 13.7 percent of states and 18.3 percent of districts, in middle or junior high schools by 15.7 percent of states and 21.3 percent of districts, and in senior high schools by 18 percent of states and 20.4 percent of districts (Burgeson et al., 2001).

[6]In 2001, 12.1 percent of Americans aged 19 years or younger—9.2 million children and youth—were without health insurance all year (Bhandari and Gifford, 2003).

TABLE 7-2 States and Districts Requiring Student Screening and Follow-Up

	States		Districts	
	% Requiring Screening	% Requiring Parental Notification	% Requiring Screening	% Requiring Parental Notification
Height and weight or BMI	26.0	61.5	38.4	81.1
Hearing	70.6	91.4	88.4	98.5
Vision	70.6	91.4	90.4	98.5
Oral health	17.6	87.5	31.1	98.3
Scoliosis	45.1	100.0	68.8	98.6
Tuberculosis	20.0	80.0	17.1	93.7

SOURCE: Brener et al., 2001.

United States whose families do not have health insurance (Bhandari and Gifford, 2003) and who may not be seen on a regular basis by a medical practitioner. Additionally, many children, particularly in their mid-childhood and teen years, do not have annual health-care visits. Parents often do not recognize that their child is overweight or obese, or they may believe that the child will outgrow his or her excess weight (Etelson et al., 2003; Maynard et al., 2003). If children were weighed and measured annually, the history of a particular child could be tracked and any increase in his or her gender- and age-specific BMI percentile would be detected, allowing for actions designed to prevent further increases and perhaps even lower the BMI.

Some states and school systems have begun providing an individualized health "report card" focused on conveying weight-status information to parents (Box 7-4) (Chomitz et al., 2003; Scheier, 2004). Concerns have been raised about unintended consequences of this approach, including potential stigmatization of children, misinterpretation of BMIs, and placement of children on harmful diets (Scheier, 2004). However, such measures are routinely collected at many schools (Table 7-2) and in health-care providers' clinics. Furthermore, many intervention studies have obtained weight and height measurements on large numbers of students. For example, CATCH collected weight, height, blood pressure, skinfold thickness, aerobic fitness, dietary intake, and physical activity data on 4,019 students in 96 schools in third grade and again in fifth grade (Luepker et al., 1996).

BOX 7-4
Arkansas BMI Initiative

Arkansas Act 1220, approved by the Arkansas General Assembly and Governor in 2003, established a multipronged state initiative to improve the health of Arkansas children (ACHI, 2004). The act mandated that parents be provided with their child's annual BMI, as well as an explanation of the BMI measure and information on health effects associated with obesity.

This mandate is being implemented in three phases using a confidential health report. Eleven schools participated in Phase I in which measurement methodologies, equipment, and reporting forms were developed and tested for validity and accuracy. Phase II consisted of field testing in a second round of schools. The final phase involves the statewide rollout of the program which began in Spring 2004 (ACHI, 2004). Community health nurses are an important part of this effort, because they are first certified in height and weight research measurements at Arkansas Children's Hospital and subsequently train school nurses and other school personnel (ACHI, 2004). Training of health-care professionals involved in pediatric and adolescent development is also a part of this initiative.

The reports being sent to parents include the child's BMI as well as information to assist them in contacting local resources for additional information. Data also will be aggregated at the school, district, and state levels. Evaluation of the program is ongoing and will include focus groups with parents.

Participant safety was continuously monitored by an independent data and safety monitoring board. A study of elementary school students and their parents in Cambridge, Massachusetts, found that, among parents of overweight children, those who received the health report card intervention were more likely to begin or consider looking into clinical services, dieting, or physical activity than those parents who received general information or no information (Chomitz et al., 2003). Evaluation of the report card approach is ongoing, but further research is needed on alternate methods for conducting weight-status assessments and conveying the information thus obtained to parents and to the students themselves (as age appropriate).

Schools should measure yearly each student's weight, height, and gender- and age-specific BMI percentile and make this information available to parents and to the student (when age appropriate). Implementation of yearly measures may be resource-intensive for schools that are currently conducting such measures. However, it is important for parents to have information about their child's BMI and other weight-status and physical fitness measures, just as they need information about other health or academic matters.

The committee recognizes that providing follow-up health-care services for children identified as being obese or at high risk for obesity will present a number of challenges including the lack of a standardized referral system; pediatricians' general lack of training in how to counsel parents and children on nutrition, physical activity, or weight management (Chapter 6); and the limited availability of nutrition education and physical activity programs to absorb the potential demand. Therefore, efforts on this issue will require working with health-care providers and others to provide the appropriate follow-up information and services.

There are sensitivities and concerns that surround this issue, and it is important that the data on each student are collected and reported validly and appropriately, with the utmost attention to privacy concerns, and with information on referrals available if further evaluation is needed. The committee urges CDC and other relevant federal, state, and local agencies to develop guidelines that assist schools in developing protocols that are not only reliable and useful, but that sensitively collect and communicate this information.

AFTER-SCHOOL PROGRAMS AND
SCHOOLS AS COMMUNITY CENTERS

Organized after-school programs, both public and private, are daily opportunities for engaging many children and youth in physical activity and promoting healthy food choices. In addition to serving students shortly after the school day is over, school facilities can also offer similar services during other nonschool hours to the wider community.

An estimated 19 percent of 5- to 14-year-old children—some seven million—care for themselves on a regular basis after school without adult supervision (Smith, 2002). Approximately 14 percent of children ages 5 to 12 with employed mothers attend after-school center programs, and another 15 percent are involved in lessons and other enrichment activities (Vandell and Shumow, 1999). These programs may be school- or community-based and can vary widely in their content, opportunities for physical activity, nature and focus, class size, staff education, and child-staff ratios (Vandell and Shumow, 1999; NRC, 2003).

Some after-school programs concentrate on homework help and tutoring; others emphasize enrichment opportunities (e.g., computer skills, art, and music programs); and some, focused on providing safe havens to children during after-school hours, offer a spectrum of options (NRC, 2000). Given the varied nature of these programs and the range of school or community groups that are responsible, a broad-reaching infrastructure does not exist for disseminating new initiatives in general. However, these programs are often readily amenable to implementing or expanding nutritional and physical activity information and to providing venues for engaging in physical activity as well (Ross et al., 1985).

In that spirit, discussions are ongoing about how best to organize and structure after-school programs, particularly regarding the balance between academic and other pursuits (NRC, 2003). The 21st Century Community Learning Centers program is an example of successfully involving schools and communities in working together to address after-school needs. Funded by the U.S. Department of Education, the program's centers now serve 1.2 million children and 400,000 adults in 6,800 schools (in all 50 states and in more than 1,400 communities) (U.S. Department of Education, 2004). These centers focus on academic improvement but also involve programs in music and other arts and use of computers. Incorporating physical activity programs and an emphasis on good nutrition into the 21st Century Community Learning Centers program and other similar efforts is recommended.

As discussed in Chapter 6, research has shown that access to opportunities for physical activity is associated with *increased* physical activity. In recognition of the positive effects of family activities and parental modeling of healthful behaviors, schools with physical activity facilities that currently go unused during nonschool hours should explore ways of making them available for community use. Expanding the use of school facilities during afternoons, evenings, weekends, and vacation periods is particularly important in communities that do not have publicly supported community recreation centers. For public schools, this objective would also expand the use of public funding.

It is important to take advantage of opportunities for improving nutrition and increasing physical activity for the large number of children who attend after-school programs. Furthermore, communities with limited recreational facilities would benefit from access to school facilities during nonschool hours. **After-school programs should encourage and enable daily physical activity, provide healthful nutritional choices, and provide students with the information to foster a better understanding of energy balance. Schools and communities should use school facilities as community centers that provide opportunities for physical activity and for programs that promote energy balance. Such programs are particularly important for children in areas where neighborhood safety concerns may present a barrier to outside physical activity.**

The committee acknowledges that there are hurdles to overcome in implementing these recommendations, particularly in obtaining the funding for their increased staffing and maintenance implications. Coordinating the logistics of the use of equipment and facilities could also be a challenge (Dryfoos, 1999). However, there are numerous benefits of expanding the use of school facilities and offering programs for youth and families— including improved social skills, a heightened sense of community, and reduction in youth crime. Given that a large number of schools in the United States are now being built or refurbished, communities have an opportunity to design these schools with facilities that can best accommodate after-school or community center programs.

As these programs are pursued, it is critical that the effects of changes in after-school programs and other after-school uses of school facilities (e.g., in the form of community centers) be evaluated. Innovations to encourage children and youth to participate in physical activities and learn about nutrition are particularly encouraged, because they have the potential to help prevent childhood overweight and obesity. Pilot results for after-school obesity prevention programs in low-income African-American communities are already showing promise in this regard (Beech et al., 2003; Robinson et al., 2003), though further research and evaluation is needed.

EVALUATION OF SCHOOL PROGRAMS AND POLICIES

In most if not all states, schools are mandated to perform periodic academic testing to compare student performance against established standards. The committee recommends extending these assessments to include parameters related to healthful eating, physical activity, and other factors related to the risk for obesity.

Recognizing that the school environment is one of the many influences on a child's dietary intake or energy expenditure, it is important to develop effective school-based programs. Thus, schools, school districts, state boards of education, and regional and national institutions have already begun to promote and implement innovative approaches for addressing the rising rates of obesity in children and youth and for promoting their health and fitness. Although these programs can be costly in terms of finances, personnel, and other resources, they have the potential to enhance the educational process.

Without systematic and widespread assessments of obesity-related behaviors and physical activity measures, however, there will be no way to identify which of the many possible strategies are potentially effective, much less the most cost-effective. Specific cause-and-effect inferences will not always be possible, but the availability of pertinent local data will enable schools, parents, school districts, states, policy makers, and researchers to identify some of the more promising approaches for further testing and development.

Many schools now use the School Health Index developed by CDC as a school self-assessment tool (CDC, 2004a). This measure incorporates physical and nutritional education components into evaluations as well as assesses other areas, particularly school health, counseling, health policies, health promotion, and family and community involvement. The committee encourages schools to use the School Health Index or similar school-specific assessments to identify areas to improve the school's health and safety promotion policies and practices.

In addition, some schools may want to assess more direct measures (such as students' gender- and age-specific BMI percentile, physical fitness, and dietary intake) to help determine whether or not the school's policy and programming changes are reducing the levels of overweight and obesity. Commitment to performing these evaluations will require legislators and other policy makers to allocate sufficient funding, employ professional staffing, and develop statewide mechanisms for reporting these assessments' results to the public.

State and local education authorities should perform periodic assessments of each school's policies and practices related to nutrition and physical activity. These assessments should address curriculum, instructional methods, school environment, extracurricular programming, and relationships with the community. Other components that could be considered based on the needs of the schools are assessments of physical activity, physical fitness, dietary intake, and BMI percentile distribution of a representative sample of students. Results of school evaluations should be reported periodically to the public. If data are collected on a representative sample of students, the results should be publicly reported only in the aggregate.

Research is needed to determine optimum ways to assess the impacts of school programs, policies, and environments on obesity prevention. Research is also needed to explore program adaptations that may be needed to accommodate schools with high levels of cultural diversity.

Potential hurdles in implementing these actions will need to be addressed. In particular, if schools and school districts are to develop valid and easy-to-use assessment measures and protocols, provide sufficient staff training to ensure reliable data collection, and then implement and report the results of these assessments, they will need sufficient funding. If schools were to meet the School Health Index standards under current economic conditions, there would likely be increased financial burden on most school systems.

The committee acknowledges that there is limited published information on schools that have implemented this type of schoolwide evaluation. However, based on the public attention paid to standardized academic testing by parents, teachers, administrators, and policy makers, it is the belief of the committee that assessment and public reporting of health-related outcomes will prove to be an incentive for schools to innovate and adopt more effective health promotion curricula, improved food-service options, and other health and fitness programming (e.g., after-school activities, family-oriented physical activities).

RECOMMENDATION

Schools offer the opportunity for reaching large numbers of young people, during a significant part of their day, and throughout much of the year. Furthermore, schools present opportunities, both in and out of the classroom, for the concepts of energy balance to be taught and put into practice. As discussed throughout the chapter, several large-scale, well-designed school-based intervention studies have shown that multicomponent changes in the school environment can improve the food and beverage selections by students, the nutritional quality of foods offered, and the duration and extent of students' physical activity while at school.

Schools should not only provide educational messages about nutrition, physical activity, and reducing sedentary behaviors, but should reinforce and support these concepts throughout the school environment. Changes that can make the school environment more supportive of healthful eating and physical activity behaviors begin with the development of nutritional standards for all food and beverage items sold in the schools and improvements in the federal school meal programs. Furthermore, opportunities for physical activity need to be expanded through ensuring daily PE, as well as increasing the options for both competitive and noncompetitive sports and activities, enhancement of after-school programs, and the opening of school facilities for use during other nonschool hours. It is also important to develop and implement curricula that will encourage students to move beyond an awareness of energy balance to the routine incorporation of good nutrition and physical activity into their daily lives.

There are numerous innovative programs and changes relevant to obesity prevention that are being implemented in schools throughout the country, and it is important to adequately evaluate these efforts to determine whether they should be continued, expanded, or refined. Furthermore, preschools and child-care centers should be included in these efforts.

The goal is for schools to implement evidence-based programs and approaches that promote healthful physical activity and nutrition behaviors for all components of school interventions, including health education, physical education, after-school programs, and walk-/bike-to-school programs. Adequate training and support for teachers, food-service personnel, and other leaders will be needed, along with adequate supplies and equipment. Federal and state agencies need to provide the resources for research and evaluation of school programs and interventions and work to disseminate those that are found to be effective in improving physical activity and nutrition behaviors.

Next steps for making progress on this issue will involve discussions of the relevant stakeholders in schools, communities, regions, and states so that action plans can be tailored to best address the issues and high-risk populations in the area.

Recommendation 9: *Schools*
Schools should provide a consistent environment that is conducive to healthful eating behaviors and regular physical activity.

To implement this recommendation:

USDA, state, and local authorities, and schools should:

• Develop and implement nutritional standards for all competitive foods and beverages sold or served in schools
• Ensure that all school meals meet the Dietary Guidelines for Americans
• Develop, implement, and evaluate pilot programs to extend school meal funding in schools with a large percentage of children at high risk of obesity

State and local education authorities and schools should:

• Ensure that all children and youth participate in a minimum of 30 minutes of moderate to vigorous physical activity during the school day
• Expand opportunities for physical activity through physical education classes; intramural and interscholastic sports programs and other physical activity clubs, programs, and lessons; after-school use of school facilities; use of schools as community centers; and walking- and biking-to-school programs
• Enhance health curricula to devote adequate attention to nutrition, physical activity, reducing sedentary behaviors, and energy balance, and to include a behavioral skills focus
• Develop, implement, and enforce school policies to create schools that are advertising-free to the greatest possible extent
• Involve school health services in obesity prevention efforts
• Conduct annual assessments of each student's weight, height, and gender- and age-specific BMI percentile and make this information available to parents
• Perform periodic assessments of each school's policies and practices related to nutrition, physical activity, and obesity prevention

Federal and state departments of education and health and professional organizations should:

- Develop, implement, and evaluate pilot programs to explore innovative approaches to both staffing and teaching about wellness, healthful choices, nutrition, physical activity, and reducing sedentary behaviors. Innovative approaches to recruiting and training appropriate teachers are also needed

REFERENCES

AAP (American Academy of Pediatrics), Committee on Sports Medicine and Fitness and Committee on School Health. 2000. Physical fitness and activity in schools. *Pediatrics* 105(5):1156-1157.

ACHI (Arkansas Center for Health Improvement). 2004. *BMI Initiative.* [Online]. Available: http://www.achi.net/BMI_Stuff/bmi.asp [accessed June 10, 2004].

Bachen CM. 1998. Channel One and the education of American youths. *Ann Am Acad Pol Soc Sci* 557:132-147.

Bandura A. 1986. *Social Foundations of Thought and Action: A Social Cognitive Theory.* Prentice-Hall Series in Social Learning Theory. Englewood Cliffs, NJ: Prentice-Hall.

Beech BM, Klesges RC, Kumanyika SK, Murray DM, Klesges L, McClanahan B, Slawson D, Nunnally C, Rochon J, McLain-Allen B, Pree-Cary J. 2003. Child- and parent-targeted interventions: The Memphis GEMS pilot study. *Ethn Dis* 13(1):S40-S53.

Bhandari S, Gifford E. 2003. *Children with Health Insurance: 2001.* Current Population Reports P60-224. Washington, DC: U.S. Census Bureau.

Biddle S, Sallis JF, Cavill N. 1998. *Young and Active? Young People and Health Enhancing Physical Activity. Evidence and Implication.* London: Health Education Authority.

Brener ND, Burstein GR, DuShaw ML, Vernon ME, Wheeler L, Robinson J. 2001. Health services: Results from the School Health Policies and Programs Study 2000. *J Sch Health* 71(1):294-304.

Burgeson CR, Wechsler H, Brener ND, Young JC, Spain CG. 2001. Physical education and activity: Results from the School Health Policies and Programs Study 2000. *J Sch Health* 71(7):279-293.

Buzby J, Guthrie JF, Kantor LS. 2003. *Evaluation of the USDA's Fruit and Vegetable Pilot Program: Report to Congress.* Washington, DC: USDA. [Online]. Available: http://www.ers.usda.gov/publications/efan03006/ [accessed March 15, 2004].

Caballero B, Davis S, Davis CE, Ethelbah B, Evans M, Lohman T, Stephenson L, Story M, White J. 1998. Pathways: A school-based program for the primary prevention of obesity in American Indian children. *J Nutr Biochem* 9(9):535-543.

Caballero B, Clay T, Davis SM, Ethelbah B, Rock BH, Lohman T, Norman J, Story M, Stone EJ, Stephenson L, Stevens J, Pathways Study Research Group. 2003. Pathways: A school-based, randomized controlled trial for the prevention of obesity in American Indian schoolchildren. *Am J Clin Nutr* 78(5):1030-1038.

Cavill N, Biddle S, Sallis JF. 2001. Health enhancing physical activity for young people: Statement of the United Kingdom Expert Consensus Conference. *Pediatr Exer Sci* 13:12-25.

CDC (Centers for Disease Control and Prevention). 1997. Guidelines for school and community programs to promote lifelong physical activity among young people. *MMWR Recomm Rep* 46(RR-6):1-36.

CDC. 2003. *Health, United States, 2003.* [Online]. Available: http://www.cdc.gov/nchs/hus.htm [accessed May 17, 2004].

CDC. 2004a. *School Health Index.* [Online]. Available: http://www.cdc.gov/HealthyYouth/shi/index.htm [accessed May 18, 2004].

CDC. 2004b. Youth risk behavior surveillance—United States, 2003. *MMWR Surveill Summ* 53(2):1-96.

Chomitz VR, Collins J, Kim J, Kramer E, McGowan R. 2003. Promoting healthy weight among elementary school children via a health report card approach. *Arch Pediatr Adolesc Med* 157(8):765-772.

Consumers Union. 1990. *Selling America's Kids: Commercial Pressures on Kids of the 90's.* Yonkers, NY: Consumers Union Education Services. [Online]. Available: http://www.consumersunion.org/other/sellingkids/index.htm [accessed February 6, 2004].

Consumers Union. 1995. *Captive Kids: Commercial Pressures on Kids at School.* Yonkers, NY: Consumers Union Education Services. [Online]. Available: http://www.consumersunion.org/other/captivekids [accessed June 18, 2004].

Cullen KW, Zakeri I. 2004. Fruits, vegetables, milk, and sweetened beverages consumption and access to à la carte/snack bar meals at school. *Am J Public Health* 94(3):463-467.

Cullen KW, Eagan J, Baranowski T, Owens E, de Moor C. 2000. Effect of à la carte and snack bar foods at school on children's lunchtime intake of fruits and vegetables. *J Am Diet Assoc* 100(12):1482-1486.

Davis SM, Going SB, Helitzer DL, Teufel NI, Snyder P, Gittelsohn J, Metcalfe L, Arviso V, Evans M, Smyth M, Brice R, Altaha J. 1999. Pathways: A culturally appropriate obesity-prevention program for American Indian schoolchildren. *Am J Clin Nutr* 69(4S):796S-802S.

DHHS (U.S. Department of Health and Human Services). 2000. *Healthy People 2010: Understanding and Improving Health.* 2nd ed. Washington, DC: U.S. Government Printing Office. [Online]. Available: http://www.healthypeople.gov/document/tableofcontents.htm [accessed April 9, 2004].

Di Bona J, Chaudhuri R, Jean-Baptiste J, Menachem P, Wurzburg M. 2003. Commercialism in North Carolina high schools: A survey of principals' perceptions. *Peabody J Educ* 78(2):41-62.

Dishman RK, Motl RW, Saunders R, Felton G, Ward DS, Dowda M, Pate RR. 2004. Self-efficacy partially mediates the effect of a school-based physical-activity intervention among adolescent girls. *Prev Med* 38(5):628-636.

Donnelly JE, Jacobsen DJ, Whatley JE, Hill JO, Swift LL, Cherrington A, Polk B, Tran ZV, Reed G. 1996. Nutrition and physical activity program to attenuate obesity and promote physical and metabolic fitness in elementary school children. *Obes Res* 4(3):229-243.

Dryfoos JG. 1999. The role of the school in children's out-of-school time. *Future Child* 9(2):117-134.

Dwyer T, Coonan WE, Leitch DR, Hetzel BS, Baghurst RA. 1983. An investigation of the effects of daily physical activity on the health of primary school students in South Australia. *Int J Epidemiol* 12(3):308-313.

Dwyer T, Sallis JF, Blizzard L, Lazarus R, Dean K. 2001. Relation of academic performance to physical activity and fitness in children. *Pediatr Exerc Sci* 13(3):225-237.

Edible Schoolyard. 2004. *The Edible Schoolyard.* [Online]. Available: http://www.edibleschoolyard.org [accessed June 4, 2004].

Etelson D, Brand DA, Patrick PA, Shirali A. 2003. Childhood obesity: Do parents recognize this health risk? *Obes Res* 11(11):1362-1368.

Ewart CK, Young DR, Hagberg JM. 1998. Effects of school-based aerobic exercise on blood pressure in adolescent girls at risk for hypertension. *Am J Public Health* 88(6):949-951.

Fardy PS, White REC, Haltiwanger-Schmitz K, Magel JR, McDermott KJ, Clark LT, Hurster MM. 1996. Coronary disease risk factor reduction and behavior modification in minority adolescents: The PATH program. *J Adolesc Health* 18(4):247-253.

Flores R. 1995. Dance for health: Improving fitness in African American and Hispanic adolescents. *Public Health Rep* 110(2):189-193.

FNS/USDA (Food and Nutrition Service/U.S. Department of Agriculture). 2003. National School Lunch, Special Milk, and School Breakfast Programs: National average payments/maximum reimbursement rates. *Fed Regist* 68(130):40623-40626.

French SA, Stables G. 2003. Environmental interventions to promote vegetable and fruit consumption among youth in school settings. *Prev Med* 37(6):593-610.

French SA, Story M, Jeffery RW, Snyder P, Eisenberg M, Sidebottom A, Murray D. 1997. Pricing strategy to promote fruit and vegetable purchase in high school cafeterias. *J Am Diet Assoc* 97(9):1008-1010.

French SA, Jeffery RW, Story M, Breitlow KK, Baxter JS, Hannan P, Snyder MP. 2001. Pricing and promotion effects on low-fat vending snack purchases: The CHIPS study. *Am J Public Health* 91(1):112-117.

French SA, Story M, Fulkerson JA. 2002. School food policies and practices: A state-wide survey of secondary school principals. *J Am Diet Assoc* 102(12):1785-1789.

French SA, Story M, Fulkerson JA, Faricy Gerlach A. 2003. Food environment in secondary schools: À la carte, vending machines, and food policies and practices. *Am J Public Health* 93(7):1161-1168.

French SA, Story M, Fulkerson JA, Hannan P. 2004. An environmental intervention to promote lower fat food choices in secondary schools: Outcomes of the TACOS study. *Am J Public Health* 94(9):1507-1512.

GAO (U.S. General Accounting Office). 2000. *Commercial Activities in Schools*. GAO/HEHS-00-156. Washington, DC: U.S. General Accounting Office. [Online]. Available: http://www.gao.gov/archive/2000/he00156.pdf [accessed February 23, 2004].

GAO. 2003. *School Lunch Program: Efforts Needed to Improve Nutrition and Encourage Healthy Eating*. GAO-03-506. Washington, DC: U.S. General Accounting Office. [Online]. Available: http://www.gao.gov/new.items/d03506.pdf [accessed February 23, 2004].

GAO. 2004. *School Meal Programs: Competitive Foods Are Available in Many Schools; Actions Taken to Restrict Them Differ by State and Locality*. GAO-04-673. Washington, DC: U.S. General Accounting Office.

Gortmaker SL, Peterson K, Wiecha J, Sobol AM, Dixit S, Fox MK, Laird N. 1999. Reducing obesity via a school-based interdisciplinary intervention among youth: Planet Health. *Arch Pediatr Adolesc Med* 153(4):409-418.

Greenberg BS, Brand JE. 1993. Television news and advertising in schools: The Channel One controversy. *J Community* 43(1):143-151.

Hannan P, French SA, Story M, Fulkerson JA. 2002. A pricing strategy to promote sales of lower fat foods in high school cafeterias: Acceptability and sensitivity analysis. *Am J Health Promot* 17(1):1-6, ii.

Harnack L, Snyder P, Story M, Holliday R, Lytle L, Neumark-Sztainer D. 2000. Availability of à la carte food items in junior and senior high schools: A needs assessment. *J Am Diet Assoc* 100(6):701-703.

Harrell JS, McMurray RG, Gansky SA, Bangdiwala SI, Bradley CB. 1999. A public health vs. a risk-based intervention to improve cardiovascular health in elementary school children: The Cardiovascular Health in Children Study. *Am J Public Health* 89(10):1529-1535.

Hastings G, Stead M, McDermott L, Forsyth A, MacKintosh A, Rayner, M, Godfrey C, Caraher M, Angus K. 2003. *Review of Research on the Effects of Food Promotion to Children.* Glasgow, UK. Center for Social Marketing, University of Strathclyde. Final report prepared for the Food Standards Agency. [Online]. Available: http://www.foodstandards.gov.uk/multimedia/pdfs/foodpromotiontochildren1.pdf [accessed November 22, 2003].

Hearn MD, Baranowski T, Baranowski J, Doyle C, Lin LS, Smith M, Wang DT, Resnicow K. 1998. Environmental determinants of behavior among children: Availability and accessibility of fruits and vegetables. *J Health Educ* 29:26-32.

Hopper CA, Gruber MB, Munoz KD, Herb RA. 1992. Effect of including parents in a school-based exercise and nutrition program for children. *Res Q Exerc Sport* 63(3):315-321.

Hopper CA, Munoz KD, Gruber MB, MacConnie SE, Schonfeldt B, Shunk T. 1996. A school-based cardiovascular exercise and nutrition program with parent participation: An evaluation study. *Child Health Care* 25(3):221-235.

IOM (Institute of Medicine). 2002. *Dietary Reference Intakes for Energy, Carbohydrate, Fiber, Fat, Fatty Acids, Cholesterol, Protein, and Amino Acids.* Washington, DC: The National Academies Press.

Jago R, Baranowski T. 2004. Non-curricular approaches for increasing physical activity in youth: A review. *Prev Med* 39(1):157-163.

Joint Committee on National Health Education Standards, American Cancer Society. 1995. *National Health Education Standards: Achieving Health Literacy.* Atlanta, GA: American Cancer Society.

Kahn EB, Ramsey LT, Brownson RC, Heath GW, Howze EH, Powell KE, Stone EJ, Rajab MW, Corso P. 2002. The effectiveness of interventions to increase physical activity. A systematic review. *Am J Prev Med* 22(4S):73-107.

Kann L, Brener ND, Allensworth DD. 2001. Health education: Results from the School Health Policies and Programs Study 2000. *J Sch Health* 71(7):266-278.

Killen JD, Telch MJ, Robinson TN, Maccoby N, Taylor B, Farquhar JW. 1988. Cardiovascular disease risk reduction for tenth graders: A multiple-factor school-based approach. *J Am Med Assoc* 260(12):1728-1733.

Kubik MY, Lytle LA, Hannan PJ, Perry CL, Story M. 2003. The association of the school food environment with dietary behaviors of young adolescents. *Am J Public Health* 93(7):1168-1173.

Levine J. 1999. Food industry marketing in elementary schools: Implications for school health professionals. *J Sch Health* 69(7):290-291.

Lopiano DA. 2000. Modern history of women in sports. Twenty-five years of Title IX. *Clin Sports Med* 19(2):163-73, vii.

Los Angeles Unified School District. 2004. *Healthy Beverage.* [Online]. Available: http://cafe-la.lausd.k12.ca.us/healthy.htm [accessed May 28, 2004].

Luepker RV, Perry CL, McKinlay SM, Nader PR, Parcel GS, Stone EJ, Webber LS, Elder JP, Feldman HA, Johnson CC, Kelder SH, Wu M. 1996. Outcomes of a field trial to improve children's dietary patterns and physical activity. The Child and Adolescent Trial for Cardiovascular Health. CATCH Collaborative Group. *J Am Med Assoc* 275(10):768-776.

Manios Y, Moschandreas J, Hatzis C, Kafatos A. 1999. Evaluation of a health and nutrition education program in primary school children of Crete over a three-year period. *Prev Med* 28(2):149-159.

Maynard LM, Galuska DA, Blanck HM, Serdula MK. 2003. Maternal perceptions of weight status of children. *Pediatrics* 111(5 Pt 2):1226-1231.

McKenzie TL, Nader PR, Strikmiller PK, Yang M, Stone EJ, Perry CL, Taylor WC, Epping JN, Feldman HA, Luepker RV, Kelder SH. 1996. School physical education: Effect of the Child and Adolescent Trial for Cardiovascular Health. *Prev Med* 25(4):423-431.

McKenzie TL, Sallis JF, Kolody B, Faucette N. 1997. Long term effects of a physical education curriculum and staff development program: SPARK. *Res Q Exerc Sport* 68(4):280-291.

McKenzie TL, Li D, Derby CA, Webber LS, Luepker RV, Cribb P. 2003. Maintenance of effects of the CATCH physical education program: Results from the CATCH-ON study. *Health Educ Behav* 30(4):447-462.

Misako A, Fisher A. 2002. *Healthy Farms, Healthy Kids: Evaluating the Barriers and Opportunities for Farm-to-School Programs.* Venice, CA: Community Food Service Coalition (CFSC). [Online]. Available: http://www.foodsecurity.org/healthy [accessed April 21, 2004].

Molnar, A. 2003. *No Student Left Unsold: The Sixth Annual Report on Trends in Schoolhouse Commercialism 2002-2003.* [Online]. Available: http://www.asu.edu/educ/epsl/CERU/CERU_Annual_Report.htm [accessed November 20, 2003].

Morris J, Zidenberg-Cherr S. 2002. Garden-enhanced nutrition curriculum improves fourth-grade school children's knowledge of nutrition and preferences for some vegetables. *J Am Diet Assoc* 102(1):91-93.

Nader PR, Stone EJ, Lytle LA, Perry CL, Osganian SK, Kelder S, Webber LS, Elder JP, Montgomery D, Feldman HA, Wu M, Johnson C, Parcel GS, Luepker RV. 1999. Three-year maintenance of improved diet and physical activity: The CATCH cohort. Child and Adolescent Trial for Cardiovascular Health. *Arch Pediatr Adolesc Med* 153(7):695-704.

NASBE (National Association of State Boards of Education). 1990. *National Commission on the Role of the School and Community in Improving Adolescent Health. Code Blue: Uniting for Healthier Youth.* Alexandria, VA: NASBE.

NASPE (National Association for Sport and Physical Education). 2004. *Physical Activity for Children: A Statement of Guidelines for Children Ages 5-12.* Reston, VA: NASPE.

Nestle M. 2000. Soft drink "pouring rights": Marketing empty calories. *Public Health Rep* 115(4):308-319.

NRC (National Research Council). 1999. *Making Money Matter: Financing America's Schools.* Washington, DC: National Academy Press.

NRC. 2000. *After-School Programs to Promote Child and Adolescent Development: Summary of a Workshop.* Washington, DC: National Academy Press.

NRC. 2003. *Working Families and Growing Kids: Caring for Children and Adolescents.* Washington, DC: The National Academies Press.

Pate RR, Long BJ, Heath G. 1994. Descriptive epidemiology of physical activity in adolescents. *Pediatr Exerc Sci* 6(4):434-447.

Pate RR, Heath GW, Dowda M, Trost SG. 1996. Associations between physical activity and other health behaviors in a representative sample of US adolescents. *Am J Public Health* 86(11):1577-1581.

Perry CL, Bishop DB, Taylor G, Murray DM, Mays RW, Dudovitz BS, Smyth M, Story M. 1998. Changing fruit and vegetable consumption among children: The 5-A-Day Power Plus program in St. Paul, Minnesota. *Am J Public Health* 88(4):603-609.

Perry CL, Bishop DB, Taylor GL, Davis M, Story M, Gray C, Bishop SC, Mays RA, Lytle LA, Harnack L. 2004. A randomized school trial of environmental strategies to encourage fruit and vegetable consumption among children. *Health Educ Behav* 31(1):65-76.

Resnicow K, Robinson TN. 1997. School-based cardiovascular disease prevention studies: Review and synthesis. *Ann Epidemiol* 7(7S):S14-S31.

Reynolds KD, Franklin FA, Binkley D, Raczynski JM, Harrington KF, Kirk KA, Person S. 2000. Increasing the fruit and vegetable consumption of fourth-graders: Results from the high 5 project. *Prev Med* 30(4):309-319.

Robinson TN. 1999. Reducing children's television viewing to prevent obesity: A randomized controlled trial. *J Am Med Assoc* 282(16):1561-1567.

Robinson TN, Killen JD, Kraemer HC, Wilson DM, Matheson DM, Haskell WL, Pruitt LA, Powell TM, Owens AS, Thompson NS, Flint-Moore NM, Davis GJ, Emig KA, Brown RT, Rochon J, Green S, Varady A. 2003. Dance and reducing television viewing to prevent weight gain in African-American girls: The Stanford GEMS pilot study. *Ethn Dis* 13(1S1):S65-S77.

Ross JG, Dotson CO, Gilbert GG, Katz SJ. 1985. After physical education: Physical activity outside of school physical education programs. *J Phys Educ Recr Dance* 56(1):77-81.

Sallis JF. 1993. Epidemiology of physical activity and fitness in children. *Crit Rev Food Sci Nutr* 33(4/5):403-408.

Sallis JF, McKenzie TL, Alcaraz JE, Kolody B, Faucette N, Hovell MF. 1997. The effects of a 2-year physical education program (SPARK) on physical activity and fitness in elementary school students. Sports, Play and Active Recreation for Kids. *Am J Public Health* 87(8):1328-1334.

Sallis JF, McKenzie TL, Conway TL, Elder JP, Prochaska JJ, Brown M, Zive MM, Marshall SJ, Alcaraz JE. 2003. Environmental interventions for eating and physical activity. A randomized controlled trial in middle schools. *Am J Prev Med* 24(3):209-217.

Scheier LM. 2004. School health report cards attempt to address the obesity epidemic. *J Am Diet Assoc* 104(3):341-344.

Shephard RJ. 1997. Curricular physical activity and academic performance. *Pediatr Exerc Sci* 9(2):113-126.

Simons-Morton BG, Parcel GS, Baranowski T, Forthofer R, O'Hara NM. 1991. Promoting physical activity and a healthful diet among children: Results of a school-based intervention study. *Am J Public Health* 81(8):986-991.

Simons-Morton BG, Taylor WC, Snider SA, Huang IW. 1993. The physical activity of fifth-grade students during physical education classes. *Am J Public Health* 83(2):262-265.

Simons-Morton BG, McKenzie TJ, Stone E, Mitchell P, Osganian V, Strikmiller PK, Ehlinger S, Cribb P, Nader PR. 1997. Physical activity in a multiethnic population of third graders in four states. *Am J Public Health* 87(1):45-50.

Smith K. 2002. Who's minding the kids? Child care arrangements: Spring 1997. *Current Population Reports* 70-86. Washington, DC: U.S. Census Bureau.

Stone M. 2002. A food revolution in Berkeley: Fighting malnutrition and disease, teaching ecological literacy, and giving hope to family farmers begins with kids growing their own food. *Whole Earth* (107):38-47.

Story M, Hayes M, Kalina B. 1996. Availability of foods in high schools: Is there cause for concern? *J Am Diet Assoc* 96(2):123-126.

Stuhldreher WL, Koehler AN, Harrison MK, Deel H. 1998. The West Virginia standards for school nutrition. *J Child Nutr Management* 22:79-86.

Trost SG, Pate RR, Sallis JF, Freedson PS, Taylor WC, Dowda M, Sirard J. 2002. Age and gender differences in objectively measured physical activity in youth. *Med Sci Sports Exerc* 34(2):350-355.

United Kingdom Department of Health. 2002. *The National School Fruit Scheme: Evaluation Summary*. London: Wellington House. [Online]. Available: www.doh.gov.uk/schoolfruitscheme [accessed April 6, 2004].

USDA. 2001a. *Foods Sold in Competition with USDA School Meal Programs: A Report to Congress*. Washington, DC: USDA. [Online]. Available: http://www.fns.usda.gov/cnd/Lunch/CompetitiveFoods/report_congress.htm [accessed November 19, 2003].

USDA. 2001b. *School Nutrition Dietary Assessment Study. II: Summary of Findings.* Nutrition Assistance Program Report Series. CN-01-SNDAIIFR. Alexandria, VA: USDA.

USDA. 2002. *School Lunch Salad Bars.* Nutrition Assistance Program Report Series. Food and Nutrition Service. CN-02-SB. Alexandria, VA: USDA.

USDA. 2003. *The Food Assistance Landscape.* Food Assistance and Nutrition Research Report Number 28-4. Washington, DC: USDA.

USDA. 2004a. *National School Lunch Program.* [Online]. Available: http://www.fns.usda.gov/cnd/lunch/AboutLunch/NSLPFactSheet.htm [accessed May 18, 2004].

USDA. 2004b. *Menu Planner for Healthy School Meals.* [Online]. Available: http://schoolmeals.nal.usda.gov/Recipes/menuplan/menuplan.html [accessed April 6, 2004].

USDA. 2004c. *The School Meals Implementation Study. Third Year Report.* [Online]. Available: http://www.fns.usda.gov/oane/ [accessed April 6, 2004].

USDA (U.S. Department of Agriculture), DHHS (U.S. Department of Health and Human Services). 2000. *Nutrition and Your Health: Dietary Guidelines for Americans.* Home and Garden Bulletin No. 232, 5th ed. Washington, DC: Government Printing Office.

U.S. Department of Education. 2002. *Projections of Education Statistics to 2012.* National Center for Education Statistics Report 2002-030. Washington, DC: U.S. Department of Education. [Online]. Available: http://nces.ed.gov/pubs2002/2002030.pdf [accessed May 27, 2004].

U.S. Department of Education. 2004. *21st Century Community Learning Centers.* [Online]. Available: http://www.ed.gov/programs/21stcclc/index.html [accessed April 6, 2004].

Vandell DL, Shumow L. 1999. After-school child care programs. *Future Child* 9(2):64-80.

Vandongen R, Jenner DA, Thompson C, Taggart AC, Spickett EE, Burke V, Beilin LJ, Milligan RA, Dunbar DL. 1995. A controlled evaluation of a fitness and nutrition intervention program on cardiovascular health in 10- to 12-year-old children. *Prev Med* 24(1):9-22.

Walter HJ, Hofman A, Connelly PA, Barrett LT, Kost KL. 1985. Primary prevention of chronic disease in childhood: Changes in risk factors after one year of intervention. *Am J Epidemiol* 122(5):772-781.

Wechsler H, Devereaux RS, Davis M, Collins J. 2000. Using the school environment to promote physical activity and healthy eating. *Prev Med* 31(2 Part 2):S121-S137.

Wechsler H, Brener ND, Kuester S, Miller C. 2001. Food service and foods and beverages available at school: Results from the School Health Policies and Programs Study 2000. *J Sch Health* 71(7):313-324.

Whitaker RC, Wright JA, Finch AJ, Psaty BM. 1993. An environmental intervention to reduce dietary fat in school lunches. *Pediatrics* 91(6):1107-1111.

Whitaker RC, Wright JA, Koepsell TD, Finch AJ, Psaty BM. 1994. Randomized intervention to increase children's selection of low-fat foods in school lunches. *J Pediatr* 125(4):535-540.

Wilcox BL, Kunkel D, Cantor J, Dowrick P, Linn S, Palmer E. 2004. *Report of the APA Task Force on Advertising and Children.* Washington, DC: American Psychological Association.

Zive MM, Elder JP, Prochaska JJ, Conway TL, Pelletier RL, Marshall S, Sallis JF. 2002. Sources of dietary fat in middle schools. *Prev Med* 35(4):376-382.

8

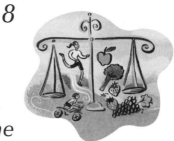

Home

A child's health and well-being are fostered by a home environment with engaged and skillful parenting that models, values, and encourages sensible eating habits and a physically active lifestyle. By promoting certain values and attitudes, by rewarding or reinforcing specific behaviors, and by serving as role models, parents can have a profound influence on their children. It is not surprising, therefore, that sedentary behaviors, obesity, and other chronic disease risk factors tend to cluster within families. Although some of these risk factors may have a genetic component, most have strong behavioral aspects. The family is thus an appropriate and important target for interventions designed to prevent obesity in children through increasing physical activity levels and promoting healthful eating behaviors.

In the United States in the 21st century, there are a great many pressures on parents and children that can adversely affect daily family life. For example, with the frequent need for both parents to work long hours, it has become more difficult for many parents to play with or monitor their children and to prepare home-cooked meals for them. Of two-parent households, 62.4 percent have both parents in the labor force; in one-parent homes, 77.1 percent of the mothers and 88.7 percent of fathers are working (Fields, 2003). Because the school day is shorter than the work day, many children come home to an empty house, where they may be unsupervised for several hours (Smith, 2002). In a national survey, parents report being well aware of the need to spend more time with their children but believe they do not have such time available (Hewlett and West, 1998). Parents from diverse socioeconomic categories actually cite a "parental time famine"—insufficient time to spend with their children. Economic and time constraints, as well as the stresses and challenges of daily living, may make healthful eating and increased physical activity a difficult reality on a day-to-day basis for many families (Devine et al., 2003).

The committee has adopted an ecological framework that considers children and youth as being influenced primarily by the family, particularly in the younger years, though other micro-environments—including the neighborhood, workplace, and school—also have important impacts on parenting and on individual and family functioning (see Chapter 3). In this ecological framework, parenting is influenced by the larger (macro) economic, political, social, and physical environments, as well as by socioeconomic status, parental goals, personal resources, and child characteristics (Parke and Buriel, 1998). Cultural norms are also an important factor. For example, parents may feel pressured to contribute cookies or soft drinks to the classroom or child-care setting if the other children are bringing in similar foods and beverages. On the other hand, if new values about what constitutes appropriate food choices for children become normative, this can produce positive changes in individual families and in their children's daytime environments.

The ecological perspective leads to strategies that target parents directly, as well as to other strategies designed to influence contextual factors that might otherwise serve to undermine healthful family values and practices. Therefore, a number of the committee's recommendations focus on promoting changes in nonhome settings (e.g., schools, communities, the built environment, the media) in order to support parents in their efforts to serve as positive models for children's eating and physical activity and to allow them to provide children with appropriate environments for preventing obesity. This is particularly important for families from high-risk populations who live in conditions that are not supportive of healthful lifestyles.

From a practical standpoint, parents play a fundamental role as household policy makers. They make daily decisions on recreational opportunities, food availability at home, and children's allowances; they determine the setting for foods eaten in the home; and they implement countless other rules and policies that influence the extent to which various members of the family engage in healthful eating and physical activity.

The committee acknowledges the broad and diverse nature of families in the United States. According to a recent U.S. Census Bureau report, in 2002 there were more than 72 million children (under 18 years of age) in the United States (Fields, 2003). Approximately 69 percent of them lived with two parents, 23 percent lived with only their mother, approximately 5 percent lived with their father, and 4 percent lived with other family members, usually grandparents, or in other situations (Fields, 2003). This report uses the term "parents" in its broadest sense to incorporate all those who are primary caregivers to children in the home.

Although treatment of childhood obesity is beyond the scope of this report, treatment studies have demonstrated that intensive involvement of parents in interventions to change obese children's dietary and physical activity behaviors has contributed to success in weight loss and long-term weight maintenance (Coates et al., 1982; Kirschenbaum et al., 1984; Epstein et al., 1990, 1994; Golan et al., 1998; Golan and Crow, 2004). It is plausible that family-based strategies that prevent weight re-gain in these studies are likely to be informative in the prevention of obesity. The fundamental influence of parents on the eating behavior of their children has also been demonstrated in the prevention of eating disorders (Graber and Brooks-Gunn, 1996). Finally, a 10-year longitudinal study conducted in Denmark has identified parental neglect as a powerful predictor of the subsequent development of obesity (as compared to putative biological predictors such as obesity in one or both parents) (Lissau and Sorensen, 1994).

While the home is an influential setting, it is also the least accessible for health promotion efforts. Mechanisms for parent education are varied and many provide only brief opportunities for health-care professionals, teachers, or others to interact with parents and share information and resources. As discussed throughout the report, there are resources in the school and the broader community that can support and inform parents and caregivers, children, and youth (see Chapters 6 and 7).

In the remainder of this chapter, the committee explores some of the ways in which parents and families can encourage healthful eating behaviors and increased physical activity. This report is not the place for an exhaustive discussion of diet and physical activity, nor is it meant to be the definitive source for parental advice; rather, the committee sought to present some actionable steps that can be taken by parents, families, children, and youth. It is important to note that many families are already quite physically active and put time and effort into providing healthful meals. It is important that parents and children extend these efforts and priorities to their schools, neighborhoods, and communities (Chapters 6 and 7) and become involved in ensuring that opportunities are made available and expanded for all families.

PROMOTING HEALTHFUL EATING BEHAVIORS

For decades, scientists have suggested that there are critical periods in the brain development of animals and humans that may profoundly affect food intake and body weight (in particular, body fat) beginning in utero—when many of the systems that regulate food intake and body weight initially develop. The factors that influence the quantity and quality of the maternal diet at the time of conception and throughout pregnancy—some of which may be within the control of the mother, while others result from social and economic environments—are thus important to consider. A recent study of 8,494 low-income children found that maternal obesity in the first trimester of pregnancy more than doubled the risk of the child being obese at 2 to 4 years of age (Whitaker, 2004). Furthermore, there are concerns that the offspring of mothers with gestational diabetes mellitus may be at higher risk for obesity, but the results are inconsistent (Silverman et al., 1998; Whitaker et al., 1998; Gillman et al., 2003). Needless to say, women of child-bearing years should pursue a healthful lifestyle that emphasizes sound dietary and physical activity habits, and because of the importance of a healthy maternal body weight at conception and adequate weight gain during pregnancy, these goals should be embraced and nurtured by the entire family.

Infancy

Researchers are examining early determinants of obesity, including factors during infancy; however, much remains to be learned. Issues being explored include the combined effects of low birthweight followed by rapid weight gain during early infancy (Stettler et al., 2002, 2003).

The associations between various feeding methods during infancy and childhood obesity have been the most thoroughly explored. Epidemiological data suggest that breastfeeding, even as it is generally practiced in the United States—that is, as a nonexclusive source of nutrition, usually of short duration—confers a small but significant degree of protection from childhood obesity, although it is not certain why this is so or the extent to which other factors may confound this finding. A recent review of 11 epidemiologic studies with adequate sample size[1] found that eight of the studies showed breastfed children to be at a lower risk of overweight after controlling for potential confounders (Dewey, 2003). Studies published since that review have generally confirmed that finding but not in all subpopulations. For example, Bergmann and colleagues (2003) examined the weight status of a cohort of children at 6 years of age and found that those who were bottle fed as infants had a higher prevalence of obesity than those who were breastfed. Other risk factors for adiposity at 6 years of age

---

[1]Criteria for studies in this review were (1) sample size of greater than 100 children per feeding group (in most cases breastfeeding versus formula feeding); (2) age at follow-up of over 3 years; and (3) measured outcomes includes percentage of children who were overweight (Dewey, 2003).

included overweight of the mother, maternal smoking during pregnancy, and low social status. In research on the weight status of 12,587 children in the United States at 4 years of age, Grummer-Strawn and Mei (2004) found that greater duration of breastfeeding showed a protective effect on the risk of overweight among non-Hispanic whites, but not among non-Hispanic blacks or Hispanics. The reasons for differences among ethnic groups are not clear; the study did not examine supplementation by formula or foods or varying dietary or physical activity patterns. A study by Bogen and colleagues (2004) also found no association between breastfeeding and obesity among 20,518 low-income black children (the study sample did not include Hispanics).

Breastfeeding is thought to promote the infant's ability to regulate energy intake, allowing him or her to eat in response to internal hunger and satiety cues—that is, to assume greater control in determining meal size (Fisher et al., 2000). In contrast, a caregiver who is formula feeding an infant may use visual information about how much remains in the bottle to "encourage" the infant to finish the bottle, potentially fostering overfeeding. Even if the caregiver makes no such effort, the uniform composition of formula, both during a single feeding and over the duration of infancy, may not provide the infant with the same metabolic/hormonal cues that are supplied with breast milk. Because the composition of breast milk changes during each feed and from one feeding to the next over the course of lactation, the full effects of this variation are not experienced when breastfeeding is nonexclusive or of short duration (Lederman et al., 2004).

Factors in breast milk may elicit metabolic programming effects that contribute to the protective association between breastfeeding and childhood obesity. There is the possibility that other parental lifestyle factors and behaviors, not yet identified, may undermine or overwhelm that protection (Dewey, 2003). Lifestyle and cultural factors may also explain the discrepant findings among different ethnic groups. It is worth emphasizing that a protective effect of breastfeeding was found in the majority of studies reviewed although not in all. But in none of the 11 studies reviewed by Dewey (2003) or those published since that review has breastfeeding been associated with increased risk for childhood obesity; breastfeeding was found to be either protective or neutral. None of the studies have found formula feeding to be protective against childhood obesity.

Research indicates that many flavors from the mother's diet are transmitted to her breast milk (Mennella and Beauchamp, 1991; Mennella, 1995). By the time complementary foods are introduced, therefore, the breastfed infant has already had experience with a variety of flavors from the adult diet, which may promote acceptance of foods during weaning (Sullivan and Birch, 1994; Mennella et al., 2001; Lederman et al., 2004). Experience with numerous flavors in breast milk (as opposed to the lack of variety experienced by the formula-fed infant) may also have more general effects, promoting the infant's acceptance of a wide range of new foods as he or she matures; further research is needed in this area (Mennella and Beauchamp, 1998; Lederman et al., 2004).

Much remains to be learned about the extent of the association between breastfeeding and childhood obesity. Nonetheless, breastfeeding is likely to be at least weakly protective against obesity, and despite the fact that the protective effects may be overwhelmed by events and environmental factors that occur later in childhood, there are numerous ancillary benefits of breastfeeding (AAP, 2004). **Breastfeeding is recommended for all infants. Exclusive breastfeeding is recommended for the first 4 to 6 months of life and breastfeeding, along with the age-appropriate introduction of complementary foods, is encouraged for the first year of life.** This is in accordance with the American Academy of Pediatrics (2004) statement recommending breastfeeding and stating that in developed countries "complementary foods may be introduced between 4 and 6 months" and the World Health Organization (2003) recommendation that encourages exclusive breastfeeding for the first 6 months of life, to the extent that this is practical for the mother and family.

Another issue that is discussed regarding infant feeding is serving size— ensuring that infants receive the appropriate amounts of milk or foods. Research has shown that early in life, infants are responsive to the energy density of food and are capable of controlling the volume taken during a feeding. Thus, even by about 6 weeks of age, infants can adjust the volume of formula consumed based on the energy density of the formula, so that total energy intake remains relatively constant (Fomon et al., 1975). Nonetheless, there is the possibility that infants can be coaxed to eat beyond satiety and that has been postulated by several researchers as a potential contributor to childhood obesity (Bergmann et al., 2003; Dewey, 2003; Lederman et al., 2004). Concern has been expressed that precocious introduction of sweetened beverages and high-fat/sweet-tasting foods may be important contributors to childhood obesity by possibly developing early preferences for such foods and beverages (Fox et al., 2004; Lederman et al., 2004). Documentation that such concerns are well founded are the findings from the Feeding Infants and Toddlers Study (FITS) that soft drinks and French fries are being fed to infants as young as 7 months of age (Fox et al., 2004).

Toddlers and Young Children

Children tend to avoid new foods. But during the transition from the exclusive milk diet of infancy to consuming a varied, modified adult diet, virtually all foods are new to the child. Fortunately, it has been found that if children have opportunities to try new foods without being coerced to eat them, many of these foods, even if initially rejected, will become part of their diet (Birch and Marlin, 1982; Loewen and Pliner, 1999). Such early experience with new options will be especially important in learning to accept fruits, vegetables, and other nutrient-rich foods later on in life (Birch, 1999; Skinner et al., 2002).

Food flavor preferences are powerful determinants of intake for children. Because infants are predisposed to prefer sweet and salty tastes, they tend to readily accept foods that are sweet or salty (Cowart, 1981; Beauchamp and Cowart, 1985; Mennella and Beauchamp, 1998). In contrast, preferences for foods that lack such tastes are learned, requiring repeated positive experiences.

Initial rejection of new foods is expected and normal. As many as five to ten exposures may be needed before certain new foods are accepted, and repeated experience is most critical during the first few years of life. Recent findings reveal that parent-led exposure can increase children's acceptance of vegetables (Wardle et al., 2003; Lederman et al., 2004), and that childcare and preschool settings are also effective locations for promoting children's acceptance of new foods (Nicklas et al., 2001). Research also shows that increasing the school based availability and accessibility of fruits and vegetables in particular can promote children's intake, at school as well as at home (Baranowski et al., 2000; Weber Cullen et al., 2000).

Of course, children can be equally responsive to less healthful options when made available. Because their preferences for high-fat, energy-dense foods are, in part, learned, providing children with frequent exposure to such foods may reinforce their liking for them (Johnson SL et al., 1991). In the 2002 FITS, which examined the dietary intake of 3,022 infants and toddlers, parents reported that 23 percent of infants and 33 percent of toddlers had not consumed any fruit during the preceding 24 hours; similarly 18 percent and 33 percent of infants and toddlers, respectively, had not consumed any vegetables (Fox et al., 2004). This study also reported changes in intake from 4 to 8 months of age when deep yellow vegetables (e.g., carrots, sweet potatoes, squash) were the vegetables consumed most often, to the patterns at 15 to 18 months, when French fries or other fried potatoes were the predominant vegetables (Fox et al., 2004). **Parents should promote healthful food choices among toddlers and young children by making a variety of nutritious, low-energy-dense foods, such as fruits and vegetables, available to them. Encouraging toddlers and young children to try a variety of foods, including fruits and vegetables, often involves offering new foods multiple times.**

Beyond quality is the issue of quantity. Limited empirical evidence suggests that children, especially those in the toddler years, have a physiological sense of satiety that guides them to eat only until they are full.

McConahy and colleagues (2002) found that the food portion sizes consumed by children 1 to 2 years of age have been consistent over the past 20 years. However, as children develop, they become increasingly responsive to environmental cues such as portion size; by the age of 5 years, larger portions can lead to increased food intake (Rolls et al., 2000). This issue is discussed further below.

Older Children and Youth

As children develop, they play an expanding role in determining the foods that are available to them. They make their own choices at school and in other out-of-home settings, and they increasingly influence family food purchases. Furthermore, as they begin to be influenced by their peers and the broader culture, they may make certain food choices based on popular appeal. It is also important to note, however, that parents are important role models and their dietary intake influences that of their children (see section below on role models).

Food and Beverage Selection and Availability

Parents can promote wise food selections and a wholesome overall diet by making nutritious options available to children. Research has shown that children's consumption of fruit, 100 percent fruit juice, and vegetables are positively influenced by the availability and accessibility of these foods in the home (Nicklas et al., 2001; Cullen et al., 2003). Similarly, parents can limit the types and quantity of energy-dense high-calorie foods (e.g., cookies, chips) that are available in the home, particularly those that have low nutrient content. Improved consumer nutrition information in restaurants and on food labels (see Chapter 5) will provide parents and young people with enhanced information on which to base their dietary decisions.

Parents are responsive to children's attempts to influence food purchases (Galst and White, 1976). Interviews with 500 children and youth aged 8 to 17 years found that 78 percent of respondents noted that they influence family food purchases (Roper ASW, 2003). For their part, 84 percent of the parents stated that their children do indeed influence such purchases.

The Dietary Guidelines for Americans and the Food Guide Pyramid provide information on the types of foods that make up a balanced and nutritious diet (USDA and DHHS, 2000; USDA, 2004). Although it is not the purpose of this report to duplicate that information, **the committee wishes to emphasize the responsibilities of children (particularly older children), youth, and parents in choosing and providing a balanced diet. Parents should promote healthful food choices by school-age children and** youth by making a variety of nutritious, low-energy-dense foods, such as fruits and vegetables, available in the home. Because nutrient quality should be a major consideration in selecting the family's foods and beverages, parents should limit their purchases of items characterized by high caloric content and low nutrient density.

The mealtime setting has been shown to affect diet quality in children and youth. Several studies have shown that increased frequency of family dinners is positively associated with older children's and adolescents' consumption of fruits and vegetables, grains, and calcium-rich foods, and negatively associated with their consumption of fried food and soft drinks (Gillman et al., 2000; Neumark-Sztainer et al., 2003a). The influence of watching television during mealtime is another area for further research. Coon and colleagues (2001) found that watching television during mealtime was associated with consumption of fewer fruits and vegetables and increased consumption of soft drinks, salty snacks, pizza, and red meat.

One of the issues that has been raised regarding childhood obesity is the potential role of sweetened beverages, such as soft drinks and "flavored drinks" (not 100 percent juices). These beverages do not provide nutrients that are needed by growing children, but do increase the caloric intake. Nevertheless, soft drink consumption more than tripled among adolescent boys between 1977-1978 and 1994, rising from 7 to 22 ounces per day (Guthrie and Morton, 2000; French et al., 2003). By the time they are 14 years of age, 32 percent of adolescent girls and 52 percent of boys are consuming three or more eight-ounce servings of soft drinks daily (Gleason and Suitor, 2001). FITS reported that infants as young as 7 months of age are consuming soft drinks as well (Fox et al., 2004). There are concerns about the effect of increased soft drink consumption on reducing micronutrient intakes and increasing energy intake (IOM, 2002) and on displacing the intake of more nutrient-rich options such as milk (ADA, 2004). Milk consumption by adolescents declined 36 percent from 1965 to 1996 (Cavadini et al., 2000). An analysis of data from the 1994-1996, 1998 Continuing Survey of Food Intakes by Individuals (CSFII) found that children and adolescents (>12 years of age) drank more soft drinks than milk, 100 percent juices, or fruit drinks (Rampersaud et al., 2003).

The link between beverage consumption and body mass index (BMI) is not definitive. In an analysis of CSFII data, Forshee and Storey (2003) reported that BMI calculated from self-reported height and weight had little or no cross-sectional association with beverage consumption. In contrast, in a prospective study of middle schoolers in which height and weight were measured directly, Ludwig and colleagues (2001) reported significant positive associations between sweetened beverage consumption and increases in BMI and obesity incidence. In a recent randomized controlled trial of a 1-year classroom-based intervention focused on carbonated beverages, dental health, and dietary intake, James and colleagues (2004) reported a significant decrease in the prevalence of overweight and obesity in the group of children receiving the intervention compared to controls. However, methodological limitations prevent conclusions regarding whether reducing soft drink consumption led to the observed changes in obesity prevalence (French et al., 2004). Further, experimental studies of the effects of reducing sweetened beverage intakes are needed to examine the potential efficacy of this approach for reducing weight gain, as well as the hypothesized causal link between sweetened beverage consumption and obesity.

Much remains to be learned about whether a unique association exists between intake of sweetened beverages and changes in BMI. Because of concerns about excessive consumption of sweetened options and the displacement of more nutrient-rich or lower calorie alternatives, children should be encouraged to avoid high-calorie, nutrient-poor beverages.

Portion Control and Eating in the Absence of Hunger

In addition to ensuring the quality of children's diets, it is important for parents to consider the quantity of food being consumed. Researchers examining the recent increases in portion sizes have found that Americans consumed larger portion sizes of nearly one-third of 107 widely consumed foods when comparing 1989-1991 with 1994-1996 data (Nestle, 2003; Smiciklas-Wright et al., 2003).

Although long-term studies investigating the effects of portion size on weight gain are lacking, short-term studies confirm that larger portions do increase intake, especially among adults and children aged 5 years and older. In research involving a range of foods that included sandwiches, macaroni and cheese, popcorn, and cookies, the larger the portion size offered, the larger the amount consumed (reviewed by Rolls, 2003; Diliberti et al., 2004).

While evidence shows that infants and toddlers can self-regulate their energy intake (discussed earlier), a series of studies found that by the age of 5 many children eat what they are served; physiological satiety cues, if they are present, are overridden by environmental cues (such as larger portion sizes) that stimulate them to eat more, even if they are not hungry (Rolls et al., 2000). In this research, 3- to 5-year-olds were fed a standard lunch on two different days in their usual preschool setting. Lunches differed only in the portion size of the entrée. Older preschoolers responded in much the same way that adults do; when given a larger portion, they ate more. But younger children were relatively unresponsive to portion size, providing more indirect support that they are still eating primarily in response to internal signals of hunger and satiety (Rolls et al., 2000; see Rolls, 2003 for a review of the adult literature).

In subsequent research, Orlet-Fisher and colleagues (2003) explored the effects of children's chronic exposure to large portions. Results indicated that when served larger portions, children ate substantially more food—but giving them the opportunity to serve themselves mitigated these effects because they tended to self-select smaller portions. In one study, they consumed 25 percent less of the lunch entrée when they served themselves, as compared to other occasions when a larger portion was served to them (Orlet-Fisher et al., 2003). The portion sizes that the children self-selected and consumed were more similar to standard, recommended serving sizes than to the large portions they had been offered, suggesting that giving children control over portion size may prevent overeating or eating in the absence of hunger.

The goal for parents is to promote the normal and effective development of internal satiety cues so that children learn to rely on their own sense of fullness. However, research suggests that restricting palatable foods can lead to increased preference for these foods and that pressuring children to "clean the plate" can encourage overeating. Such practices can prompt children to attend to external cues, such as the availability of food or the amount remaining on the plate, and divert them from internal cues of hunger and satiety (Birch et al., 1987; Fisher and Birch, 1999; Orlet-Fisher et al., 2003). Golan and Crow (2004) point out the impact of parenting styles on children's eating behaviors: "authoritative parenting (in which parents are both firm and supportive and assume a leadership role in the environmental change with appropriate granting of child's autonomy) rather than authoritarian style (which controls child-feeding practices) was found to be the effective parental child-feeding modality" (p. 358).

Child characteristics influence the choice of these feeding practices; overweight children tend to elicit higher levels of parental restriction, and thinner children are more likely to be pressured to eat. Pressure and restriction tend to be used with different foods (pressure with perceived "healthful foods" that parents want to encourage; restriction with some snack foods that parents want to limit), but a parent who uses one tactic is likely to use the other as well (Fisher et al., 2002). However, one of the limitations of this research to date is that it has been conducted with middle-class white families and sometimes only with one gender, severely limiting the ability to generalize.

Research has also shown that using foods as rewards or in other positive contexts can result in greater preference for and intake of those foods (Birch et al., 1980; Birch, 1981). Furthermore, this practice dissociates eating from hunger. Parents should avoid using food as a reward.

More research is also needed to understand developmental progression—the neural and physiological underpinnings of hunger and satiety—and the regulation of food intake and energy balance. It is also important to learn more about how the timing of snacks and meals influence eating and weight status.

Meanwhile, research results that have been obtained thus far should prompt parents to consider making constructive family policies that move away from pressures and restrictions and more toward positive practices regarding what, where, and when foods and beverages can be consumed. Such practices, by which parents can help children learn to regulate their own energy intake, include the following:

- Allow children to determine their own portions at meals.
- Encourage children to pay attention to their own internal signals of fullness and permit them to decide when they have finished eating a meal. Do not insist on their "cleaning the plate."
- Avoid using food as a reward. This practice dissociates eating from hunger and clearly establishes preferences for foods used as rewards.
- Make fruits and vegetables readily available in the home to encourage selection of these foods as snacks and desserts.
- Offer smaller portions of foods (e.g., smaller cookies or slices of pizza).
- Carefully consider the quality of and the possible need to limit the types of snack foods and beverages that are available and accessible to children in the home.

Parents should educate their children, from a young age, about making decisions regarding dietary intake, so that as they get older, the children can take on increasing responsibility for decisions regarding the types and amounts of foods and beverages they consume. While permitting children to determine portion sizes for themselves, parents should encourage smaller portions with an option for seconds. For children too young to serve themselves, parents should offer age-appropriate portion sizes.

PROMOTING PHYSICAL ACTIVITY

There is still much to be learned about the determinants of physical activity and fitness in children and adolescents and how to influence their level of activity throughout the developmental stages. As discussed throughout the report, physical activity can influence the body-fat level of children (Gutin et al., 2004).

Correlates of Physical Activity

Developmental, Biological, and Psychosocial Correlates

Children's gender and age are both important factors to consider in examining physical activity levels. Boys are generally more involved in moderate to vigorous physical activity than are girls (DHHS, 1996; Sallis et al., 2000). Explanations may include differential development of motor skills, body composition differences during growth, variations in socialization regarding sports and physical activity, and other social and environmental factors (Sallis et al., 1992; Kohl and Hobbs, 1998). From a developmental perspective, unstructured gross motor play is important in young children for optimal brain development and is important for social, emotional, and cognitive development (Butcher and Eaton, 1989; Pica, 1997). As children get older they are generally less physically active, although this may be more true for girls than for boys (Goran et al., 1999). The social, psychological, and behavioral effects of puberty may play an important role in physical activity levels (Lindquist et al., 1999), although more research is needed, particularly research that focuses on measured physical activity (e.g., using accelerometry) rather than self-report or other indirect methods of documenting physical activity.

The personal psychosocial factors that influence physical activity differ somewhat between children and adolescents. Intention to be physically active, preference for physical activity, positive beliefs about physical activity, enjoyment of physical activity, and enjoyment of physical education classes have been shown to be positively associated with physical activity in children (Stucky-Ropp and DiLorenzo, 1993; Pate et al., 1997; Trost et al., 1997, 1999; DiLorenzo et al., 1998; Sallis et al., 2000). Perceived barriers to physical activity (including not enough time or the activity is too hard) have been found to be negatively associated with physical activity behavior in children (Sallis et al., 2000).

In adolescents, correlates of physical activity include perceived activity competence, intention to be active, sensation seeking, perception of academic rank and academic expectations, and depression (an inverse correlate) (Sallis et al., 2000; Motl et al., 2002; Schmitz et al., 2002). Perceived self-worth, perceived time constraints, and value placed on health and appearance may influence prevalence of physical activity or change in physical activity levels in adolescent girls (Schmitz et al., 2002; Neumark-Sztainer et al., 2003b).

Physical activity self-efficacy (confidence in one's ability to participate in exercise) has been widely studied as a potential psychosocial correlate of increased levels of physical activity, but the association is not clear in children and adolescents (CDC, 1997).

Social Environment Correlates

The social environment in which children live strongly influences their health behaviors in general and levels of physical activity in particular, and the primary social influences on young people are their family and peers. But although it is intuitively attractive to hypothesize that parents' physical activity behavior correlates with that of their children, research does not definitively support that hypothesis. Sallis and colleagues (2000), in a review of correlational studies, reported that parents' physical activity had an indeterminate relationship to children's physical activity. Kohl and Hobbs (1998), however, reported that children whose parents are physically active are much more likely than other children to be physically active.

In any case, parents' *support* for a child or adolescent's physical activity, and the perceptions of their parents' physical activity behavior, do appear to be important correlates of physical activity in children and youth. Parental support can include a wide range of actions, from encouraging the child or adolescent to try or to continue a new activity, to providing transportation to an activity class, to purchasing sports equipment.

Researchers have identified several family variables, including support for physical activity, mother's perception of barriers to physical activity, and parental modeling of physical activity, to be associated with physical activity levels in fifth- and sixth-grade boys and girls (Stucky-Ropp and DiLorenzo, 1993; DiLorenzo et al., 1998). Trost and colleagues (1997, 1999) found that perception of mother's physical activity level was a correlate of vigorous physical activity in fifth-grade girls and that active sixth-grade boys were more likely than nonactive boys to report that their mothers were physically active. Other studies have also identified family support for physical activity as a correlate of children's physical activity (Sallis et al., 2000; Zakarian et al., 1994).

Although the focus of influence in adolescence shifts from family to peers, parents and other family members continue to influence teenagers' physical activity. In the studies reviewed by Sallis and colleagues (2000), parental support, direct help from parents in being physically active, and siblings' physical activity were consistently correlated with adolescents' physical activity. McGuire and colleagues (2002) found a significant, though modest, relationship between parents' reported encouragement and physical activity levels in female adolescents of all racial and ethnic groups and in African-American and white boys. In a population of inactive adolescent girls, social support from parents, peers, and teachers was consistently and positively associated with change in physical activity over time (Neumark-Sztainer et al., 2003b). Researchers did not find a clear positive correlation between parents' reported physical activity behaviors and those of their teenage children (McGuire et al., 2002).

Although Schmitz and colleagues (2002) found that young adolescents who received free or reduced-price lunches reported higher levels of physical activity, most studies report a positive correlation between parents' education and socioeconomic status (SES) and children's physical activity (Pate et al., 1996; Gordon-Larsen et al., 2000). Parents who have the time and resources to participate in physical activity themselves may be better able to encourage their children to do likewise, and they are more apt to have the resources to enroll their children in sporting activities and provide sports equipment and the associated transport (Koivisto et al., 1994; Sallis et al., 1999). Researchers have identified other barriers faced by low-income families with regard to healthful physical activity behaviors, including a lack of safe places for physical activity (AAP, 2003).

Physical Environment Correlates

As discussed in Chapters 6 and 7 on communities and schools, there are many factors—including safety and access to physical activity opportunities—that play important roles in determining when, where, and how children engage in physical activity. One of the strongest correlates of physical activity in children is the amount of time spent outside (Klesges et al., 1990; Baranowski et al., 1993; Sallis et al., 1993). In most homes, after all, there are limited options for physical activity inside the home, and it is outdoors where children are generally more physically active and where more energy is expended.

Family-Based Interventions

A recent comprehensive review of physical activity interventions identified 11 studies that were family-based and met the methodological criteria of the Task Force on Community Preventive Services (Kahn et al., 2002). Most of these interventions were implemented as parts of multicomponent school-based studies such as the Child and Adolescent Trial for Cardiovascular Health (described in Chapter 7) and generally involved parent-child activities that were completed at home (Johnson CC et al., 1991; Hopper et al., 1992, 1996; Davis et al., 1995; Edmundson et al., 1996; Sallis et al., 1997; Manios et al., 1999). Four other family-based studies (Nader et al., 1983, 1989; Bishop and Donnelly, 1987; Baranowski et al., 1990) examined interventions to educate families on nutrition and physical activity through sessions at community centers or schools. The interventions that were part of a school-based program were marginally more effective in increasing physical activity or improving indicators of cardiovascular fitness, but it was not possible to differentiate the effects of the family intervention from those of the other study components. In another study, Taggart and colleagues (1986) demonstrated that a program that used parent training and family contracting increased physical activity in children with low fitness levels.

More remains to be learned about developmentally appropriate interventions to encourage physical activity, as well as about the changes in the nature and duration of physical activity throughout childhood and adolescence. The development of better tools for measuring physical activity will help to eliminate some of the inconsistencies found in the data and is an important research need. It is also important to learn more about the factors during childhood and adolescence that foster lifelong habits of daily physical activity.

Promoting Physical Activity

Parents should promote physical activity by supporting and encouraging children and youth to be active and play outdoors and participate in opportunities for physical activity. This may increase the time that parents spend outdoors interacting with their children or ensuring their safety or going with their children to the park, playground, gymnasium, or other appropriate location for physical activity. The ancillary benefits of physical activity and outdoor play and interaction are numerous. For children, youth, and parents, the time spent interacting outdoors increases opportunities for social contact, nurturing, bonding, and maturational guidance. In some residential areas, where safety is such a concern that parents cannot let their children play outside the home, there is a particular need for the community to develop and foster opportunities for outside play—including parks, playgrounds, and recreational facilities (see Chapter 6).

There are numerous ways in which parents can help to increase their child's or adolescent's physical activity levels by supporting and engaging in a range of recreational or utilitarian (e.g., walking to the grocery store) activities that may promote lifelong habits of regular physical activity (Shape Up America, 2004). Examples include:

- Walking or bicycling (with proper safety measures including helmets) to run errands or as a regular means of transport
- Encouraging and monitoring outdoor play
- Assessing the community for opportunities for physical activity and supporting participation by the child and family (e.g., parks, baseball fields, soccer fields, lakes, pools, gyms, community and youth programs, recreational leagues, and camps)
- Engaging in family outings and vacations that are centered around physical activity
- Giving gifts (e.g., jump ropes, balls, sports equipment) that encourage activity.

Not every parent has the skills to coach a child in a particular physical activity, but parents can still function as "cheerleaders" for their child and adolescent. This type of emotional support is not only meaningful and rewarding to the child but also may encourage still more physical activity.

Furthermore, parents can be effective advocates in their schools and communities for increased recess, physical education, recreational facilities, playgrounds, parks, and sidewalks.

It is also important for parents, children, and youth to take advantage of the opportunities for physical activity that come along throughout the day and to realize that not all physical activity has to be a planned event. Examples include walking to do errands or having children walk at the grocery store or mall rather than ride in shopping carts or strollers.

DECREASING INACTIVITY

A complementary strategy for promoting physical activity among children and youth is to decrease their *in*activity. Of the sedentary behaviors that may be linked to the upsurge in childhood obesity, television watching has been most widely studied. Other types of screen time (such as computer use and video game playing) have not been researched as extensively with regard to obesity, though they share many similarities in principle; various combinations, in fact, are often examined along with television in studies of media use and obesity. One study found that the time spent watching television, taped television shows, or commercial videos averaged per day: 2.5 hours for children between the ages of 2 and 7, 4.5 hours for 8- to 13-year-olds, and 3.3 hours for 14- to 18-year-olds (Roberts et al., 1999). The 2003 Youth Risk Behavior Surveillance nationwide survey found that 38.2 percent of high school students reported watching television three hours or longer on an average school day; 67.2 percent of African-American students, 45.9 percent of Hispanic students, and 29.3 percent of white students reported three or more hours of television viewing (CDC, 2004c).

Television viewing may have a negative effect on both sides of the energy balance equation. It may displace active play and physical activity time, and it is associated with increased food and calorie intake—as an accompaniment of television viewing, as a result of food advertising, or both (Robinson, 2001a). Many epidemiological studies have found positive associations between increased prevalence of obesity or overweight and greater lengths of television viewing time, although comparing the results is difficult due to differences in methods and reporting (reviewed by Robinson, 2001b). Gortmaker and colleagues (1996) found a strong positive association between parent or child reports of children's television watching time and prevalence of obesity. This study of 746 children and youths (ages 10 to 15 years) found that those who watched more than five hours of television per day were 4.6 times as likely to be obese as those watching zero to two hours. This observation held when adjusted for maternal overweight, SES, and other factors.

Similarly, Crespo and colleagues (2001) found that in a sample of

4,069 children and adolescents aged 8 to 16 years, the prevalence of obesity was highest for those watching four or more hours of television a day and lowest among those watching one hour or less. Other studies have reported associations that were not statistically significant, but all have generally found associations of similar magnitude (reviewed by Robinson, 2001b). Dennison and colleagues (2002) found in a cross-sectional survey that children with televisions in their bedrooms spent an additional 4.6 hours per week watching television or videos. Furthermore, the investigators observed that the prevalence of BMIs greater than the 85th percentile was higher in children with a television in their bedroom than in those without one.

In attempting to determine how television viewing may promote childhood obesity, studies have examined the advertising of foods (particularly high-calorie, high-fat, or high-sugar foods and beverages), eating while watching television, decreased physical activity levels while viewing television, and the potential for physical activity that is lost due to time spent watching. An analysis of commercial advertising during children's programming time (Saturday morning television, in this study) found that more than half of the commercials (56.5 percent) were for food (Kotz and Story, 1994). A recent review of the literature on food advertising to children found that the four primary categories of food items advertised are breakfast cereals, snacks, candy, and soft drinks (Hastings et al., 2003). Additionally, the authors found a recent trend towards increased advertising by fast food restaurants. Research has shown that television advertising influences children's food knowledge, choices, and consumption of particular food products, as well as influencing purchase-related behavior and purchasing decisions (Gorn and Goldberg, 1982; Hastings et al., 2003).

Also, as noted earlier in this chapter, watching television during mealtime is associated with decreased intake of fruits and vegetables and increased consumption of soft drinks, salty snacks, pizza, and red meat (Coon et al., 2001). Children report consuming a large proportion of their daily calories while watching television, although there has not been evidence to date that the types or energy densities of foods that children eat while watching television differ significantly from those eaten when not watching (Matheson et al., 2004).

Studies of the nature and extent of associations between increased television viewing and decreased physical activity have produced inconsistent findings—possibly due, in part, to the known limitations of self- and parent-reporting on how children spend their time (Robinson, 2001b). A review by Sallis and colleagues (2000) noted that studies of children ages 4 to 12 had mixed results regarding the associations of sedentary behaviors (specifically, watching television and playing video games) with extent of physical activity, while in teenagers ages 13 to 18, there appeared to be no association. In one study of 191 3- to 4-year-olds that used direct observations of physical activity and television watching, physical activity levels were lowest during the longest periods of television watching (DuRant et al., 1994). In a study of sixth- and seventh-grade-girls, more hours of television watching was significantly but weakly associated with less reported physical activity (Robinson et al., 1993). Additionally, one experimental study of 13 8- to 12-year-old nonobese children did not find significant changes in short-term physical activity or energy expenditure when sedentary behavior (including television viewing) was decreased by 50 percent from baseline (Epstein et al., 2002). Natural experiments have found some evidence that introduction of television into communities where it did not exist previously does displace other more physical activities (Brown et al., 1974; Williams and Hanford, 1986). Thus, although a link between more screen time and less physical activity has face validity, clarification of this relationship must await the results of additional experimental studies with more objective measures.

Other factors that have been considered in the association of sedentary behaviors and obesity include computer use and video game play, parental patterns of sedentary behavior, parental monitoring of television viewing hours, and neighborhood characteristics such as safety of the area for outside play (Davison and Birch, 2001). Research has also been conducted to examine the possibility that television watching is associated with a decrease in children's metabolic rates, but results from those studies have been mixed (Klesges et al., 1993; Dietz et al., 1994; Buchowski and Sun, 1996).

A few family-based interventions have focused on reducing sedentary behaviors, particularly television watching, to influence eating and activity patterns, and ultimately to produce weight loss. Early results from these studies have shown promise, but are still too preliminary for making conclusions about their efficacy (Robinson et al., 2003). Indirect evidence supporting this approach, however, has come from two studies by Epstein and colleagues (1995, 2000) that tested the effect of reducing sedentary behaviors as part of an intensive, family-based weight-loss program for children who were already overweight. The program showed effects on weight loss that were at least comparable to efforts that targeted increasing physical activity directly or targeted the combination of decreasing sedentary behavior and increasing physical activity. This study demonstrates the validity of targeting decreased inactivity as a potentially effective strategy that is distinct from strategies seeking to increase physical activity.

Of most direct relevance to recommendations for preventing obesity are experimental studies showing that reducing the amount of television viewing and other sedentary behaviors reduces weight gain and prevalence of obesity both among population-based samples of children and adolescents (Gortmaker et al., 1999; Robinson, 1999) and groups of overweight children (Epstein et al., 1995). From a primary prevention perspective, two school-based interventions with population-based samples of children and adolescents demonstrated that reductions in screen time, whether alone (Robinson, 1999) or as part of a more comprehensive obesity prevention program (Gortmaker et al., 1999), resulted in decreased gain in BMI and body fatness and reduced prevalence of obesity.

Although the specific mechanism(s) of how reducing television viewing influences weight gain is, as yet, undetermined, these demonstrated effects on reduced weight gain and obesity provide sufficient rationale for the recommendation to reduce children's screen time. The committee concludes that reducing children's and youth's screen time is an important population-based strategy for preventing obesity in children and youth, and that a time-limit recommendation would be most useful to parents, policy makers, and child health and education advocates and professionals. The committee notes that there are many ancillary reasons for recommending limits on children's television viewing time (despite the demonstrated benefits of some media content). The American Academy of Pediatrics has recommended that televisions not be placed in children's bedrooms, and it urges parents to limit their children's television viewing time to no more than one to two hours of quality programming per day; it also recommends that television viewing among children younger than 2 years be discouraged altogether (AAP, 2001). Many other child and health advocacy organizations and agencies have made comparable recommendations for reductions in television and other screen viewing time for a variety of reasons including violent media content (APA and AAP, 1995; AMA, 1996; NEA, 1999; DHHS, 2000; AACAP, 2001; National PTA, 2001).

The committee recommends that parents should limit their children's television viewing and recreational screen time to less than two hours per day. This specific time limit is derived from the evidence provided by the two school-based primary prevention intervention studies that demonstrated reductions in body weight, body fat, and prevalence of obesity. The interventions in those trials set goals to limit television, videotape, and video game use to no more than seven hours per week (Robinson, 1999) and to limit television viewing to less than two hours in any one day (Gortmaker et al., 1999). (It should be noted that a key word here is "recreational." The committee's recommendation does not preclude the use of computers and other media for educational purposes.)

An important part of parenting involves monitoring children's behaviors and setting and enforcing limits on those behaviors. Such family policies should be set for a variety of reasons, including the protection of young children (e.g., keeping them from playing in the street) and assurance of their healthy development. Naturally, there is great variation in the nature and extent to which parents set limits and how those limits change as the child matures. One challenge for parents of older children is knowing how to involve them in decision-making so that they learn to apply limits for themselves; they should come to realize, for example, that they are responsible for their own health and need to practice health-promoting behaviors. But in the current food and activity environment—where palatable, energy-dense, and inexpensive foods are readily available and opportunities for sedentary behaviors are abundant—a degree of parental monitoring and limit setting is still needed to support eating and physical activity patterns that can maintain children's energy balance at a healthy weight.

PARENTS AS ROLE MODELS

Parents' eating behaviors can serve as models for children's behavior (Fisher and Birch, 1995; Cutting et al., 1999). Such models, however, can be either positive or negative. The current epidemic of adult obesity and the epidemiological data on adults' dietary and physical activity patterns suggest cause for concern (CDC, 2004a,b). But the public's growing awareness of the obesity epidemic and of the health consequences of obesity, in children and adults alike, may change these patterns. When parents adopt a healthier lifestyle, they may foster the development of healthful behaviors and patterns in their children, in addition to positively affecting their own well-being. Researchers have provided evidence that modeling and enhanced familiarity have independent significant effects on food intake (Cullen et al., 2000, 2003). With respect to physical activity, the provision of instrumental support for children's sports participation is associated with greater levels of physical activity among children (Davison et al., 2003).

Parents who consume fruits and vegetables, for example, have children who do the same (Cullen et al., 2001; Nicklas et al., 2001; Fisher et al., 2002). Comparable patterns are seen with milk intake, at least for mothers and daughters (Fisher et al., 2001). Similarly, parents who display their mastery of portion control can provide positive influences. Hill and colleagues have reported that mothers who diet or are restrained eaters tend to have daughters who show the same kinds of patterns (Hill et al., 1990; Pike and Rodin, 1991). Abramovitz and Birch (2000) found that mothers' dieting is the best predictor of their 5-year-old daughters' knowledge of dieting. Cutting and colleagues (1999) showed that familial similarities in mothers' and daughters' overweight status are mediated by similarities in "disinhibited overeating" (overeating in the absence of hunger).

As discussed earlier in this chapter, parents who are supportive of physical activity have children who are more physically active (Sallis et al., 1988; Davison et al., 2003). However, evidence for a direct effect of parent modeling on youth physical activity is inconsistent at best. This is in contrast to the stronger evidence for modeling regarding eating patterns. The discrepant findings may be explained by different mediators. If parents are eating fruits and vegetables and drinking milk, it means those foods are readily available to the child. However, parents often engage in different types of physical activities than children or in different settings, so the parent going to a health club or on a run may not facilitate the child's physical activity and could serve as a barrier.

Researchers have compared the effects of different families' eating and activity patterns on their children. Families can be categorized as either "obesogenic," where physical activity is relatively low and energy and fat intakes are high, or nonobesogenic, where parents show higher levels of activity and lower energy intakes. For example, in one study, girls living in obesogenic families gained more weight from age 5 to 7 than girls from nonobesogenic families, and the former were more likely to be overweight at age 7 (Davison and Birch, 2002). These effects were mediated by similarities in mother-daughter eating patterns and father-daughter physical activity patterns, suggesting that while mothers were effective models for daughters' eating habits, fathers' levels of physical activity influenced their daughters in that area.

It is not known to what extent the observed effects of modeling reflect modeling per se or result simply from the fact that parents either do or do not establish routine access to healthful options so that these options are familiar to their children. That is, parents who eat a healthful diet and are active typically provide access to healthful food and opportunities for physical activity for their children as well. As discussed in Chapter 3, guidance regarding a balanced diet and regular physical activity is available through the Dietary Guidelines for Americans.

Parents should provide positive role models of eating and physical activity behaviors for their children. The committee urges parents to be positive role models for their children by decreasing the amount of time they engage in sedentary activities such as watching TV, increasing the amount of time they engage in physical activity each day, and modeling eating habits that include balance and variety in their food choices and portion control.

RAISING AWARENESS OF WEIGHT AS A HEALTH ISSUE

It is critically important that parents view childhood obesity as a health issue and realize that obesity can have a deleterious impact on physical as well as mental health, both during childhood and later in life. Yet parents of overweight or obese children do not always recognize their child's weight status and many are not fully aware of its adverse consequences (Young-Hyman et al., 2000; Etelson et al., 2003; Maynard et al., 2003).

Because children often exhibit idiosyncratic growth patterns, it is important to evaluate a child within the context of his or her own particular growth history as well as relative to a healthy and appropriate reference population. For individuals under 20 years of age, BMI is a complex concept; not only do weight and height change as the body grows, but body-fat content and muscular development are also changing, and there are significant gender differences in the pattern of change. Thus it is important to use gender- and age-specific BMI percentiles to determine whether a particular child has excess weight.

During infancy, parents tend to be well aware of their child's weight and height, and it is not unusual for them to know where his or her measurements fall on the health-care provider's growth curves, which are derived from reference populations of healthy children of the same age and sex. However, as children grow, and particularly in the late elementary and middle- and high school years, this information often is *not* familiar to parents—unless they think their child is failing to grow, which may sensitize them to the need for careful monitoring and tracking. Parents may also notice particular periods of height change, as when the child rapidly outgrows his or her clothes. Because of the variable timing of growth spurts, and the sometimes dramatic changes in body composition with age, continued monitoring of growth on an annual basis is warranted; if concerns arise about the child's growth trajectory, parents should then discuss these issues with a qualified health-care professional.

Routine determination of children's BMI percentile, and regular communication between parents and health-care providers regarding their child's BMI-percentile history and current status, are crucial to increasing the knowledge base of parents regarding their child's growth pattern and weight status. Parents also need to be aware of the strong connection between good nutrition and physical activity to the child's weight—and to his or her health. If excessive weight gain is observed, it is important for parents to discuss follow-up steps and behavior changes with their child's health-care provider (see Chapter 6). These discussions should be sensitive to parental concerns about the stigma of obesity and its potential impact on the child's self-esteem and should take care to allay concerns about eating disorders (Borra et al., 2003).

Just as vaccination schedules require parental intervention during childhood, parents should be discussing the prevention of obesity with their health-care providers to make sure that the child is on a healthy growth track. **Parents should consider the weight of their children to be a critically important indicator of health. They should ensure that a trained professional routinely (at least once a year) measures their child's height and weight in order to track his or her age- and gender-specific BMI percentile.**

But given that many families do not have the health insurance to cover preventive services, and these types of health-care visits may therefore impose a financial burden, the committee also recommends (in Chapter 7) that schools conduct periodic assessments of students' weight status and provide the resulting information to parents—and to the children themselves, as age-appropriate.

RECOMMENDATION

Home environments that support healthful eating and physical activity are important in helping children maintain energy balance at a healthy weight. Preventing childhood obesity starts with a healthful diet and lifestyle at conception and throughout pregnancy and is promoted by exclusive breastfeeding during infancy. As discussed throughout this chapter, parents can ensure that healthful foods are available in the home and that healthful eating behaviors (e.g., family meals, limited snacking, and portion control) are promoted. Older children and youth must be aware of their own eating habits and activity patterns and engage in health-promoting behaviors. By being supportive of their children's athletic and other interests in physical activity and by encouraging children to play outside, parents can enhance opportunities for moderate to vigorous physical activity and promote physical fitness. Furthermore, parents can set a good example for their children by modeling healthful eating behaviors and being physically active. Parents can also be effective advocates by becoming involved in efforts in their neighborhoods, schools, and community to improve neighborhood safety and to expand the access and availability of opportunities such as recreational facilities, playgrounds, sidewalks, bike paths, and farmers' markets (Chapters 6 and 7).

Recommendation 10: *Home*
Parents should promote healthful eating behaviors and regular physical activity for their children.

To implement this recommendation parents can:

- Choose exclusive breastfeeding as the method for feeding infants for the first four to six months of life
- Provide healthful food and beverage choices for children by carefully considering nutrient quality and energy density
- Assist and educate children in making healthful decisions regarding types of foods and beverages to consume, how often, and in what portion size
- Encourage and support regular physical activity
- Limit children's television viewing and other recreational screen time to less than two hours per day

- Discuss weight status with their child's health-care provider and monitor age- and gender-specific BMI percentile
- Serve as positive role models for their children regarding eating and physical activity behaviors

REFERENCES

AACAP (American Academy of Child and Adolescent Psychiatry). 2001. *Children and Watching TV*. Facts for Families, No. 54. [Online]. Available: http://www.aacap.org/publications/factsfam/tv.htm [accessed June 7, 2004].

AAP (American Academy of Pediatrics). 2001. Children, adolescents, and television. *Pediatrics* 107(2):423-426.

AAP. 2003. Prevention of pediatric overweight and obesity. *Pediatrics* 112(2):424-430.

AAP. 2004. *Pediatric Nutrition Handbook*. 5th ed. Washington, DC: AAP.

Abramovitz BA, Birch LL. 2000. Five-year-old girls' ideas about dieting are predicted by their mothers' dieting. *J Am Diet Assoc* 100(10):1157-1163.

ADA (American Dietetic Association). 2004. Position of the American Dietetic Association: Dietary guidance for healthy children ages 2 to 11 years. *J Am Diet Assoc* 104(4):660-677.

AMA (American Medical Association). 1996. *Physician Guide to Media Violence*. Chicago, IL: AMA.

APA (American Psychological Association), AAP (American Academy of Pediatrics). 1995. *Raising Children to Resist Violence: What You Can Do*. Washington, DC: APA and AAP.

Baranowski T, Simons-Morton B, Hooks P, Henske J, Tiernan K, Dunn JK, Burkhalter H, Harper J, Palmer J. 1990. A center-based program for exercise change among black-American families. *Health Educ Q* 17(2):179-196.

Baranowski T, Thompson WO, DuRant RH, Baranowski J, Puhl J. 1993. Observations on physical activity in physical locations: Age, gender, ethnicity, and month effects. *Res Q Exerc Sport* 64(2):127-133.

Baranowski T, Davis M, Resnicow K, Baranowski J, Doyle C, Lin LS, Smith M, Wang DT. 2000. Gimme 5 fruit, juice, and vegetables for fun and health: Outcome evaluation. *Health Educ Behav* 27(1):96-111.

Beauchamp GK, Cowart BJ. 1985. Congenital and experiential factors in the development of human flavor preferences. *Appetite* 6(4):357-372.

Bergmann KE, Bergmann RL, von Kries R, Bohm O, Richter R, Dudenhausen JW, Wahn U. 2003. Early determinants of childhood overweight and adiposity in a birth cohort study: Role of breast-feeding. *Int J Obes Relat Metab Disord* 27(2):162-172.

Birch LL. 1981. Generalization of a modified food preference. *Child Dev* 52:755-758.

Birch LL. 1999. Development of food preferences. *Annu Rev Nutr* 19:41-62.

Birch LL, Marlin DW. 1982. I don't like it; I never tried it: Effects of exposure on two-year-old children's food preferences. *Appetite* 3(4):353-360.

Birch LL, Zimmerman S, Hind H. 1980. The influence of social-affective context on preschool children's food preferences. *Child Dev* 51:856-861.

Birch LL, McPhee L, Shoba BC, Pirok E, Steinberg L. 1987. What kind of exposure reduces children's food neophobia? Looking vs. tasting. *Appetite* 9(3):171-178.

Bishop P, Donnelly JE. 1987. Home based activity program for obese children. *Am Correct Ther J* 41(1):12-19.

Bogen DL, Hanusa BH, Whitaker RC. 2004. The effect of breast-feeding with and without concurrent formula use on the risk of obesity at 4 years of age. *Obes Res* 12:1528-1536.

Borra ST, Kelly L, Shirreffs MB, Neville K, Geiger CJ. 2003. Developing health messages: Qualitative studies with children, parents, and teachers help identify communications opportunities for healthful lifestyles and the prevention of obesity. *J Am Diet Assoc* 103(6):721-728.

Brown JR, Cramond JK, Wilde RJ. 1974. Displacment effects of television and the child's functional orientation to the media. In: Blumler JG, Katz E, eds. *The Uses of Mass Communications: Current Perspectives on Gratifications Research.* Beverly Hills, CA: Sage Publications. Pp. 93-112.

Buchowski MS, Sun M. 1996. Energy expenditure, television viewing and obesity. *Int J Obes* 20(3):236-244.

Butcher JE, Eaton WO. 1989. Gross motor proficiency in preschoolers: Relationships with free play behavior and activity level. *J Hum Movement Stud* 16:27-36.

Cavadini C, Siega-Riz AM, Popkin BM. 2000. US adolescent food intake trends from 1965 to 1996. *Arch Dis Child* 83(1):18-24.

CDC (Centers for Disease Control and Prevention). 1997. Guidelines for school and community programs to promote lifelong physical activity among young people. *MMWR Recomm Rep* 46(RR-6):1-36.

CDC. 2004a. Prevalence of no leisure-time physical activity—35 states and the District of Columbia, 1988-2002. *MMWR* 53(4):82-86.

CDC. 2004b. Trends in intake of energy and macronutrients—United States, 1971-2000. *MMWR* 53(4):80-82.

CDC. 2004c. Youth risk behavior surveillance—United States, 2003. *MMWR Surveill Summ* 53(SS-2):1-96.

Coates TJ, Killen JD, Slinkard LA. 1982. Parent participation in a treatment program for overweight adolescents. *Int J Eat Disord* 1(3):37-48.

Coon KA, Goldberg J, Rogers BL, Tucker KL. 2001. Relationships between use of television during meals and children's food consumption patterns. *Pediatrics* 107(1):E7.

Cowart BJ. 1981. Development of taste perception in humans: Sensitivity and preference throughout the life span. *Psychol Bull* 90:43-73.

Crespo CJ, Smit E, Troiano RP, Bartlett SJ, Macera CA, Andersen RE. 2001. Television watching, energy intake, and obesity in US children: Results from the third National Health and Nutrition Examination Survey, 1988-1994. *Arch Pediatr Adolesc Med* 155(3):360-365.

Cullen KW, Baranowski T, Rittenberry L, Olvera N. 2000. Social-environmental influences on children's diets: Results from focus groups with African-, Euro- and Mexican-American children and their parents. *Health Educ Res* 15(5):581-590.

Cullen KW, Baranowski T, Rittenberry L, Cosart C, Hebert D, de Moor C. 2001. Child-reported family and peer influences on fruit, juice and vegetable consumption: Reliability and validity of measures. *Health Educ Res* 16(2):187-200.

Cullen KW, Baranowski T, Owens E, Marsh T, Rittenberry L, de Moor C. 2003. Availability, accessibility, and preferences for fruit, 100% fruit juice, and vegetables influence children's dietary behavior. *Health Educ Behav* 30(5):615-626.

Cutting TM, Fisher JO, Grimm-Thomas K, Birch LL. 1999. Like mother, like daughter: Familial patterns of overweight are mediated by mothers' dietary disinhibition. *Am J Clin Nutr* 69(4):608-613.

Davis SM, Lambert LC, Gomez Y, Skipper B. 1995. Southwest Cardiovascular Curriculum Project: Study findings for American Indian elementary students. *J Health Educ* 26(Suppl):S72-S81.

Davison KK, Birch LL. 2001. Childhood overweight: A contextual model and recommendations for future research. *Obes Rev* 2(3):159-171.

Davison KK, Birch LL. 2002. Obesigenic families: Parents' physical activity and dietary intake patterns predict girls' risk of overweight. *Int J Obes Relat Metab Disord* 26(9):1186-1193.

Davison KK, Cutting TM, Birch LL. 2003. Parents' activity-related parenting practices predict girls' physical activity. *Med Sci Sports Exerc* 35(9):1589-1595.

Dennison BA, Erb TA, Jenkins PL. 2002. Television viewing and television in bedroom associated with overweight risk among low-income preschool children. *Pediatrics* 109(6):1028-1035.

Devine CM, Connors MM, Sobal J, Bisogni CA. 2003. Sandwiching it in: Spillover of work onto food choices and family roles in low- and moderate-income urban households. *Soc Sci Med* 56(3):617-630.

Dewey KG. 2003. Is breastfeeding protective against child obesity? *J Hum Lact* 19(1):9-18.

DHHS (U.S. Department of Health and Human Services). 1996. *Physical Activity and Health: A Report of the Surgeon General.* Atlanta, GA: CDC.

DHHS, Agency for Health Care Policy and Research. 2000. *Child Health Guide: Put Prevention into Practice.* Rockville, MD: Agency for Health Care Policy and Research. [Online]. Available: http://www.ahrq.gov/ppip/childguide/ [accessed June 10, 2004].

Dietz WH, Bandini LG, Morelli JA, Peers KF, Ching PL. 1994. Effect of sedentary activities on resting metabolic rate. *Am J Clin Nutr* 59(3):556-559.

Diliberti N, Bordi PL, Conklin MT, Roe LS, Rolls BJ. 2004. Increased portion size leads to increased energy intake in a restaurant meal. *Obes Res* 12(3):562-568.

DiLorenzo TM, Stucky-Ropp RC, Vander Wal JS, Gotham HJ. 1998. Determinants of exercise among children II. A longitudinal analysis. *Prev Med* 27(3):470-477.

DuRant RH, Baranowski T, Johnson M, Thompson WO. 1994. The relationship among television watching, physical activity, and body composition of young children. *Pediatrics* 94(4 Pt 1):449-455.

Edmundson E, Parcel GS, Feldman HA, Elder J, Perry CL, Johnson CC, Williston BJ, Stone EJ, Yang M, Lytle L, Webber L. 1996. The effects of the Child and Adolescent Trial for Cardiovascular Health upon psychosocial determinants of diet and physical activity behavior. *Prev Med* 25(4):442-454.

Epstein LH, Valoski A, Wing RR, McCurley J. 1990. Ten-year follow-up of behavioral, family-based treatment for obese children. *J Am Med Assoc* 264(19):2519-2523.

Epstein LH, Valoski A, Wing RR, McCurley J. 1994. Ten-year outcomes of behavioral family-based treatment for childhood obesity. *Health Psychol* 13(5):373-383.

Epstein LH, Valoski AM, Vara LS, McCurley J, Wisniewski L, Kalarchian MA, Klein KR, Shrager LR. 1995. Effects of decreasing sedentary behavior and increasing activity on weight change in obese children. *Health Psychol* 14(2):109-115.

Epstein LH, Paluch RA, Gordy CC, Dorn J. 2000. Decreasing sedentary behaviors in treating pediatric obesity. *Arch Pediatr Adolesc Med* 154(3):220-226.

Epstein LH, Paluch RA, Consalvi A, Riordan K, Scholl T. 2002. Effects of manipulating sedentary behavior on physical activity and food intake. *J Pediatr* 140(3):334-339.

Etelson D, Brand DA, Patrick PA, Shirali A. 2003. Childhood obesity: Do parents recognize this health risk? *Obes Res* 11(11):1362-1368.

Fields J. 2003. *Children's Living Arrangements and Characteristics: March 2002.* Current Population Reports. Washington, DC: U.S. Census Bureau.

Fisher JO, Birch LL. 1995. Fat preferences and fat consumption of 3- to 5-year-old children are related to parental adiposity. *J Am Diet Assoc* 95(7):759-764.

Fisher JO, Birch LL. 1999. Restricting access to foods and children's eating. *Appetite* 32(3):405-419.

Fisher JO, Birch LL, Smiciklas-Wright H, Picciano MF. 2000. Breast-feeding through the first year predicts maternal control in feeding and subsequent toddler energy intakes. *J Am Diet Assoc* 100(6):641-646.

Fisher JO, Mitchell DC, Smiciklas-Wright H, Birch LL. 2001. Maternal milk consumption predicts the tradeoff between milk and soft drinks in young girls' diets. *J Nutr* 131(2):246-250.

Fisher JO, Mitchell DC, Smiciklas-Wright H, Birch LL. 2002. Parental influences on young girls' fruit and vegetable, micronutrient, and fat intakes. *J Am Diet Assoc* 102(1):58-64.

Fomon SJ, Filer LJ, Thomas LN, Anderson TA, Nelson SE. 1975. Influence of formula concentration on caloric intake and growth of normal infants. *Acta Paediatr Scand* 64(2):172-181.

Forshee RA, Storey ML. 2003. Total beverage consumption and beverage choices among children and adolescents. *Int J Food Sci Nutr* 54(4):297-307.

Fox MK, Pac S, Devaney B, Jankowski L. 2004. Feeding infants and toddlers study: What foods are infants and toddlers eating? *J Am Diet Assoc* 104(1 Suppl 1):S22-S30.

French SA, Lin BH, Guthrie JF. 2003. National trends in soft drink consumption among children and adolescents age 6 to 17 years: Prevalence, amounts, and sources, 1977/1978 to 1994/1998. *J Am Diet Assoc* 103(10):1326-1331.

French SA, Hannan PJ, Story M. 2004. School soft drink intervention study. *Br Med J* 329(7462):E315-E316.

Galst J, White M. 1976. The unhealthy persuader: The reinforcing value of television and children's purchase influencing attempts at the supermarket. *Child Dev* 47:1089-1096.

Gillman MW, Rifas-Shiman SL, Frazier AL, Rockett HR, Camargo CA Jr, Field AE, Berkey CS, Colditz GA. 2000. Family dinner and diet quality among older children and adolescents. *Arch Fam Med* 9(3):235-240.

Gillman MW, Rifas-Shiman S, Berkey CS, Field AE, Colditz GA. 2003. Maternal gestational diabetes, birth weight, and adolescent obesity. *Pediatrics* 111(3):e221-e226.

Gleason P, Suitor C. 2001. *Children's Diets in the Mid-1990's: Dietary Intake and Its Relationship with School Meal Participation*. Report No. CN-01-CD1. Alexandria, VA: USDA.

Golan M, Crow S. 2004. Targeting parents exclusively in the treatment of childhood obesity: Long-term results. *Obes Res* 12(2):357-361.

Golan M, Weizman A, Apter A, Fainaru M. 1998. Parents as the exclusive agents of change in the treatment of childhood obesity. *Am J Clin Nutr* 67(6):1130-1135.

Goran MI, Reynolds KD, Lindquist CH. 1999. Role of physical activity in the prevention of obesity in children. *Int J Obes Relat Metab Disord* 23(Suppl 3):S18-S33.

Gordon-Larsen P, McMurray RG, Popkin BM. 2000. Determinants of adolescent physical activity and inactivity patterns. *Pediatrics* 105(6):E83.

Gorn GJ, Goldberg ME. 1982. Behavioral evidence for the effects of televised food messages on children. *J Consumer Res* 9:200-205.

Gortmaker SL, Must A, Sobol AM, Peterson K, Colditz GA, Dietz WH. 1996. Television viewing as a cause of increasing obesity among children in the United States, 1986-1990. *Arch Pediatr Adolesc Med* 150(4):356-362.

Gortmaker SL, Peterson K, Wiecha J, Sobol AM, Dixit S, Fox MK, Laird N. 1999. Reducing obesity via a school-based interdisciplinary intervention among youth: Planet Health. *Arch Pediatr Adolesc Med* 153(4):409-418.

Graber JA, Brooks-Gunn J. 1996. Prevention of eating problems and disorders: Including parents. *Eat Disord* 4(4):348-363.

Grummer-Strawn LM, Mei Z. 2004. Does breastfeeding protect against pediatric overweight? Analysis of longitudinal data from the Centers for Disease Control and Prevention Pediatric Nutrition Surveillance System. *Pediatrics* 113(2):e81-e86.

Guthrie JF, Morton JF. 2000. Food sources of added sweeteners in the diets of Americans. *J Am Diet Assoc* 100(1):43-51.

Gutin B, Barbeau P, Yin Z. 2004. Exercise interventions for prevention of obesity and related disorders in youths. *Quest* 56:120-141.

Hastings G, Stead M, McDermott L, Forsyth A, MacKintosh A, Rayner, M, Godfrey C, Caraher M, Angus K. 2003. *Review of Research on the Effects of Food Promotion to Children.* Glasgow, UK: Center for Social Marketing, University of Strathclyde. Available: http://www.food.gov.uk/multimedia/pdfs/foodpromotiontochildren1.pdf [accessed November 22, 2003].

Hewlett SA, West C. 1998. *The War Against Parents.* New York: Houghton Mifflin.

Hill AJ, Weaver C, Blundell JE. 1990. Dieting concerns of 10-year-old girls and their mothers. *Br J Clin Psychol* 29(Pt 3):346-348.

Hopper CA, Gruber MB, Munoz KD, Herb RA. 1992. Effect of including parents in a school-based exercise and nutrition program for children. *Res Q Exerc Sport* 63(3):315-321.

Hopper CA, Munoz KD, Gruber MB, MacConnie SE, Schonfeldt B, Shunk T. 1996. A school-based cardiovascular exercise program with parent participation: An evaluation study. *Child Health Care* 25(3):221-235.

IOM (Institute of Medicine). 2002. *Dietary Reference Intakes for Energy, Carbohydrate, Fiber, Fat, Fatty Acids, Cholesterol, Protein, and Amino Acids.* Washington, DC: The National Academies Press.

James J, Thomas P, Cavan D, Kerr D. 2004. Preventing childhood obesity by reducing consumption of carbonated drinks: Cluster randomized controlled trial. *Br Med J* 328(7450):1237.

Johnson CC, Nicklas TA, Arbeit ML, Harsha DW, Mott DS, Hunter SM, Wattigney W, Berenson GS. 1991. Cardiovascular intervention for high-risk families: The Heart Smart Program. *South Med J* 84(11):1305-1312.

Johnson SL, McPhee L, Birch LL. 1991. Conditioned preferences: Young children prefer flavors associated with high dietary fat. *Physiol Behav* 50(6):1245-1251.

Kahn EB, Ramsey LT, Brownson RC, Heath GW, Howze EH, Powell KE, Stone EJ, Rajab MW, Corso P. 2002. The effectiveness of interventions to increase physical activity. A systematic review. *Am J Prev Med* 22(4 Suppl):73-107.

Kirschenbaum DS, Harris ES, Tomarken AJ. 1984. Effects of parental involvement in behavioral weight loss therapy for preadolescents. *Behav Ther* 15(5):485-500.

Klesges RC, Eck LH, Hanson CL, Haddock CK, Klesges LM. 1990. Effects of obesity, social interactions, and physical environment on physical activity in preschoolers. *Health Psychol* 9(4):435-449.

Klesges RC, Shelton ML, Klesges LM. 1993. Effects of television on metabolic rate: Potential implications for childhood obesity. *Pediatrics* 91(2):281-286.

Kohl HW, Hobbs KE. 1998. Development of physical activity behaviors among children and adolescents. *Pediatrics* 101(3 Pt 2):549-554.

Koivisto UK, Fellenius J, Sjoden PO. 1994. Relations between parental mealtime practices and children's food intake. *Appetite* 22(3):245-257.

Kotz K, Story M. 1994. Food advertisements during children's Saturday morning television programming: Are they consistent with dietary recommendations? *J Am Diet Assoc* 94(11):1296-1300.

Lederman SA, Akabas S, Moore BJ, Bentley ME, Devaney B, Gillman MW, Kramer MS, Mennella JA, Ness A, Wardle J. 2004. Summary of the presentations at the Conference on Preventing Childhood Obesity, December 8, 2003. *Pediatrics* 114:1146-1173.

Lindquist CH, Reynolds KD, Goran MI. 1999. Sociocultural determinants of physical activity among children. *Prev Med* 29(4):305-312.

Lissau I, Sorensen TI. 1994. Parental neglect during childhood and increased risk of obesity in young adulthood. *Lancet* 343(8893):324-327.

Loewen R, Pliner P. 1999. Effects of prior exposure to palatable and unpalatable novel foods on children's willingness to taste other novel foods. *Appetite* 32(3):351-366.

Ludwig DS, Peterson KE, Gortmaker SL. 2001. Relation between consumption of sugar-sweetened drinks and childhood obesity: A prospective, observational analysis. *Lancet* 357(9255):505-508.

Manios Y, Moschandreas J, Hatzis C, Kafatos A. 1999. Evaluation of a health and nutrition education program in primary school children of Crete over a three-year period. *Prev Med* 28(2):149-159.

Matheson DM, Killen JD, Wang Y, Varady A, Robinson TN. 2004. Children's food consumption during television viewing. *Am J Clin Nutr* 79(6):1088-1094.

Maynard LM, Galuska DA, Blanck HM, Serdula MK. 2003. Maternal perceptions of weight status of children. *Pediatrics* 111(5 Pt 2):1226-1231.

McConahy KL, Smiciklas-Wright H, Birch LL, Mitchell DC, Picciano MF. 2002. Food portions are positively related to energy intake and body weight in early childhood. *J Pediatr* 140(3):340-347.

McGuire MT, Hannan PJ, Neumark-Sztainer D, Cossrow NH, Story M. 2002. Parental correlates of physical activity in a racially/ethnically diverse adolescent sample. *J Adolesc Health* 30(4):253-261.

Mennella JA. 1995. Mother's milk: A medium for early flavor experiences. *J Hum Lact* 11(1):39-45.

Mennella JA, Beauchamp GK. 1991. Maternal diet alters the sensory qualities of human milk and the nursling's behavior. *Pediatrics* 88(4):737-744.

Mennella JA, Beauchamp GK. 1998. Early flavor experiences: Research update. *Nutr Rev* 56(7):205-211.

Mennella JA, Jagnow CP, Beauchamp GK. 2001. Prenatal and postnatal flavor learning by human infants. *Pediatrics* 107:E88.

Motl RW, Dishman RK, Ward DS, Saunders RP, Dowda M, Felton G, Pate RR. 2002. Examining social-cognitive determinants of intention and physical activity among black and white adolescent girls using structural equation modeling. *Health Psychol* 21(5):459-467.

Nader PR, Baranowski T, Vanderpool NA, Dunn K, Dworkin R, Ray L. 1983. The Family Health Project: Cardiovascular risk reduction education for children and parents. *J Dev Behav Pediatr* 4(1):3-10.

Nader PR, Sallis JF, Patterson TL, Abramson IS, Rupp JW, Senn KL, Atkins CJ, Roppe BE, Morris JA, Wallace JP, Vega WA. 1989. A family approach to cardiovascular risk reduction: Results from the San Diego Family Health Project. *Health Educ Q* 16(2):229-244.

National PTA (National Parent Teachers Association), Cable in the Classroom, National Cable and Telecommunications Association. 2001. *Taking Charge of Your TV: A Guide to Critical Viewing for Parents and Children.* [Online]. Available: http://www.ciconline.com/Enrichment/MediaLiteracy/TakingCharge/ParentsGuide/default.htm [accessed July 6, 2004].

NEA (National Education Association). 1999. *52 Ways to Help Your Child Learn.* Washington, DC: NEA.

Nestle M. 2003. Increasing portion sizes in American diets: More calories, more obesity. *J Am Diet Assoc* 103(1):39-40.

Neumark-Sztainer D, Hannan PJ, Story M, Croll J, Perry C. 2003a. Family meal patterns: Associations with sociodemographic characteristics and improved dietary intake among adolescents. *J Am Diet Assoc* 103(3):317-322.

Neumark-Sztainer D, Story M, Hannan PJ, Tharp T, Rex J. 2003b. Factors associated with changes in physical activity: A cohort study of inactive adolescent girls. *Arch Pediatr Adolesc Med* 157(8):803-810.

Nicklas TA, Baranowski T, Baranowski JC, Cullen K, Rittenberry L, Olvera N. 2001. Family and child-care provider influences on preschool children's fruit, juice, and vegetable consumption. *Nutr Rev* 59(7):224-235.

Orlet-Fisher J, Rolls BJ, Birch LL. 2003. Children's bite size and intake of an entree are greater with large portions than with age-appropriate or self-selected portions. *Am J Clin Nutr* 77(5):1164-1170.

Parke RD, Buriel R. 1998. Socialization in the family: Ethnic and ecological perspectives. In: Damon W, ed. *Handbook of Child Psychology.* 5th ed. New York: Wiley.

Pate RR, Heath GW, Dowda M, Trost SG. 1996. Associations between physical activity and other health behaviors in a representative sample of US adolescents. *Am J Public Health* 86(11):1577-1581.

Pate RR, Trost SG, Felton GM, Ward DS, Dowda M, Saunders R. 1997. Correlates of physical activity behavior in rural youth. *Res Q Exerc Sport* 68(3):241-248.

Pica R. 1997. Beyond physical development: Why young children need to move. *Young Child* 52(6):4-11.

Pike KM, Rodin J. 1991. Mothers, daughters, and disordered eating. *J Abnorm Psychol* 100(2):198-204.

Rampersaud GC, Bailey LB, Kauwell GPA. 2003. National survey beverage consumption data for children and adolescents indicate the need to encourage a shift toward more nutritive beverages. *J Am Diet Assoc* 103(1):97-100.

Roberts D, Foehr U, Rideout V, Brodie M. 1999. *Kids and Media at the New Millennium.* Menlo Park, CA: The Henry J. Kaiser Family Foundation. [Online]. Available: http://www.kff.org/content/1999/1535/KidsReport%20FINAL.pdf [accessed April 15, 2004].

Robinson TN. 1999. Reducing children's television viewing to prevent obesity: A randomized controlled trial. *J Am Med Assoc* 282(16):1561-1567.

Robinson TN. 2001a. Population-based obesity prevention for children and adolescents. In: Johnston FE, Foster GD, eds. *Obesity, Growth and Development.* London: Smith-Gordon. Pp. 129-141.

Robinson TN. 2001b. Television viewing and childhood obesity. *Pediatr Clin North Am* 48(4):1017-1025.

Robinson TN, Hammer LD, Killen JD, Kraemer HC, Wilson DM, Hayward C, Taylor CB. 1993. Does television viewing increase obesity and reduce physical activity? Cross-sectional and longitudinal analyses among adolescent girls. *Pediatrics* 91(2):273-280.

Robinson TN, Killen JD, Kraemer HC, Wilson DM, Matheson DM, Haskell WL, Pruitt LA, Powell TM, Owens AS, Thompson NS, Flint-Moore NM, Davis GJ, Emig KA, Brown RT, Rochon J, Green S, Varady A. 2003. Dance and reducing television viewing to prevent weight gain in African-American girls: The Stanford GEMS pilot study. *Ethn Dis* 13(1 Suppl 1):S1.65-S1.77.

Rolls BJ. 2003. The supersizing of America. Portion size and the obesity epidemic. *Nutr Tod* 38(2):42-53.

Rolls BJ, Engell D, Birch LL. 2000. Serving portion size influences 5-year-old but not 3-year-old children's food intakes. *J Am Diet Assoc* 100(2):232-234.

Roper ASW. 2003. *2003 Roper Youth Report.* New York. [Online]. Available: http://www.roperasw.com/newsroom/press/p0310002.html [accessed May 3, 2004].

Sallis JF, Patterson TL, Buono MJ, Atkins CJ, Nader PR. 1988. Aggregation of physical activity habits in Mexican-American and Anglo families. *J Behav Med* 11(1):31-41.

Sallis JF, Simons-Morton BG, Stone EJ, Corbin CB, Epstein LH, Faucette N, Iannotti RJ, Killen JD, Klesges RC, Petray CK, Rowland TW, Taylor WC. 1992. Determinants of physical activity and interventions in youth. *Med Sci Sports Exerc* 24(6 Suppl):S249-S257.

Sallis JF, Nader PR, Broyles SL, Berry CC, Elder JP, McKenzie TL, Nelson JA. 1993. Correlates of physical activity at home in Mexican-American and Anglo-American preschool children. *Health Psychol* 12(5):390-398.

Sallis JF, McKenzie TL, Alcaraz JE, Kolody B, Faucette N, Hovell MF. 1997. The effects of a 2-year physical education program (SPARK) on physical activity and fitness in elementary school students. Sports, Play and Active Recreation for Kids. *Am J Public Health* 87(8):1328-1334.

Sallis JF, Alcaraz JE, McKenzie TL, Hovell MF. 1999. Predictors of change in children's physical activity over 20 months. Variations by gender and level of adiposity. *Am J Prev Med* 16(3):222-229.

Sallis JF, Prochaska JJ, Taylor WC. 2000. A review of correlates of physical activity of children and adolescents. *Med Sci Sports Exerc* 32(5):963-975.

Schmitz KH, Lytle LA, Phillips GA, Murray DM, Birnbaum AS, Kubik MY. 2002. Psychosocial correlates of physical activity and sedentary leisure habits in young adolescents: The Teens Eating for Energy and Nutrition at School study. *Prev Med* 34(2):266-278.

Shape Up America! 2004. *99 Tips for Family Fitness Fun*. [Online]. Available: http://www.shapeup.org/pubs/99tips/index.html [accessed June 24, 2004].

Silverman BL, Cho NH, Rizzo TA, Metzger BE. 1998. Long-term effects of the intrauterine environment: The Northwestern University Diabetes in Pregnancy Center. *Diab Care* 21(S2):B142-B149.

Skinner JD, Carruth BR, Bounds W, Ziegler P, Reidy K. 2002. Do food-related experiences in the first 2 years of life predict dietary variety in school-aged children? *J Nutr Educ Behav* 34(6):310-315.

Smiciklas-Wright H, Mitchell D, Mickle S, Goldman J, Cook A. 2003. Foods commonly eaten in the United States, 1989-1991 and 1994-1996: Are portion sizes changing? *J Am Diet Assoc* 103(1):41-47.

Smith K. 2002. *Who's Minding the Kids? Child Care Arrangements: Spring 1997*. Current Population Reports P70-86. Washington, DC: U.S. Census Bureau.

Stettler N, Zemel BS, Kumanyika S, Stallings VA. 2002. Infant weight gain and childhood overweight status in a multicenter, cohort study. *Pediatrics* 109(2):194-199.

Stettler N, Kumanyika SK, Katz SH, Zemel BS, Stallings VA. 2003. Rapid weight gain during infancy and obesity in young adulthood in a cohort of African Americans. *Am J Clin Nutr* 77(6):1374-1378.

Stucky-Ropp RC, DiLorenzo TM. 1993. Determinants of exercise in children. *Prev Med* 22(6):880-889.

Sullivan SA, Birch LL. 1994. Infant dietary experience and acceptance of solid foods. *Pediatrics* 93(2):271-277.

Taggart AC, Taggart J, Siedentop D. 1986. Effects of a home-based activity program. A study with low fitness elementary school children. *Behav Modif* 10(4):487-507.

Trost SG, Pate RR, Saunders R, Ward DS, Dowda M, Felton G. 1997. A prospective study of the determinants of physical activity in rural fifth-grade children. *Prev Med* 26(2):257-263.

Trost SG, Pate RR, Ward DS, Saunders R, Riner W. 1999. Correlates of objectively measured physical activity in preadolescent youth. *Am J Prev Med* 17(2):120-126.

USDA. 2004. *Food Guide Pyramid for Young Children*. Washington, DC: USDA, CNPP. [Online]. Available: http://www.usda.gov/cnpp/KidsPyra/ [accessed April 15, 2004].

USDA (U.S. Department of Agriculture), DHHS (U.S. Department of Health and Human Services). 2000. *Nutrition and Your Health: Dietary Guidelines for Americans.* Home and Garden Bulletin No. 232, 5th ed. Washington, DC: Government Printing Office.

Wardle J, Cooke LJ, Gibson EL, Sapochnik M, Sheiham A, Lawson M. 2003. Increasing children's acceptance of vegetables: A randomized trial of parent-led exposure. *Appetite* 40(2):155-162.

Weber Cullen K, Baranowski T, Rittenberry L, Cosart C, Owens E, Hebert D, de Moor C. 2000. Socioenvironmental influences on children's fruit, juice and vegetable consumption as reported by parents: Reliability and validity of measures. *Public Health Nutr* 3(3):345-356.

Whitaker RC. 2004. Predicting preschooler obesity at birth: The role of maternal obesity in early pregnancy. *Pediatrics* 114(1):e29-36.

Whitaker RC, Pepe MS, Seidel KD, Wright JA, Knopp RH. 1998. Gestational diabetes and the risk of offspring obesity. *Pediatrics* 101(2):e9.

WHO (World Health Organization). 2003. *Global Strategy for Infant and Young Child Feeding.* Geneva: WHO.

Williams TM, Handford AG. 1986. Television and other leisure activities. In: Williams TM, ed. *The Impact of Television: A Natural Experiment in Three Communities.* Orlando, FL: Academic Press. Pp. 143-213.

Young-Hyman D, Herman LJ, Scott DL, Schlundt DG. 2000. Care giver perception of children's obesity-related health risk: A study of African American families. *Obes Res* 8(3):241-248.

Zakarian JM, Hovell MF, Hofstetter CR, Sallis JF, Keating KJ. 1994. Correlates of vigorous exercise in a predominantly low SES and minority high school population. *Prev Med* 23(3):314-321.

9

Confronting the Childhood Obesity Epidemic

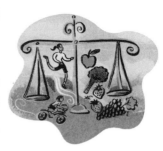

besity in U.S. children and youth is an epidemic characterized by an unexpected and excess number of cases on a steady increase in recent decades. The epidemic is relatively new but widespread, and one that is disproportionately affecting those with the fewest resources to prevent it. Although it does not have the exotic nature or immediate mortality of severe acute respiratory syndrome, anthrax, or Ebola virus, it is harming a much broader cross section of our young people and may significantly undermine their health and well-being throughout their lives. Obesity can affect a child's health immediately through physical or psychological conditions such as type 2 diabetes, hypertension, steatohepatitis, depression, and stigma. Obesity can also affect a child's health in the longer term with additional illnesses that include arthritis, cancer, and cardiovascular disease.

Infectious disease epidemics require and usually receive immediate high-level attention, with resources invested to control the problem and prevent its recurrence. Childhood obesity must be treated with comparable urgency. As with other emerging health problems, our degree of knowledge and arsenal of effective interventions are quite limited. But we do not have the luxury of waiting to accumulate large bodies of evidence. Therefore, it behooves us to chart our course of action wisely based on what evidence we have—drawing from our dealings with analogous problems and the outcomes of natural experiments—and learn as we proceed. Complicating the process will be the multiple causes and correlates of childhood obesity and the need for many concurrent actions and interventions. Nevertheless, as we carefully evaluate our programs and policies in terms of efficacy, effectiveness, and cost utility, we can devise new and innovative approaches based on our experience, discard those that are less useful, promote those that work, and follow through accordingly.

Childhood obesity is complex because it has biological, behavioral, social, economic, environmental, and cultural causes, which collectively have created over decades an adverse environment for maintaining a healthy weight. This environment is characterized by:

- Urban and suburban designs that discourage walking and other physical activities
- Pressures on families to minimize food costs and acquisition and preparation time, resulting in frequent consumption of energy-dense convenience foods that are high in calories and fat
- Reduced access and affordability in some communities to fruits, vegetables, and other nutritious foods
- Decreased opportunities for physical activity at school and after school, and reduced walking or biking to and from school
- Competition for leisure time that was once spent playing outdoors with sedentary screen time—including watching television or playing computer and video games.

The result is that obesity from unhealthful eating and inactivity has rapidly become the social norm in many communities across America. In that respect, the nation is moving away from—instead of toward—the "healthy people in healthy communities" vision of *Healthy People 2010*. Although assigning blame for this situation may be easy, it is unlikely to be accurate or productive. In general, the average person does not make the conscious choice to become obese, despite the adverse health and social consequences. No industry aims to promote weight gain among its customers. Nonetheless, excess weight is gained slowly over time as companies develop and market foods and beverages to maximize revenues; community zoning and street-design decisions are influenced by numerous social and financial pressures; schools face scheduling constraints in fitting everything into the school day while facing the reality of budgetary limits; and individuals make small but cumulative behavioral decisions daily about eating and physical activity in the obesogenic environment that surrounds them.

Now that the nation has begun to realize the significant health, psychological, and societal costs of an unhealthy weight, it is time to re-examine its way of thinking and revise the social norms that are now accepted. This process should span virtually the entire spectrum of society, from corporate board rooms to federal agencies, from elected officials to health insurers and employee unions, from health and medical professionals to teachers and school administrators, from foundations and public service organizations to medical and public health researchers, and of course, it must involve entire communities and families, including parents, relatives, friends, and the children themselves. Although this challenge may appear to be overwhelming, there have been many examples over the past century—relating to smoking, seatbelts, and children's car seats, for example—of substantial shifts in the American culture, society's outlook, and, most important, in people's behavior and their health outcomes. Culture is not a static set of values and practices. It is continuously recreated as people adapt and redefine their values and behaviors to changing realities. These changes have occurred once there has been a collective understanding of the severity of the problem, its impact on health, and mobilization around the potential for improvement. Similar conditions now apply to childhood obesity, and the need for change should be particularly compelling in that the health of America's children is at stake.

As institutions, organizations, and individuals across the nation begin to make changes, social norms are also likely to change, so that obesity in children and youth will be acknowledged as an important and preventable health outcome and healthful eating and regular physical activity will be the accepted and encouraged standard.

Changing the social norms toward healthful lifestyles will have amplified benefits. Individual-level changes toward nutritious diets and increases in physical activity levels have short- and long-term potential for improved health and well-being. Likewise, the enhancements and improvements made to the built and social environments in our communities to improve access to healthful foods and opportunities for physical activity may also improve the safety of neighborhoods and street crossings and strengthen community cohesion.

Preventing childhood obesity should become engrained as a collective responsibility requiring individual, family, community, corporate, and governmental commitments. The key will be to bring changes to bear on this issue from many directions, at multiple levels, and through collaboration within and between many sectors. For example, shared responsibilities on issues such as increasing outdoor play opportunities and walking- or biking-to-school programs will require attention from zoning and planning commissions, public works departments, public safety and police agencies, school boards, parks commissions, community members, and parents.

This is a major societal health problem that will be minimally affected by isolated measures or selectively assigned responsibilities. It will also require a long-term commitment spanning many years and possibly decades because the epidemic has taken years to develop and will require persistent efforts and the investment of sustained resources to effectively ameliorate.

As with many health issues, there are high-risk populations, including low-income and ethnic minority communities, for which obesity prevention initiatives will need to be particularly focused. Resources will need to address a range of issues such as safety, language barriers, limited access to food and health services, income differentials, and the influence of culture on food selection and preferences for available physical activities.

Tough choices will have to be made at all levels of society. There will be trade-offs in convenience, in cost, in what's "easy," in pushing one's self and one's organization, in choosing between priorities, in devising new laws and regulations, and in setting limits on individuals and on industries.

Science can best help by integrating a traditional biomedical approach to such health concerns with behavioral and social science research. Effective solutions lie not in a magical "eat all you want" pill but rather in intensive, often laborious, and long-term improvements in the environments that surround children in their homes, schools, communities, commercial markets, and modes of entertainment. While biology may often encourage us to eat more than we need to, biological solutions are not the answer from an ethical or practical perspective. Nor is genetics the primary problem or the sole determinant. Rather, it is the complex interplay among an individual's knowledge, attitudes, values, behaviors, and environments that play the most influential roles in promoting obesity.

In reviewing the available evidence to inform this report, there was an abundance of scientific studies on the causes and correlates of obesity but few studies testing potential solutions within diverse and complex social and environmental contexts, and no proven effective population-based solutions. Moreover, a concern of the committee is that even if many of the recommended actions are implemented, research should contain a better balance between studies that continue to address the underlying causes of the obesity epidemic and studies that test potential *solutions*—that is, identifying appropriate methodologies for effectively promoting healthful eating and physical activity and reducing sedentary behaviors that will support obesity prevention in children and youth.

NEXT STEPS FOR ACTION AND RESEARCH

Recognizing the multifactorial nature of the problem, the committee deliberated on how best to prioritize the next steps for the nation in preventing obesity in children and youth. The traditional method of prioritizing recommendations of this nature would be to base these decisions on the strength of the scientific evidence demonstrating that specific interventions have a direct impact on reducing obesity prevalence and to order the evidence-based approaches based on the balance between potential benefits and associated costs including potential risks. However, a robust evidence base is not yet available. Instead, we are in the midst of compiling that much needed evidence at the same time that there is an urgent need to respond to this epidemic of childhood obesity. Therefore, the committee used the best scientific evidence available—including studies with obesity as the outcome measure and studies on improving dietary behaviors, increasing physical activity levels, and reducing sedentary behaviors as well as years of experience and study on what has worked in addressing similar public health challenges—to develop the recommendations presented in this report. These recommendations constitute the committee's priorities and the recommended steps to achieve them.

As evidence was limited, yet the health concerns are immediate and warrant preventive action, it is an explicit part of the committee's recommendations that obesity prevention actions and initiatives should include evaluation efforts to help build the evidence base that continues to be needed to more effectively fight this epidemic.

From the report's ten recommendations, the committee has identified a set of immediate steps based on the short-term feasibility of the actions and the need to begin a well-rounded set of changes that recognize the diverse roles of multiple stakeholders (Table 9-1). In discussions and interactions that have already begun and will follow with this report, each community and stakeholder group will determine their own set of priorities and next steps. Furthermore, action is urged for all areas of the 10 recommendations, as the list in Table 9-1 is only meant as a starting point.

The committee was also asked to set forth research priorities. There is still much to be learned about the causes, correlates, prevention, and treatment of obesity in children and youth. Because the focus of this study is on prevention, the committee concentrated its efforts throughout the report on identifying areas of research that are priorities for progress toward preventing childhood obesity. The three research priorities discussed throughout the report are:

• Evaluation of obesity prevention interventions—The committee encourages the evaluation of interventions that focus on preventing obesity, improving dietary behaviors, increasing physical activity levels, and reducing sedentary behaviors. Specific policy, environmental, social, clinical, and behavioral intervention approaches should be examined for their feasibility, efficacy, effectiveness, and sustainability. Evaluations may be in the form of randomized controlled trials and quasi-experimental trials. Cost effectiveness research should be an important component of evaluation efforts.

• Behavioral research—The committee encourages experimental research examining the fundamental factors involved in changing dietary behaviors, physical activity levels, and sedentary behaviors. This research

TABLE 9-1 Immediate Steps

Federal government	• Establish an interdepartmental task force and coordinate federal actions • Develop nutrition standards for foods and beverages sold in schools • Fund state-based nutrition and physical activity grants with strong evaluation components • Develop guidelines regarding advertising and marketing to children and youth by convening a national conference • Expand funding for prevention intervention research, experimental behavioral research, and community-based population research; strengthen support for surveillance, monitoring, and evaluation efforts
Industry and media	• Develop healthier food and beverage product and packaging innovations • Expand consumer nutrition information • Provide clear and consistent media messages
State and local governments	• Expand and promote opportunities for physical activity in the community through changes to ordinances, capital improvement programs, and other planning practices • Work with communities to support partnerships and networks that expand the availability of and access to healthful foods
Health-care professionals	• Routinely track body mass index in children and youth and offer appropriate counseling and guidance to children and their families
Community and nonprofit organizations	• Provide opportunities for healthful eating and physical activity in existing and new community programs, particularly for high-risk populations
State and local education authorities and schools	• Improve the nutritional quality of foods and beverages served and sold in schools and as part of school-related activities • Increase opportunities for frequent, more intensive and engaging physical activity during and after school • Implement school-based interventions to reduce children's screen time • Develop, implement, and evaluate innovative pilot programs for both staffing and teaching about wellness, healthful eating, and physical activity
Parents and families	• Engage in and promote more healthful dietary intakes and active lifestyles (e.g., increased physical activity, reduced television and other screen time, more healthful dietary behaviors)

should inform new intervention strategies that are implemented and tested at individual, family, school, community, and population levels. This would include studies that focus on factors promoting motivation to change behavior, strategies to reinforce and sustain improved behavior, identification and removal of barriers to change, and specific ethnic and cultural influences on behavioral change.

•   Community-based population-level research—The committee encourages experimental and observational research examining the most important established and novel factors that drive changes in population health, how they are embedded in the socioeconomic and built environments, how they impact obesity prevention, and how they affect society at large with regard to improving nutritional health, increasing physical activity, decreasing sedentary behaviors, and reducing obesity prevalence.

The recommendations that constitute this report's action plan to prevent childhood obesity commence what is anticipated to be an energetic and sustained effort. Some of the recommendations can be implemented immediately and will cost little, while others will take a large economic investment and require a longer time to implement and to see the benefits of the investment. Some will prove useful, either quickly or over the longer term, while others will prove unsuccessful. Knowing that it is impossible to produce an optimal solution a priori, we more appropriately adopt surveillance, trial, measurement, error, success, alteration, and dissemination as our course, to be embarked on immediately. Given that the health of today's children and future generations is at stake, we must proceed with all due urgency and vigor.

A

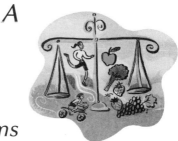

Acronyms

AAFP	American Academy of Family Physicians
AAP	American Academy of Pediatrics
ADA	American Dietetic Association; also American Diabetes Association
ALSPAC	Avon Longitudinal Study of Pregnancy and Childhood
AMA	American Medical Association
APA	American Psychological Association
ARS	Agricultural Research Service
ASSIST	American Stop Smoking Intervention Study
BLS	U.S. Bureau of Labor Statistics
BMI	Body mass index
BRFSS	Behavioral Risk Factor Surveillance System
CACFP	Child and Adult Care Food Program
Caltrans	California Department of Transportation
CARU	Children's Advertising Review Unit
CATCH	Child and Adolescent Trial for Cardiovascular Health program
CDC	Centers for Disease Control and Prevention
CFSC	Community Food Security Coalition
CHD	coronary heart disease
CHSI	Community Health Status Indicators project
CMS	Centers for Medicare & Medicaid Services

CNU	Congress for the New Urbanism
CSF	Curriculum and Standards Framework
CSFII	Continuing Survey of Food Intakes by Individuals
CSPI	Center for Science in the Public Interest
CVD	Cardiovascular disease
DALYs	Disability-adjusted life years
DHHS	U.S. Department of Health and Human Services
DRI	Dietary Reference Intake
DV	Daily Value (as in % DV)
DVD	Digital video disc
DXA	Dual energy X-ray absorptiometry
EER	Estimated Energy Requirement
EFNEP	Expanded Food and Nutrition Education Program
EPA	U.S. Environmental Protection Agency
FAO	Food and Agricultural Organization
FCC	U.S. Federal Communications Commission
FDA	U.S. Food and Drug Administration
FGP	Food Guide Pyramid
FITS	Feeding Infants and Toddlers Study
FMI	Food Marketing Institute
FMNV	Foods of minimal nutritional value
FNB	Food and Nutrition Board
FSP	Food Stamp Program
FTC	Federal Trade Commission
GAO	U.S. Government Accountability Office (previously U.S. General Accounting Office)
GEMS	Girls Health Enrichment Multi-site Study
HDL	High-density lipoprotein
HEI	Healthy Eating Index
HPDP	Health Promotion and Disease Prevention Board
IFIC	International Food Information Council
IMPACT	Improved Nutrition and Physical Activity Act
IOM	Institute of Medicine
ITE	Institute of Transportation Engineers
KEDS	Kids' Eating Disorders Survey

LDL	Low-density lipoprotein
LEAP	Lifestyle Education for Activity Program
LSRO	Life Sciences Research Organization

MEPS	Medical Expenditure Panel Survey
MHHP	Minnesota Heart Health Program
MOVE	Measurement of the Value of Exercise Project
M-SPAN	Middle-School Physical Activity and Nutrition

NACCHO	National Association of County and City Health Officials
NASPE	National Association for Sport and Physical Education
NCHS	National Center for Health Statistics
NCI	National Cancer Institute
NCQA	National Committee for Quality Assurance
NEA	National Education Association
NHANES	National Health and Nutrition Examination Survey
NHES	National Health Examination Survey
NHIS	National Health Interview Survey
NHLBI	National Heart, Lung, and Blood Institute
NHS	National Health Service (United Kingdom)
NHTS	National Household Travel Survey
NICHD	National Institute of Child Health and Human Development
NIDDK	National Institute of Diabetes and Digestive and Kidney Diseases
NIH	National Institutes of Health
NLEA	Nutrition Labeling and Education Act
NLSAH	National Longitudinal Study of Adolescent Health
NLSY	National Longitudinal Survey of Youth
NPTS	National Personal Transportation Survey
NRC	National Research Council
NSLP	National School Lunch Program

| OECD | Organization for Economic Cooperation and Development |

| PE | Physical education |
| PPHEAL | Partnership to Promote Healthy Eating and Active Living |

RCT	Randomized controlled trial
RDA	Recommended Dietary Allowance
RWJF	The Robert Wood Johnson Foundation

| SARS | Severe acute respiratory syndrome |
| SBP | School Breakfast Program |

SCT	Social cognitive theory
SES	Socioeconomic status
SHPPS	School Health Policies and Programs Study
SMART	Student Media Awareness to Reduce Television curriculum
SNDAS	School Nutrition Dietary Assessment Study
SPARK	Sports, Play, and Active Recreation for Kids program
USDA	U.S. Department of Agriculture
USPSTF	U.S. Preventive Services Task Force
VCR	video cassette recorder
WHO	World Health Organization
WIC	Special Supplemental Nutrition Program for Women, Infants, and Children
YMCLS	Youth Media Campaign Longitudinal Survey
YRBS	Youth Risk Behavior Survey
YRBSS	Youth Risk Behavior Surveillance System

B

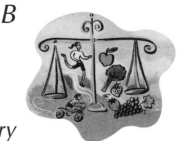

Glossary

Active living A way of life that integrates physical activity into daily routines. The two types of activities that comprise active living are recreational or leisure, such as jogging, skateboarding, and playing basketball; and utilitarian or occupational such as walking or biking to school, shopping, or running errands.

Away-from-home foods Foods categorized according to where they are obtained such as restaurants and other places with wait service; fast food establishments and self-service or carry-out eateries; schools, including day care, after-school programs, and summer camp; and other outlets, including vending machines, community feeding programs, and eating at someone else's home.

Balanced diet The overall dietary pattern of foods consumed that provide all the essential nutrients in the appropriate amounts to support life processes, such as growth in children without promoting excess weight gain.

Basal metabolism The amount of energy needed for maintenance of life when a person is at digestive, physical, and emotional rest.

Body mass index BMI is an indirect measure of body fat calculated as the ratio of a person's body weight in kilograms to the square of a person's height in meters.

BMI (kg/m^2) = weight (kilograms) ÷ height (meters)^2
BMI (lb/in^2) = weight (pounds) ÷ height (inches)^2 × 703

In children and youth, BMI is based on growth charts for age and gender and is referred to as BMI-for-age which is used to assess underweight, overweight, and risk for overweight. According to the Centers for Disease Control and Prevention (CDC), a child with a BMI-for-age that is equal to or greater than the 95th percentile is considered to be overweight. A child with a BMI-for-age that is equal to or between the 85th and 95th percentile is considered to be at risk of being overweight. In this report, the definition of obesity is equivalent to the CDC definition of overweight.

Built environment The man-made elements of the physical environment; buildings, infrastructure, and other physical elements created or modified by people and the functional use, arrangement in space, and aesthetic qualities of these elements.

Calorie A kilocalorie is defined as the amount of heat required to change the temperature of one gram of water from 14.5 degrees Celsius to 15.5 degrees Celsius. In this report, calorie is used synonymously with kilocalorie as a unit of measure for energy obtained from food and beverages.

Community A social entity that can be spatially based on where people live in local neighborhoods, residential districts, or municipalities, or relational such as people who have common ethnic or cultural characteristics or share similar interests.

Co-morbidity In relation to obesity, an associated condition such as hypertension, type 2 diabetes, or asthma that worsens with weight gain and improves with weight loss.

Competitive foods Foods and beverages offered at schools other than meals and snacks served through the federally reimbursed school lunch, breakfast and after-school snack programs. Competitive foods includes food and beverages items sold through à la carte lines, snack bars, student stores, vending machines, and school fundraisers.

Dietary Guidelines for Americans A federal summary of the latest dietary guidance for the public based on current scientific evidence and medical knowledge, issued by the U.S. Department of Health and Human Services and U.S. Department of Agriculture, and is revised every 5 years.

Dietary Reference Intakes   A set of four, distinct nutrient-based reference values that replace the former Recommended Dietary Allowances in the United States. They include Estimated Average Requirements, Recommended Dietary Allowances, Adequate Intakes, and Tolerable Upper Level Intakes.

Disability   A physical, intellectual, emotional, or functional impairment that limits a major activity, and may be a complete or partial impairment.

Disease   An impairment, interruption, disorder, or cessation of the normal state of the living animal or plant body or of any of its components that interrupts or modifies the performance of the vital functions, being a response to environmental factors (e.g., malnutrition, industrial hazards, climate), to specific infective agents (e.g., worms, bacteria, or viruses), to inherent defects of the organism (e.g., various genetic anomalies), or to combinations of these factors; conceptually, a disease (which is usually tangible or measurable but may be symptom-free) is distinct from illness (i.e., the associated pain, suffering, or distress, which is highly individual and personal).

Energy balance   A state where energy intake is equivalent to energy expenditure, resulting in no net weight gain or weight loss. In this report, energy balance in children is used to indicate equality between energy intake and energy expenditure that supports normal growth without promoting excess weight gain.
   The relation between intake of food and output of work that is positive when the body stores extra food as fat and negative when the body draws on stored fat to provide energy for work.

Energy density   The amount of energy stored in a given food per unit volume or mass. Fat stores 9 kilocalories/gram (gm), alcohol stores 7 kilocalories/gm, carbohydrate and protein each store 4 kilocalories/gm, fiber stores 1.5 to 2.5 kilocalories/gm, and water has no calories. Foods that are almost entirely composed of fat with minimal water (e.g., butter) are more energy dense than foods that consist largely of water, fiber, and carbohydrates (e.g., fruits and vegetables).

Energy expenditure   Calories used to support the body's basal metabolic needs plus those used for thermogenesis, growth, and physical activity.

Energy intake   Calories ingested as food and beverages.

Environment   The external influences on the life of an individual or community.

Epidemic   A condition that is occurring more frequently and extensively among individuals in a community or population than is expected.

Exercise   Planned, structured, and repetitive body movements done to improve or maintain one or more components of physical fitness, such as maintaining or increasing muscle tone and strength.

Fast food   Foods designed for ready availability, use, or consumption and sold at eating establishments for quick availability or take-out.

Fat   The chemical storage form of fatty acids as glycerol esters, also known as triglycerides. Fat is stored primarily in adipose tissue located throughout the body, but mainly under the skin (subcutaneously) and around the internal organs (viscerally). Fat mass is the sum total of the fat in the body while, correspondingly, the remaining, nonfat components of the body constitute the fat-free mass. Lean tissues such as muscle, bone, skin, blood, and the internal organs are the principal locations of the body's fat-free mass. In common practice, however, the terms "fat" and "adipose tissue" are often used interchangeably. Furthermore, "fat" is commonly used as a subjective or descriptive term that may have a pejorative meaning.

Fitness   A set of attributes, primarily respiratory and cardiovascular, relating to ability to perform tasks requiring physical activity.

Food Guide Pyramid   An educational tool designed for the public that translates and graphically illustrates recommendations from the Dietary Guidelines for Americans and nutrient standards such as the Dietary Reference Intakes into food-group-based advice that promotes a healthful diet.

Food security   Access by all people, at all times to sufficient food for an active and healthful life, including, at a minimum, the ready availability of nutritionally adequate and safe foods and an assured ability to acquire foods in socially acceptable ways.

Food system   The interrelated functions that encompass food production, processing, and distribution; food access and utilization by individuals, households, communities, and populations; and food recycling, composting, and disposal.

Foods of minimal nutritional value   Foods prohibited by federal regulation for sale in school food service areas during meal periods. For artificially sweetened foods, FMNV are defined as providing less than 5 percent of the Reference Daily Intake (RDI) for each of eight specified nutrients (protein, vitamin A, vitamin C, niacin, riboflavin, thiamine, calcium, iron) per serving; for all other foods, defined as providing less than 5 percent of the RDI for each of eight specified nutrients per 100 calories and less than 5 percent of the RDI for each of eight specified nutrients per serving. The four categories of foods specified in the regulation are: soda water, water ices, chewing gum, and certain candies (i.e., hard candy, jellies and gums, marshmallow candies, fondant, licorice, and spun candy).

Health   A state of complete physical, mental, and social well-being and not merely the absence of disease or infirmity.

Health promotion   The process of enabling people to increase control over and to improve their health. To reach a state of complete physical, mental, and social well-being, an individual or group must be able to identify and to realize aspirations, to satisfy needs, and to change or cope with the environment. Health is a resource for everyday life, not the objective of living, and is a positive concept emphasizing social and personal resources, as well as physical capacities.

Healthy weight   In children and youth, a level of body fat where co-morbidities are not observed. In adults, a BMI between 18.5 and 24.9 kg/m^2.

Nutrient density   The amount of nutrients that a food contains per unit volume or mass. Nutrient density is independent of energy density although, in practice, the nutrient density of a food is often described in relationship to the food's energy density. Fruits and vegetables are nutrient dense but not energy dense. Compared to foods of high-fat content, soda or soft drinks are not particularly energy dense because these are made up primarily of water and carbohydrate, but because they are otherwise low in nutrients, their energy density is high for the nutrient content.

Nutrition Facts panel   Standardized detailed nutritional information on the contents and serving sizes of nearly all packaged foods sold in the marketplace. The panel was designed to provide nutrition information to consumers and was mandated by the Nutrition Labeling and Education Act of 1994.

Obesity   An excess amount of subcutaneous body fat in proportion to lean body mass. In adults, a BMI of 30 or greater is considered obese. In this report, obesity in children and youth refers to the age- and gender-specific BMI that are equal to or greater than the 95th percentile of the CDC BMI charts. In most children, these values are known to indicate elevated body fat and to reflect the co-morbidities associated with excessive body fatness.

Obesogenic   Environmental factors that may promote obesity and encourage the expression of a genetic predisposition to gain weight.

Overweight   In children and youth, BMI is used to assess underweight, overweight, and risk for overweight. Children's body fatness changes over the years as they grow. Girls and boys differ in their body fatness as they mature, thus, BMI for children, also referred to as BMI-for-age, is gender and age specific. BMI-for-age is plotted on age- and gender-specific BMI charts for children and teens 2 to 20 years. According to CDC, at risk of overweight is defined as BMI-for-age 85th percentile to < 95th percentile. Overweight is defined as BMI-for-age $\geq$ 95th percentile.

Physical activity   Body movement produced by the contraction of skeletal muscles that result in energy expenditure above the basal level. Physical activity consists of athletic, recreational, housework, transport, or occupational activities that require physical skills and utilize strength, power, endurance, speed, flexibility, range of motion, or agility.

Physical education   Refers to a planned, sequential program of curricula and instruction that helps students develop the knowledge, attitudes, motor skills, self-management skills, and confidence needed to adopt and maintain physically active lifestyles.

Physical fitness   A set of attributes that people have or achieve that relates to the ability to perform physical activity. The ability to carry out daily tasks with vigor and alertness, without undue fatigue, and with ample energy to enjoy leisure-time pursuits and meet unforeseen emergencies.

Physical inactivity   Not meeting the type, duration, and frequency of recommended leisure-time and occupational physical activities.

Population health   The state of health of an entire community or population as opposed to that of an individual. It is concerned with the interrelated factors that affect the health of populations over the life course, and the distribution of the patterns of health outcomes.

Prevention   With regard to obesity, *primary* prevention represents avoiding the occurrence of obesity in a population; *secondary* prevention represents early detection of disease through screening with the purpose of limiting its occurrence; and *tertiary* prevention involves preventing the sequelae of obesity in childhood and adulthood.

Risk   The possibility or probability of loss, injury, disadvantage, or destruction.

Risk analysis   Risk analysis is broadly defined to include risk assessment, risk characterization, risk communication, risk management, and policy relating to risk, in the context of risks of concern to individuals, to public- and private-sector organizations, and to society at a local, regional, national, or global level.

Safety   The condition of being protected from or unlikely to cause danger, risk or injury that either may be perceived or objectively defined.

School meals   Comprises the food service activities that take place within the school setting. The federal child nutrition programs include the National School Lunch Program, School Breakfast Program, Child and Adult Care Food Program, Summer Food Service Program, and Special Milk Program.

Sedentary   A way of living or lifestyle that requires minimal physical activity and that encourages inactivity through limited choices, disincentives, and/or structural or financial barriers.

Well-being   A view of health that takes into account a child's physical, social, and emotional health.

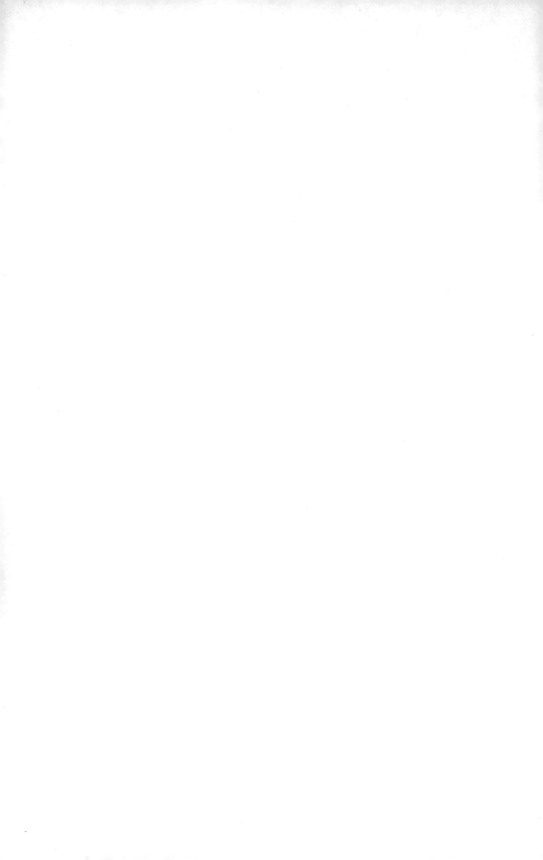

C

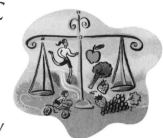

Literature Review

The committee reviewed and considered a broad array of information in its work on issues potentially involved in the prevention of obesity and overweight in children and youth. Information sources included the primary research literature in public health, medicine, allied health, psychology, sociology, education, and transportation; reports, position statements, and other resources (e.g., websites) from the federal government, state governments, professional organizations, health advocacy groups, trade organizations, and international health agencies; textbooks and other scientific reviews; federal and state legislation; and news articles.

LITERATURE REVIEW

In order to conduct a thorough review of the medical and scientific literature, the committee, Institute of Medicine (IOM) staff, and outside consultants conducted online bibliographic searches of relevant databases (Box C-1) that included Medline, AGRICOLA, CINAHL, Cochrane Database, EconLit, ERIC, PsycINFO, Sociological Abstracts, EMBASE, TRIS, and LexisNexis. To begin the process of identifying the primary literature in this field, the IOM staff at the beginning of the study conducted general bibliographic searches on topics related to prevention interventions of obesity in children and youth. These references (approximately 1,000 citations) were categorized and annotated by the staff and reference lists of key citations were provided to the committee. After examining the initial search and identifying key indexing terms in each of the databases, a comprehen-

BOX C-1
Online Databases

AGRICOLA is a bibliographic database of citations to the agricultural literature. Production of these records in electronic form began in 1970, but the database covers materials in all formats, including printed works from the 15th century. The records describe publications and resources encompassing aspects of agriculture and allied disciplines such as agricultural economics, animal and veterinary sciences, earth and environmental sciences, entomology, extension and education, farming and farming systems, fisheries and aquaculture, food and human nutrition, forestry, and plant sciences. AGRICOLA indexes more than 2,000 serials as well as books, pamphlets, conference proceedings, and other resources. This database is updated and maintained by the National Agricultural Library.

CINAHL (Cumulative Index to Nursing and Allied Health Literature) is a bibliographic database of citations of the literature related to nursing and allied health professions from 1982 to the present. Over 1,200 English language journals are indexed with online abstracts available for more than 800 of these titles. Some full-text articles are available. The database also indexes health-care books, dissertations in nursing, conference proceedings, standards of professional practice, educational software, and audiovisual media.

Cochrane Database (Cochrane Database of Systematic Reviews) is a database containing the full text of over 1,600 systematic reviews of the effects of health care. The reviews are highly structured and systematic, with evidence included or excluded on the basis of explicit quality criteria, to minimize bias. Data are often combined statistically (with meta-analysis) to increase the power of the findings of numerous studies, each too small to produce reliable results individually. It is prepared by the Cochrane Collaboration and is now published by John Wiley & Sons, Ltd. (Chichester, UK). These reviews are regularly updated.

EconLit is the American Economic Association's bibliographic database of economics literature published in the United States and other countries from 1969 to the present. EconLit contains citations and abstracts from more than 500 economics journals. Some full-text articles are available. The database also indexes books, book chapters, book reviews, dissertations, essays, and working papers. The database covers subjects including accounting, consumer economics, monetary policy, labor, marketing, demographics, modeling, economic theory, and planning. EconLit contains over 350,000 records and is updated monthly.

EMBASE (Excerpta Medica) database is a major biomedical and pharmaceutical containing more than 9 million records from 1974 to the present from over 4,000 journals; approximately 450,000 records are added annually. Over 80 percent of recent records contain full author abstracts. This bibliographic database indexes international journals in the following fields: drug research, pharmacology, pharmaceutics, toxicology, clinical and experimental human medicine, health policy and management, public health, occupational health, environmental health, drug dependence and abuse, psychiatry, forensic medicine, and biomedical engineering/instrumentation. EMBASE is produced by Elsevier Science.

ERIC (Educational Resources Information Center) is a national education database containing nearly 100,000 citations and abstracts published from 1993 to the present. ERIC contains over one million citations of research documents, journal articles, technical reports, program descriptions and evaluations, and curricular materials in the field of education. ERIC is sponsored by the U.S. Department of Education, Office of Educational Research and Improvement.

LexisNexis provides access to full-text information from over 5,600 sources, including national and regional newspapers, wire services, broadcast transcripts, international news, and non-English language sources; U.S. federal and state case law, codes, regulations, legal news, law reviews, and international legal information; and business news journals, company financial information, Securities and Exchange Commission filings and reports, and industry and market news. It is produced by Reed Elsevier, Inc.

MEDLINE is the U.S. National Library of Medicine's premier bibliographic database containing citations from the mid-1960s to the present, and covering the fields of medicine, nursing, dentistry, veterinary medicine, the health-care system, and the preclinical sciences. PubMed provides online access to over 12 million MEDLINE citations. MEDLINE contains bibliographic citations and author abstracts from more than 4,600 biomedical journals published in the United States and 70 other countries. PubMed includes links to many sites providing full-text articles and other related resources. This database can be accessed at http://www.ncbi.nlm.nih.gov/PubMed.

PsycINFO is a bibliographic database of psychological literature with journal coverage from the 1800s to the present and book coverage from 1987 to the present. It contains more than 1,900,000 records including citations and summaries of journal articles, book chapters, books, and technical reports, as well as citations to dissertations, all in the field of psychology and psychological aspects of related disciplines. Journal coverage includes full-text article links to 42 American Psychological Association journals including peer-reviewed international journals. PsycINFO is produced by the American Psychological Association.

Sociological Abstracts indexes the international literature in sociology and related disciplines in the social and behavioral sciences from 1963 to the present. This bibliographic database contains citations (from 1963) and abstracts (only after 1974) of journal articles, dissertations, conference reports, books, book chapters, and reviews of books, films, and software. Approximately 1,700 journals and 900 other serials published in the United States and other countries in over 30 languages are screened yearly and added to the database bi-monthly. The Sociological Abstracts database contained approximately 600,000 records in 2003. A limited number of full-text references are available. Sociological Abstracts is prepared by Cambridge Scientific Abstracts.

TRIS (Transportation Research Information Services) is a bibliographic database on transportation information published from 1970 to the present. The database contains more than 535,000 records and includes journal articles, government reports, technical reports, books, conference proceedings and ongoing research. Major subjects include aviation, highways, maritime, railroads, and transit; design and construction; environmental issues; finance; human factors; materials; operations; planning; transportation and law enforcement; and safety. TRIS is produced and maintained by the Transportation Research Board at the National Academies.

sive search strategy was designed in consultation with librarians at the George E. Brown Jr. Library of the National Academies. Search terms incorporated relevant MeSH (Medical Subject Headings) terms as well as terms from the EMBASE thesaurus. To maximize retrieval, the search strategy incorporated synonymous terms on the topics of obesity, overweight, or body weight; dietary patterns (including breastfeeding); and physical activity (including exercise, recreation, physical fitness, or physical education and training). The searches were limited to English language and targeted to retrieve citations related to infants, children, or youth (less than 18 years of age). The searches were not limited by date of publication. This broad search resulted in over 40,000 citations. Subsequent analysis of the resulting database focused on resources published since 1994 (approximately 19,000 citations).

As the study progressed, additional focused searches were conducted. Topics of these searches included prevention of obesity in adults (primarily meta-analyses and reviews); prevention interventions focused on co-morbidities of obesity in children (i.e., diabetes, hypertension); behaviorally focused interventions; and statistical information on trends in obesity and physical activity. Additional references were identified by reviewing the reference lists found in major review articles, key reports, prominent websites, and relevant textbooks. Committee members, workshop presenters, consultants, and IOM staff also supplied references.

The committee maintained the reference list in a searchable database that was indexed to allow searches by keywords, staff annotations, type of literature (e.g., literature review), or other criteria. Additionally, an Internet-based site was developed to facilitate the committee's access to subject bibliographies that were developed from the search as well as to full text of some of the key resources. After indexing the citations, subject bibliographies were developed for the committee on topics including definition and measurement of childhood obesity and overweight; correlates and determinants (breastfeeding, dietary patterns, physical activity, television viewing, etc.); economic issues; etiology/epidemiology; ethnology and disparities; prevention interventions (family-based, school-based, community-based, etc.); and prevalence. Bibliographies were updated throughout the study and committee members requested the full text of journal articles and other resources as needed for their information and analysis.

D

Lessons Learned from Public Health Efforts and Their Relevance to Preventing Childhood Obesity

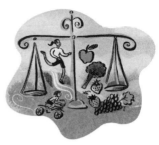

Michael Eriksen, Sc.D.[1]

INTRODUCTION

A s a nation, we are experiencing an epidemic of obesity that is unprecedented in its magnitude or rapidity. Overweight and obesity not only plague the majority of adults, but children are becoming increasingly overweight, with corresponding decrements in health status and quality of life.

While the problem clearly exists, the causes are less clear. There is little clarity about the relative importance of possible causative factors such as changes in dietary patterns, increases in fast food and soft drink consumption, increases in portion size, decreases in physical activity, increases in television viewing, or most likely, a mix of all these factors. Clearly, a thorough understanding of the precise causes of childhood obesity, and how these factors interact, would increase the probability of developing effective prevention and control strategies. In the absence of a precise understanding of the etiology of the problem, it may be useful to look at the lessons learned from other public health campaigns and to try to determine if these lessons have any relevance for the prevention of childhood obesity.

One way to better understand how to deal with a particular public health problem is to look at the experience in dealing with other public health issues, especially those where there has been a modicum of success.

[1]Professor and Director, Institute of Public Health, Georgia State University, Atlanta, GA

For the purposes of this appendix, the experience with public health programs, such as tobacco control, injury prevention, underage alcohol use, gun control, and others are qualitatively examined with particular attention to their possible relevance for the prevention of childhood obesity.

PUBLIC HEALTH LESSONS LEARNED

The purpose of this paper is not to suggest specific intervention strategies to prevent childhood obesity, but rather to learn from other public health experiences and to glean lessons that might help inform efforts to prevent childhood obesity. There is certainly no shortage of theories, models, and approaches to help guide public health program planning. There are multiple health behavior theories that are commonly used to guide public health efforts (Glanz et al., 2002), and popular planning models have been designed to help diagnose health problems (Green and Kreuter, 2000), identify the factors that contribute to these problems, and devise appropriate interventions. In general, these theories and models recommend taking a broad view of changing health behaviors and conditions, suggesting multifactorial, comprehensive interventions that address multiple aspects of the problem. Recently, the Institute of Medicine (2002) endorsed this broad approach to public health interventions, recommending the adoption of an "ecological model" for viewing public health problems and interventions, where the individual is viewed within a larger context of family, community, and society. Overall, there is increasing interest in public health interventions being comprehensive, addressing the multiple factors that influence the health problem, and striving to strike a balance between efforts directed at the individual and the social-environmental context in which people live. It is likely that this approach will be as relevant for the prevention of childhood obesity as it is for other contemporary public health challenges. However, as previously stated, the purpose here is not to propose a comprehensive intervention program for childhood obesity, but rather to identify the factors associated with success in other public health areas, both as a result of planned interventions and also corresponding to social, cultural, or temporal factors.

Despite the notable successes in public health over the past century, there are no generally agreed on approaches or interventions that can be applied to multiple public health problems, with the same intervention effect seen with different problems. There are general guidelines and recommendations, core functions for public health, but no generic model program, best practices, or common lessons learned that could be applied to most or all public health problems.

There are "best practices" for specific public health problems, but little research or insight of the extent to which these categorical approaches are generalizable to other public health challenges. For example, the Centers for Disease Control and Prevention's (CDC's) Best Practices for Comprehensive Tobacco Control Programs (CDC, 1999a) describes nine programmatic areas (i.e., community programs, school programs, statewide programs, etc.) that have been shown to be effective in reducing tobacco use.[2] In practice, these programs are typically delivered "comprehensively," and it is difficult, if not impossible, to tease out the relative impact of specific program components within these comprehensive, real-life campaigns. For this reason, program evaluations of large-scale public health campaigns tend to assess the collective effort, rather than the impact of individual program components. Because of the difficulty in teasing out the effect of one component of a comprehensive program, evaluations have tended to focus on the overall program impact and on the relationship between financial investment in program activities and changes in health behaviors. Data on the impact of comprehensive programs is strong, both in terms of changes in health behavior, as well as in terms of health outcomes (CDC, 2000). Recent analysis has confirmed that the greater the investment in comprehensive programs, composed of evidence-based programs, the larger the public health benefit (Farrelly et al., 2003).

In addition to tobacco control, recent review articles have analyzed the evidence for the effectiveness of public health interventions for a variety of public health problems, including dietary behavior, underage drinking, and motor vehicle injuries, to name just a few. For example, a recent review by Bowen and Beresford (2002) concluded that although much has been learned about trying to change dietary practices clinically, it is particularly important to learn how to transform the successes obtained from interventions aimed at the individual to community and public health settings. Gielen and Sleet (2003) reviewed the injury prevention literature and concluded that a simplistic belief that imparting information would result in behavior change and injury risk reduction resulted in an over-reliance on engineering solutions alone as the basis for injury prevention programs. These authors reinforce the need for interdisciplinary approaches to injury prevention, using behavioral science theory, coupled with engineering solutions.

These observations from other public health problems (e.g., determining how to expand clinical success to communities, combining behavioral

---

[2]For example, in 1999, the CDC's *Best Practices for Comprehensive Tobacco Control Programs* was developed to guide state health departments in planning and allocating funds from the Master Settlement Agreement. The *Best Practices* document does not explicitly recommend policy or regulatory actions, such as an increase in the excise tax on tobacco products, or clean indoor air laws, because they did not require budget expenditures.

and environmental approaches) are informative and relevant for the development of programs to prevent childhood obesity.

Ten Greatest Public Health Achievements in the 20th Century

To begin to understand the potential generalizability of "best practices" for specific health problems, it is useful to look at the evidence for the specific success stories and determine if there are any common elements, or lessons learned, that tend to span multiple problems.

In 1999, acknowledging public health successes, CDC published a list of the ten greatest public health achievements of the 20th century (CDC, 1999b) (Box D-1).

The subsequent *Morbidity and Mortality Weekly Reports (MMWR)* documented the reason these achievements were selected and described the progress made in each area in terms of death and disease prevented. Although efforts were made to account for the reasons for the progress, there was no systematic effort to attribute improvements in health status to specific interventions, and no attempt was made to determine if there were common interventions that contributed to the amelioration of multiple health problems.

A preliminary review of the *MMWR* reports reveals a pattern of categories of interventions that appear to have played a role in accomplishing multiple achievements. The goal was to identify instances, across achievements, of community intervention categories found in the past to have strong evidence of effectiveness with multiple health behaviors or problems. As Table D-1 shows, intervention categories identified most frequently included community-wide campaigns, mass-media strategies, changes to

---

BOX D-1
Ten Great Public Health Achievements
United States, 1900-1999

- Vaccination
- Motor vehicle safety
- Safer workplaces
- Control of infectious disease
- Decline in deaths from coronary heart disease and stroke
- Safer and healthier foods
- Healthier mothers and babies
- Family planning
- Fluoridation of drinking water
- Recognition of tobacco use as a health hazard

TABLE D-1 Community Intervention Categories and 10 Greatest Public Health Achievements 1900-1999

	Community-Wide Campaigns	School-Based Interventions	Mass-Media Strategies	Laws and Regulations	Provider Reminder Systems	Reducing Costs to Patients
Vaccination	X		X	X		X
Motor-vehicle safety	X	X	X	X		
Safer workplaces	X			X		
Control of infectious diseases	X		X	X		X
Decline in deaths from coronary heart disease and stroke	X		X			
Safer and healthier foods	X	X	X	X		X
Healthier mothers and babies	X		X	X		X
Family planning	X			X		X
Fluoridation of drinking water				X	X	
Recognition of tobacco use as a health hazard			X		X	

laws and regulations, and reductions in patient costs. Those categories mentioned least frequently included school-based interventions, and provider reminder systems. In addition, some contextual factors were similar across achievements. For example, in nearly all cases, policy changes were followed by the emergence of new government leadership structures that were effective enforcers of the new policies and oversaw the development and implementation of new programs. Additionally, improved surveillance methods, control measures, technologies, and treatments, and expanding systems of service delivery and provider education, were frequently cited as driving factors in these achievements.

The Guide to Community Preventive Services

Intensive effort has been devoted to reviewing the evidence of effectiveness, first for clinical preventive services (AHRQ, 2002) and now for community preventive services (CDC, 2004c), but these efforts focus on the quality of evidence for specific diseases and health behaviors, rather than drawing conclusions, or generalizing, across health problems.

The task force has completed the analysis of the evidence in nine major areas. More reports, including those central to preventing childhood obesity (e.g., school-based programs, community fruit and vegetable consumption, consumer literacy, and food and nutrition policy) have not yet been released (CDC, 2004c). Of the nine completed reports (most of which focused on adult health behaviors), the task force has determined that 34 interventions could be recommended based on "strong" scientific evidence, another 14 could be recommended as having "sufficient" scientific evidence, and for 42, there was insufficient evidence to make a recommendation. The Guide emphasizes that "...a determination that evidence is insufficient should not be confused with evidence of ineffectiveness."

There was relatively little overlap in the nearly 50 recommended interventions, primarily because the interventions studied were very specific to the health behavior or health condition studied. However, certain categories of interventions appear to have strong evidence of effectiveness for multiple health behaviors and problems. The interventions listed in Table D-2 appear to be effective in multiple areas.

Thus, there are at least seven types of macrolevel interventions that appear to have evidence supporting their effectiveness for multiple public health problems. Other interventions that are effective for multiple behaviors and conditions may be identified in future work by the task force. Similarly, some of the types of interventions that currently have insufficient evidence may in fact have relevance for multiple health problems, but the current body of research is insufficient in relation to rules of evidence. As is

TABLE D-2 Recommended Public Health Interventions Common to Multiple Health Behaviors and Conditions, *The Guide to Community Preventive Services*

Type of Intervention	Health Behavior or Condition
Community-wide campaigns	Physical activity** Motor vehicle occupant injuries* Oral health (water fluoridation)**
School-based interventions	Physical activity** Oral health (sealants)** Vaccine preventable diseases (requirement for school admission)* Skin cancer*
Mass-media strategies	Tobacco initiation and cessation** Motor vehicle occupant injuries**
Laws and regulations	Reducing exposure to secondhand smoke** Motor vehicle occupant injuries**
Provider reminder systems	Vaccine preventable diseases** Tobacco cessation*
Reducing costs to patients	Tobacco cessation* Vaccine preventable diseases**
Home visits	Vaccine preventable diseases* Violence prevention**

* Sufficient evidence.
** Strong evidence.
SOURCE: CDC, 2004c.

often the case, the requisite research is difficult to conduct, or has yet to be conducted.

Based on the experience to date from *The Guide to Community Preventive Services*, it appears that comprehensive programs that involve communities, schools, mass media, health providers, and laws and regulations are most likely to be effective for a number of health problems. It is reasonable to assume that some or all of the types of interventions may have utility in preventing childhood obesity

Lessons Learned Across Multiple Public Health Problems

The focus on "internal validity" has greatly improved the practice of public health and the implementation of evidence-based approaches shown to be effective for specific health problems. This focus on disease- or behavior-specific evidence has not, however, advanced our understanding of the "external validity" or generalizability of interventions across multiple health problems. Namely, extant research has failed to determine if there are common approaches that may be effective across a variety of health problems.

There is a clear need for "lessons learned" from public health interventions and an assessment of the generalizability of interventions, and a determination of under what conditions, and for which populations, they may work. While analysis of the same degree of rigor that has been applied to assessing the evidence for effectiveness of specific programs does not exist across multiple programs, some efforts have been made to analyze the experiences of successful public health campaigns, and to identify elements that appear to be associated with program success. Some of this work has been done by academic researchers and some advanced by the public health practice community, most notably the articulation of the Ten Essential Public Health Services (CDC, 2004a) and the National Public Health Performance Standards (CDC, 2004b). While these efforts to improve practice are noteworthy and of critical importance, the following section highlights some of the academic reviews focused on factors associated with successful health movements.

For example, based on analysis of success with lead, fluoride, auto safety, and tobacco, Isaacs and Schroeder (2001) concluded that the ingredients of success for public health programs include a mixture of (1) highly credible scientific evidence, (2) campaigns with highly effective advocates, (3) a supportive partnership with the media, and (4) laws and regulations, often, but not always, at the federal level.

Drawing on social movement and other sociological theories, Nathanson analyzed the tobacco and gun control movements and concluded that successful health-related social movements had the following elements in common: a socially and scientifically credible threat to the public health, mobilization of a diverse constituency, and "the convergence of political opportunities with target vulnerabilities."

Some researchers have looked for public health lessons that may be directly applicable to obesity or dietary change. Researchers at CDC analyzed the experience with the tobacco control movement in relation to possible implications for preventing obesity (Mercer et al., 2003). They used the intervention framework described in the 2000 Surgeon General's Report, *Reducing Tobacco Use*, and reflected on the relevance of educational, clinical, regulatory, economic, and comprehensive interventions for the prevention of obesity (DHHS, 2000).

Researchers at the World Health Organization (WHO) looked at the recently adopted Framework Convention on Tobacco Control (FCTC) in terms of its possible implications for improving global dietary and physical activity levels (Yach et al., 2003). These researchers concluded that strategies to improve diet and physical activity levels must be different from those employed for tobacco control, because the nature of the behaviors are different, but also in relation to possible private-sector interactions. According to the authors, a formal treaty approach is not warranted,[3] but that the organizing framework for the FCTC may be useful for the development of national plans and policies. In their article, Yach and colleagues (2003) draw comparisons between tobacco and food strategies, using the template of the FCTC, including a discussion of (1) price and tax measures, (2) labeling and product content, (3) educational campaigns, (4) product marketing, (5) clinical interventions, (6) product supply, (7) liability and corporate behavior, and (8) supportive and facilitative measures.

Economos and colleagues (2001) conducted a global analysis of social change models by interviewing 34 key informants. These investigators concluded that a number of factors are being associated with a successful social change. These factors included having the issue being perceived as a crisis, a persuasive science base, important economic implications, strategic leadership (spark plugs), a coalition or mobilizing network, community and media advocacy, government involvement, media involvement, policy and environmental change, and a coordinated, but flexible plan.

A synthesis of these studies suggests a set of core factors that appear to be associated with successful health-related social change efforts. These core factors include:

- A persuasive science base documenting a socially and scientifically credible threat to the public health with important economic implications;
- A supportive partnership with the media;
- Strategic leadership and a prominent champion;
- A diverse constituency of highly effective advocates; and
- Enabling and reinforcing laws, regulations, and policies.

It is not clear whether all these factors need to be present for each public health campaign, or if there is a preferred sequence of activities, although the order presented above corresponds roughly to the tobacco control movement and exhibits some face validity for these core concepts.

In summary, some of the factors associated with successful public health campaigns are formal, planned interventions (e.g., mass-media campaigns,

---

[3]However, an accompanying commentary (Daynard, 2003) suggested that consideration should be given to a treaty model for global obesity prevention, similar to the FCTC, if only for the increased awareness of civil society and governments of the problem resultant from treaty development and negotiations process.

school-based programs), while other elements associated with success are cultural or social factors (e.g., leadership, advocacy, scientific evidence). Although these social factors are less likely to be planned in the same way as formal interventions are, they can and should be cultivated and combined with more traditional intervention strategies This mix of formal interventions, typically provided by the medical and public health communities, coupled with social change strategies, typically stimulated by advocacy organizations and civil society, are most likely to result in successful and sustained health-related social change. Empirical data are lacking, but some could argue that the two types of interventions are inextricably linked, and either alone is unlikely to achieve success. If anything, anecdotal evidence suggests that social factors (those less likely to be initiated by the health community) are more likely to be associated with success in health-related social movements, if only serving to create a "tipping point" for social change (Gladwell, 2000).

AN ORGANIZING FRAMEWORK FOR PUBLIC HEALTH INTERVENTIONS

To learn from the lessons of other public health experiences and determine whether there is any utility or relevance for preventing childhood obesity, it is useful to have a conceptual framework to organize the experiences, principles, and strategies. In the 2000 Surgeon General's Report, *Reducing Tobacco Use*, a framework was developed to categorize the different types of tobacco control interventions (DHHS, 2000). This framework reviewed the evidence within the following categories: educational, clinical, legal, economic, regulatory, and comprehensive. Although it was developed for tobacco control, this framework may be useful in categorizing interventions for other types of public health problems and has already been used to analyze similarities and differences between tobacco control and the prevention of obesity (Mercer et al., 2003). Analyzing strategies to prevent underage drinking, Komro and Toomey (2002) identified six different types of alcohol prevention strategies: school, extracurricular, family, policy, community, and multicomponent.

Drawing on and expanding the framework in the 2000 Surgeon General's Report and from other sources, the next section reviews findings from a variety of public health campaigns, particularly efforts to reduce tobacco use, and other public health experiences that have commercial dimensions, or that have been politically sensitive (e.g., underage alcohol consumption, injury prevention). The following section reviews six categories of interventions that may have relevance for the prevention of childhood obesity. These categories are:

- The information environment
- Access and opportunity
- Economic factors
- The legal and regulatory environment
- Prevention and treatment programs
- The social environment

The Information Environment

The environment in which people are informed about public health issues is of critical importance, but also fraught with controversy, particularly when dealing with the marketing of commercial products. As a rule, the public health community tends to favor restrictions on commercial speech, if felt necessary to insure the public health. On the other hand, commercial interests tend to view any restrictions on marketing as infringements of their constitutional right to freedom of speech. A thorough discussion on individual speech versus commercial speech is beyond the scope of this paper; however, this tenet was a central argument in the Food and Drug Administration's (FDA's) attempt to regulate tobacco products (Kessler, 2001), and it remains an argument whenever legislators or regulators attempt to restrict the advertising for commercial products such as tobacco, alcohol, and foods.

Although product advertising may result in a public health benefit when the advertising promotes healthy products (Ippolito and Mathios, 1995), the majority of the debate about product marketing focuses on those products that may have harmful effects, particularly among children. Despite the concerns of commercial interests, governments do have the right to alter the informational environment, particularly when the information being conveyed is considered to be false, misleading, or deceptive. In the United States, the regulatory authority in this area is shared by multiple federal agencies, but particularly by the FDA and the Federal Trade Commission (FTC). Gostin (2003) notes that government's power to alter the informational environment is one of the major ways in which governments can "assure the conditions for people to be healthy." The article goes on to describe that governments can alter the informational environment in a number of ways, including by sponsoring health education campaigns and other persuasive communications, requiring product labeling, and restricting harmful or misleading advertising.

Most of the effort in altering the information environment has been done in relation to children and adolescents, particularly when it is believed that the information being conveyed may be harmful or misleading to children (Strasburger and Donnerstein, 1999). Because of this, the quality of the evidence documenting the effect of informational efforts, particularly the marketing of commercial products to children is intensely debated. As one might assume, public health advocates are convinced that marketing efforts are a substantial contributing factor to youth risk behaviors, particularly in the areas of tobacco use, underage drinking, and consumption of high-fat and calorie-dense foods. The manufacturers of these products (and their legal counsel) take just the opposite position, claiming there is insufficient empirical evidence to prove the precise role of marketing on the relevant behaviors of children. At most, manufacturers may concede that marketing may influence the selection of a particular brand of a product but that there is little evidence that marketing contributes to the initiation or use of a product, or causes an overall increase in demand for that product. Despite the lack of existence of the single, definitive, experimental study that unarguably proves that advertising affects the health behaviors of young people, including the initiation and continuation of consumption, most public health authorities agree that the overall weight of the scientific evidence points inescapably to this conclusion.

Concern about the effect of the information environment, particularly the effect of the marketing of harmful products on children, became prominent during the early 1990s corresponding to the increase in youth smoking. Discovering that very young children were more likely to recognize Joe Camel than Mickey Mouse, and that adolescents were much more likely than adults to smoke the most advertised brands, led regulators to attempt to restrict the information environment, particularly as it relates to young people (Kessler, 2001). The battles have continued over the last decade, with litigation replacing public policy as the primary vehicle to restrict advertising, or at least receive compensation for the harm caused. To a large extent, the 1998 Master Settlement Agreement (MSA) attempted to resolve this issue, combining cash payments to states and voluntary limitations on marketing practices (Schroeder, 2004). However, most believe the problem continues and marketing for tobacco products is unabated. Following the MSA agreement with the states, in 1999 the U.S. Department of Justice[4] filed suit against the tobacco industry under racketeering and organized crime statues, including the claim that tobacco companies aggressively marketed cigarettes to children. This case was scheduled to go to trial in September 2004. In February 2004, the U.S. District Court denied a motion by the tobacco companies to dismiss the section of the case related to youth marketing of tobacco products.[4]

Thus, the issue of the impact of product marketing on the health-related behaviors of young people continues to be reviewed scholarly, as

---

[4]USA v. Philip Morris USA Inc., Civil Action 99-2496.

well as legally. Overall, there is good evidence that the advertising and marketing of food products influences parental and child food choice (Food Standards Agency, 2003). Additional empirical studies clearly document the increase in the number of television commercials viewed by children (Kunkel, 2001), the increase in ads for high-fat and high-sodium convenience foods (Gamble and Cotugna, 1999), the effect of even brief exposure to television commercials on food preferences of young children (Borzekowski and Robinson, 2001), and an association between television viewing and the consumption of fast foods (French et al., 2001). Most recently, and directly related to the dietary behaviors of children, the Kaiser Family Foundation (2004) reviewed the evidence on the effect of all types of media on children's dietary behavior, and recommended the reduction or regulation of food ads targeted to children, among other policy options. The American Psychological Association (APA, 2004) recently concluded that televised advertising messages can lead to unhealthy eating habits, particularly for children under 8 years of age who are unable to critically comprehend advertised messages. The APA report went on to recommend:

> Restrict advertising primarily directed to young children of eight years and under. Policymakers need to take steps to better protect young children from exposure to advertising because of the inherent unfairness of advertising to audiences who lack the capability to evaluate biased sources of information found in television commercials.

Currently, there are no legal restrictions on the marketing of unhealthy food to children. Correspondingly, food companies are unfettered in their marketing of calorie-dense and low-nutritional-quality food to children. Some consider it to be "open season" on children, with cartoon characters, celebrities, promotional tie-ins, product placement, sponsorship, games, and toys all be used to market unhealthy foods to children. Candy, soft drinks, and high-fat and high-sodium foods are even marketed in elementary schools (Levine, 1999). None of these strategies are still used to promote tobacco products to children, mainly because it is illegal to sell tobacco products to minors, some states prohibit the use and possession of tobacco products by minors, and the tobacco companies themselves have either voluntarily agreed not to market to children, or have been prohibited from doing so as the result of the settlement of legal proceedings. There is good evidence to suggest that restrictions on the advertising of unhealthy foods, the promotion of healthy choices, and possibly paid counter-advertising campaigns will improve the information environment relative to the prevention of childhood obesity. It is unlikely, however, that such actions will be forthcoming from the federal government, especially the FTC. Recently, Tim Muris, a month after announcing he would step down as FTC Chairman, penned a commentary in *The Wall Street Journal* entitled, "Don't

Blame TV" where he stated, "Banning junk food ads on kids' programming is impractical, ineffective and illegal" (Muris, 2004).

Warning Labels, Ingredient Disclosure, and Labeling

As part of being an informed consumer, public health experts are calling for the full disclosure of ingredients. Commercially purchased food products currently have nutritional labels, which contain ingredients used in the food product, as well as nutritional information on calories, fat, and other nutritional parameters. As product packaging has increased, many nutritional labels still present the nutritional parameters for a "serving" rather than for the contents of the package. The FDA is currently investigating the need to require the provision of "whole package data" in addition to nutritional information per serving (Day, 2003; Matthews et al., 2003; Stein, 2003). Food purchased in restaurants and fast food establishments do not contain nutritional information on the menus or with the meals, although many fast food establishments have nutritional information posted or available on request.

Warning labels have been required on cigarette packages since the late 1960s; however, U.S. warning labels have not kept pace with international standards and generally are not noticed by smokers. Starting with Canada and now required by a number of other countries, graphic and vivid warning labels are required on all tobacco products. Similar labels are required by member states who are signatory to the FCTC (WHO, 2003). Graphic and vivid warning labels, similar to those used in Canada, have been shown to attract the attention of smokers, contribute to their interest in quitting smoking, and increase quit attempts (Hammond et al., 2003). They have even been associated with a reduction in cigarette smoking (Hammond et al., 2004). Currently, there are no warnings labels for food products, other than for alcoholic products, and in some instances, for certain food products that may contain a high risk of infectious disease (e.g., uncooked shellfish). The 2004 report of the APA on the effect of advertising on children concluded that any warnings, disclosures, or disclaimers about products advertised to children should be communicated in clear language comprehensible to the intended audience (APA, 2004).

Access and Opportunity

Children's and adolescents' ease of access and ready opportunity to purchase foods with high sugar, fat, and sodium content likely contribute to the increase in the prevalence of childhood overweight and obesity. Although empirical evidence on the precise contribution of easy availability and access to food products is not strong, some restrictions on access for children are appropriate, at a minimum, to establish a foundation for subsequent public health interventions.

The Community Environment

Community access to food products is ubiquitous and, before recommending restrictions or limitations on access in the community, it may be useful to examine the experience with attempting to restrict minors' access to tobacco products. Because the sale, and frequently the possession, of tobacco products by minors is illegal, various steps have been enacted to enforce tobacco access restrictions. Federal legislation has been promulgated to require states to enforce a prohibition on the sale of tobacco products to minors, and some stores voluntarily restrict access to tobacco products by keeping inventory behind the counter and requiring a personal interaction between the sales clerk and the customer to obtain the product. The evidence, however, is unclear about the effectiveness of enforcement of minors' access laws in reducing the use of tobacco products (Warner et al., 2003). Increasingly, minors have used other means (shoplifting, purchasing by friends, social acquisition) to obtain cigarettes. Whether or not these restrictions are effective by themselves, enforcement of laws to prevent the sale of tobacco products by minors sends a strong and consistent message on the hazard of tobacco use and should be considered as necessary, but not necessarily sufficient action, to prevent adolescent tobacco use.

Regarding calorie-dense or low-nutritional-quality foods, there is no restriction whatsoever on their retail and commercial availability. As is the case with cigarettes, these snack and fast food products are ubiquitously available—in vending machines, gas stations, convenience stores, and many other places. In fact, nearly every retail and commercial outlet sells gums, candies, crackers, cookies, and soft drinks. However, in reviewing the literature on the influence of availability on food choices, French and colleagues (1997) concluded that the relationship is inconsistent, particularly compared to the strong inverse relationship between price and consumption. Further research is needed to determine if restricting commercial access and availability would be effective in reducing the consumption of calorie-dense and low-nutritional-quality foods. As long as these products can be sold legally to minors, it is unlikely that widespread restriction of access to these products is feasible, and even if feasible, whether restriction would have a public health effect.

In addition to examining access to certain food products, it is perhaps more important to understand the changing patterns of consumption and how these patterns may inform interventions to reduce the risk of obesity. The published literature indicates that over the past few decades, and accelerating in the past few years, there have been increases in eating outside the home (particularly at fast food restaurants) (Guthrie et al., 2002; Nielsen et al., 2003; Bowman et al., 2004), increases in portion size (Young and Nestle, 2002; Nielsen and Popkin, 2003), and increases in soft drink consumption (AAP, 2004).

The School Environment

Schools are an important setting to encourage health-promoting behaviors, including the prevention of obesity (Dietz and Gortmaker, 2001). CDC has issued guidelines for schools to prevent nicotine addiction that include smoke-free policies, tobacco prevention policies, and smoking cessation assistance for teachers, staff, and students (CDC, 1994). Similar guidelines exist for nutrition and physical activity programs in schools (CDC, 1996). There is good scientific evidence that manipulation of the school cafeteria and physical activity environment can improve the cardiovascular health of elementary school children, including body mass index (Wechsler et al., 2000). However, the presence of vending machines, concerns about cafeteria menus, and the declining requirement for physical education in schools suggest that the school environment may need improvement.

The American Public Health Association (2003) has called for the development of school policies for the promotion of healthful eating environments and the prohibition of soft drinks and other low-nutrition foods during the school day. The American Academy of Pediatrics (2004) calls for school policies that restrict the sale of soft drinks. There has been some progress in removing soft drinks and snack foods in vending machines from elementary and middle schools particularly in California. This has been achieved by state legislation or local school board policy (e.g., Los Angeles Unified School District), with the major concerns being loss of school district revenue and commitment to long-term contracts with soft drink manufacturers. There is a clear need for additional research on the relative importance of the school environment in contributing to the problem of overweight and obesity among children, as well as the role schools may play in ameliorating this problem. Recently, the National Institutes of Health announced a new funding program to support research in this area (NIH, 2004).

Economic Factors

In addition to altering the informational environment, Gostin (2003) also notes that the government's power to tax and spend is one of the major ways in which governments can "assure the conditions for people to be healthy." He goes on to note that the power to levy taxes can provide incentives to engage in healthy behaviors and disincentives to practice risky ones, but also notes that these taxes can be inequitable and regressive.

Most of the public health experience with manipulating economic factors to encourage healthy behaviors or to discourage risky behaviors has been related to excise tax policy on products like tobacco, gasoline, and alcohol. Because of the popularity of increasing tobacco taxes as a public health strategy and the parallels that are frequently drawn between tobacco tax policy and a possible similar tax scheme for certain foods, the following section highlights some of the specific aspects of the taxation of tobacco products.

Tobacco products, like most consumer products, have been shown to be price sensitive; as price increases, consumption decreases. Children have been shown to be most price sensitive, with an approximate 7 percent decrease in consumption for every 10 percent increase in price (DHHS, 2000). As a result of this well-established price elasticity, an excise tax increases on tobacco products has been a common and popular way to reduce adolescent tobacco use, and to increase much-needed state revenue. In 2002-2003, nearly half the states increased their excise tax on tobacco products (Campaign for Tobacco Free Kids, 2004). Some states have earmarked or dedicated a portion of the excise tax increase for tobacco prevention or health promotion programs. This approach of excise tax increase and earmarking for prevention programs could be considered to help prevent childhood obesity, especially because one of the most frequently heard argument for not removing vending machines and soft drinks from schools is concerns about loss of much-needed revenue.

It is likely that the same strategy for calorie-dense and low-nutritional-quality foods would have the same effect as seen for tobacco—as price increases, consumption falls. However, it is also likely that efforts to tax these products would be even more difficult than taxing tobacco products. In California, an effort to levy a one-cent excise tax on soft drinks to compensate for the lost revenue from removing soft drinks from vending machines in schools had to be removed in order for the vending machine legislation to pass. Internationally, a plan to tax foods such as dairy products, pastries, chocolates, pizzas, and burgers at a higher rate than other food products was briefly considered, then dismissed as unworkable by the British government (Food Navigator, 2004). Jacobson and Brownell (2000) suggest that to avoid the possible negative reaction to the levying of large excise taxes on soft drinks and snack foods, municipalities should consider small tax increases, and the proceeds from these increases should be used to fund health promotion programs, including subsidizing the availability of healthier food choices. The American Public Health Association adopted a similar policy recommendation at its 2003 annual meeting (APHA, 2003).

In addition to considering excise taxes on calorie-dense or low-nutritional-quality foods, incentives or subsidies to make fruits and vegetables more available and affordable could be considered. French and colleagues (1997) reviewed the literature on the relationship between price and consumption of fruits and vegetables and found a consistent pattern, namely that lower prices are associated with higher consumption. In their own empirical work, these researchers found this same pattern among adolescents and found it to be robust across different age groups and food types.

As efforts progress in reducing tobacco use, concern has been expressed about the economic well-being of tobacco farmers and cigarette manufacturing workers and their communities. Similar concerns could be expressed if economic pressures were exerted on certain segments of the food production, manufacturing, and distribution systems.

The Legal and Regulatory Environment

Laws and regulations have become increasingly prominent and effective in improving the public health. Public health law has emerged as a strategic element in planning public health interventions (Goodman et al., 2003), and the IOM has identified law and policy as one of the eight emerging themes for the future of public health training (IOM, 2002). Laws and regulations seem to be one of the few common themes spanning multiple reports from the Ten Greatest Achievements in Public Health to *The Guide to Community Preventive Services*, and also appear to be an essential factor in successful health-related social movements. The following section discusses the importance of laws, regulations, and litigation.

Laws

Laws have played a critical role in the achievement of many public health accomplishments in the 20th century. Starting with infectious disease control, and moving to public health preparedness, the presence of laws has made the critical difference for public health authorities to safeguard the public health, and correspondingly, the absence of legal authority has consistently served as an impediment. Mensah and his colleagues (2004) reviewed the use of law as a tool for preventing chronic disease with particular attention to the impact of bans or restrictions on public smoking, laws on blood alcohol concentration, food fortification, and the FCTC. In addition to these examples, the public health literature is replete with examples of the use of laws to promote the public health.

With respect to laws related to preventing childhood obesity, there is little related federal legislation, other than efforts to provide liability protection to food and soft drink manufacturers. Therefore, most of the legislative initiatives have occurred at the state level. The Kansas Health Institute (2004) recently reviewed obesity-related legislation passed by states between 1999 and 2003.

There are a number of examples of federal legislation with relevance for the prevention of childhood obesity. Review articles attest to the importance of laws in preventing motor vehicle injuries, such as the creation of the National Highway Traffic Safety Administration in 1970, and the use of federal legislation in implementing conditional funding mechanisms that encourage state legislatures to pass injury prevention laws (IOM, 1999). With respect to firearm legislation, there is a complex structure to keep firearms out of the hands of criminals, but no federal agency has regulatory authority over gun design. A recent report from the Community Preventive Services Taskforce did not find sufficient evidence of the effectiveness of firearms laws, such as bans on specified firearms or ammunition, restrictions on firearm acquisition, waiting periods for firearm acquisition, firearm registration and licensing of firearm owners, "shall issue" concealed weapon carry laws, child access prevention laws, zero tolerance laws for firearms in schools, and combinations of firearms laws in preventing firearm-related injuries (Hahn et al., 2003). As discussed earlier, however, insufficient evidence should not be confused with evidence of ineffectiveness.

Regulation

Legislation often results in administrative actions to regulate products that might have an adverse effect on the public's health. There does not appear to be a clear relationship between potential harm from products and the level of regulation. For example, food products are relatively tightly regulated, particularly by the FDA as a result of the authority contained in the Food, Drug and Cosmetic Act. On the other hand, tobacco and gun design are virtually unregulated. The lack of regulation of tobacco products and the public health communities' call for meaningful FDA regulatory authority may provide a useful framework for the potential that product regulation may play in preventing childhood obesity.

Despite substantial progress in reducing tobacco use, tobacco products continue to be relatively unregulated, although the tobacco industry has made protestations to the contrary (Eriksen and Green, 2002). The 1990s saw unprecedented efforts to regulate tobacco products, with the FDA, under the direction of the President, exerting jurisdiction over tobacco products, only to be rebuffed by the Supreme Court, which ruled that Congress has not provided the FDA with the explicit authority to regulate tobacco products.[5]

---

[5]FDA v Brown and Williamson.

Food products, on the other hand, do come under FDA authority and are clearly regulated in terms of certain aspects of health and safety, including nutritional labeling and health claims. However, the FDA does not currently regulate the nutritional content of food products, portion size, or marketing strategies. Currently, if a food product were to make an unjustified health claim, the FDA could act. Similarly, if the advertising were deemed to be false, misleading, or deceptive, the FTC could take action. However, concerns about food product marketing are not focused primarily on health claims or deception, but rather focus on making calorie-dense and low-nutritional-quality food particularly attractive to children. So, it is unlikely that traditional FDA or FTC authority would help in the area of greatest concern regarding marketing unhealthful food products to children.

If governmental regulation is not likely or possible, mandatory industry standards could be considered to guide minimum nutrient content, portion size, and marketing of products targeted to children. In addition to federal regulation, local authorities also have the ability to regulate food products, particularly in the areas of licensing, sampling, zoning restrictions, land use (Ashe et al., 2003), and conditional use permits (Bolen and Kline, 2003). Local restrictions on advertising may be more difficult with regards to First Amendment considerations and free speech. Local efforts to regulate tobacco ads have often been stymied because of federal preemptive legislation. The same pre-emption of local authority may not exist for local control over food marketing.

Litigation

In addition to laws and regulation, litigation has recently become a powerful tool in preventing product-related injuries and ensuring the public health in areas such as tobacco, gun violence, and lead paint. In a recent review, Vernick and colleagues (2003) conclude that although litigation is not a perfect tool, it is an important one, and one that has made some products safer. Parmet and Daynard (2000) reach similar conclusions and agree that litigation can deter dangerous activities and contribute to the public health. However, both reviews agree that there is a dearth of empirical evidence on the actual impact of litigation, but litigation appears to have a modest and important role in protecting the public's health. Others argue that product liability litigation has unacceptable social costs and may diminish the role of personal responsibility. Everyone agrees, however, that litigation has played an extremely important role in tobacco control (Jacobson and Warner, 1999), and many see that experience as a model for preventing obesity (Mello et al., 2003).

For tobacco control, the 1990s were the era of tobacco litigation. A myriad of individual, class action, and state Attorney General suits transformed the tobacco control environment and resulted in lasting change in the way tobacco products are marketed and how the public views tobacco companies. Perhaps of most note, the MSA of November 1998 required the participating tobacco companies to agree to restrict certain marketing practices, disband trade associations, reform their corporate behavior, and provide hundreds of billions of dollars to settling states over the next 25 years (Schroeder, 2004). In addition to significant financial disgorgement, tobacco litigation in the 1990s also resulted in an unprecedented level of tobacco industry document disclosure that has served as a treasure trove of insight, scholarship, and, perhaps most importantly, changed the social-normative opinion of the general public toward tobacco companies (Bero, 2003).

With respect to food-related litigation, there have been some initial attempts to sue fast food restaurants based on the claim that they are at least partially responsible for the epidemic of childhood obesity, and for other reasons, such as consumer safety (e.g., excessive temperature of coffee resulting in customer harm). To date, these efforts have been less than successful, but are widely seen as the vanguard of future litigation efforts (Mello et al., 2003). In fact, attorneys experienced in tobacco litigation recently sponsored a conference to develop strategies and resources to direct individual and class action efforts toward the problems of childhood obesity.

At this point, it is not clear whether these efforts will follow the tobacco model and be successful in obtaining settlements or court victories. The process of discovery is likely to yield internal documents that could be damaging to, at least, the public's perception of food companies. On the other hand, the current cases have tended to be seen by the public as frivolous, and as disregarding the dimension of personal responsibility. In response to the increase in litigation directed against food severs and manufacturers, Senator Mitch McConnell, a pro-tobacco legislator from Kentucky, introduced "The Common Sense for Consumption Act," which seeks to stop frivolous law suits against restaurants and the food industry (Higgins, 2003). A dozen states have introduced legislation aimed at prohibiting lawsuits against food and beverage manufacturers for obesity-related health problems (Campos, 2004). This approach is consonant with the effort to provide immunity to manufacturers and distributors of potentially harmful products such as tobacco, alcohol, and guns. Congress is currently considering providing immunity to gun manufacturers and dealers from civil suits by victimized families and local governments (*New York Times*, 2004). Public attitudes toward suing fast food restaurants, documents obtained through discovery, and federal efforts at tort reform are all likely to shape the litigation environment over the next few years.

Prevention and Treatment Programs

In addition to the effects of product marketing, different environments, economic factors, and laws on health-related behaviors, there is also the strong and direct role played by individual efforts and planned interventions to improve health behaviors. The impact of specific interventions on public health success stories is described earlier in this paper. It is not the intent here to review the literature on the quality of the scientific evidence for changing dietary behaviors, but rather to highlight lessons from other public health areas that may have some utility for multiple health problems, and may be generalizable to preventing childhood obesity.

School-Based Interventions

As previously discussed, school-based programs appear to have robust and generalizable benefits to a number of public health programs, including oral health, motor vehicle safety, and tobacco control. With respect to tobacco use prevention programs, evidence has found them to be effective, especially those that have been conducted in coordination with comprehensive community and mass-media prevention programs (DHHS, 1994; Jago and Baranowski, 2004). It is likely that school-based nutrition and physical activity programs could be even more effective in preventing childhood obesity than school tobacco programs are in reducing tobacco use (Dietz and Gortmaker, 2001). This opinion is due to the fact that nutrition and physical activity behaviors are a normal part of every school day and public health approaches could be fairly easily adopted and implemented. Vending machine policies, school breakfast and lunch programs, and required physical activity programs are all significant components to childhood obesity prevention programs in which schools can play a constructive role.

Media Campaigns

Mass-media efforts that build on sophisticated marketing approaches can also be effective in improving dietary behavior and increasing physical activity levels among young people. In tobacco control, themes of tobacco industry manipulation, the health effects of involuntary smoking on nonsmokers, and graphic depictions of the harm of smoking among real people have proven to be effective (Hersey et al., 2004; Sowden and Arblaster, 2004). It is not clear whether these themes will be relevant for preventing childhood obesity, particularly the extent to which the practices and behavior of food companies will be exploited.

Individual and Clinical Efforts

Historically, the mainstay of efforts to reduce the burden of obesity has focused on individual and clinical efforts. There are well-established interventions for both preventing and controlling obesity, but the challenge now is take the individual and clinical efforts and to extend them so as to have a population effect. The same is the case with helping smokers quit smoking (Fiore et al., 2004). Most smokers would like to quit and wish they had never started, but overcoming nicotine addiction is difficult, with most successful quitters making multiple attempts before achieving success. Smoking cessation is extremely important in order to make public health progress during the next few decades. The public health benefit from cessation is almost immediate, while the benefit from keeping children from starting to smoke will not be reaped for decades. While both prevention and treatment are important, the benefits from treatment or cessation will accrue more quickly. The same is likely to be true for obesity and its sequelae.

Most successful smoking cessation is achieved through individual self-help efforts. Pharmacologic interventions are assuming increasing importance, as is physician counseling, but still, most smokers quit on their own. Similarly, it is important to understand the relative importance of self-help versus medical or health professions intervention in the prevention and treatment of childhood obesity. Because of the lifestyle behaviors associated with obesity (diet and physical activity), it is likely that individual, self-help interventions will be common, but also that the role of the health-care professional is critical, particularly that of the pediatrician (Dietz and Gortmaker, 2001; AAP, 2003).

Efforts to quit smoking may be initially successful, but after a few days or weeks they are plagued by relapse. In fact, after a year, only about 30 percent of short-term quitters have achieved long-term abstinence. Again, a similar situation exists for obesity prevention and treatment, where long-term success in weight loss is often even more elusive than that for smoking cessation.

The Social Environment

The social environment—the way in which citizens, communities, the private sector, and governments interact to create norms and expectations—is a subtle but essential dimension of health-related social movements. Concern about the increase in alcohol-related motor vehicle fatalities created an environment receptive to increases in public involvement and support for public policies to reduce the harm caused by alcohol-impaired driving (DeJong and Hingson, 1998; Shults et al., 2001). The popularity of designated drivers, minimum legal drinking age, blood alcohol concentration laws, community traffic safety programs, and other interventions are a direct result of changing social norms. The desire of nonsmokers to be protected from exposure to secondhand smoke is a critical element in changing the tobacco control environment and how smoking is perceived in society. As a result of nonsmokers' rights advocacy, most workplaces are smoke-free, serum cotinine levels have been reduced by nearly 75 percent in the last decade (CDC, 2003), and the social norms associated with smoking have been permanently changed. It is not clear, however, that the prevention of childhood obesity has a dimension that can serve as a parallel to nonsmokers' exposure to secondhand smoke.

There are a number of possible ways to engage the interest and involvement of society in the issue of childhood obesity in a similar way that it has been secured by other public health problems. One way, which is already happening, is the increasing public concern about the magnitude of the problem and the need for collective action. Given the rapid increase in the prevalence of childhood obesity, the "visibility" of the problem, and the seriousness of the problem for the affected individuals, social and normative change is already beginning to occur. Further, the social costs of obesity that are being borne by society as a whole, suggest the appropriateness of collective and policy interventions.

One of the biggest changes in the social environment for tobacco control is that some tobacco companies are beginning to acknowledge that their products are harmful and addicting. Despite the decades of scientific evidence on the adverse health effects of tobacco use, tobacco companies, primarily for legal reasons, have denied the harm and addictiveness of tobacco products. As a result of the MSA, tobacco companies have begun to become more candid about the harm caused by their products, both in public statements and on their websites. But the level of candor is not consistent among all companies, nor is it consistent in all instances, especially in litigation, where companies tend to continue to deny that their product contributed to the harm claimed by the plaintiff.

At this point in time, it is not clear how the food industry will respond to social and public health pressures to limit marketing of unhealthful products to children and to assume at least partial responsibility for the epidemic of childhood obesity in this country and around the world (Daynard, 2003). However, some change has already begun, with companies such as Kraft announcing changes in portion size and fat content in some of the products most popular with children. Like tobacco companies, it is likely that the food industry will not respond monolithically. Instead those market leaders that can afford to have market share frozen, or those companies that want to be perceived as a leader, or can carve out a "health" niche with their customers, will likely respond differently from other companies.

If the tobacco experience is any guide, it is likely that the food companies will act just enough to avoid government regulation, but will fall short on making structural changes in product design or marketing that will fundamentally alter their marker position. To date, companies have been much more comfortable with educational campaigns emphasizing personal responsibility and the need for increased physical activity than with proposing major policy or structural changes.[6]

In trying to anticipate possible changes in corporate behavior, it should be remembered that marketing and selling unhealthy food, as opposed to tobacco for minors, is completely legal. On the other hand, document discovery has not yet taken place, and if it does, it may change public perceptions pertaining to the legality versus morality of marketing to children those products with known adverse health effects.

The recognition for collaborative approaches to preventing obesity has already begun, and various governments are beginning to launch broad-based national strategies for tackling obesity (Mayor, 2004). In fact, the WHO approved a Global Strategy for Diet, Physical Activity and Health (WHO, 2004) that calls for multisectoral collaboration to address the increasing global prevalence of obesity.

SUMMARY

Efforts to address contemporary public health problems are often difficult to evaluate for a number of reasons including the urgency and need for a rapid response, the lack of classical experimental design, often not having an unexposed control group, difficulty in measuring social factors, and not understanding the dynamics between social forces and health behaviors (McQueen, 2002).

While difficult, it is important to understand the factors that contribute to public health advances and the reasons for the failure of unsuccessful public health programs. This is particularly true as we face new problems that have complex, multifactorial, and often commercially linked dimensions. Rather than "reinventing the wheel," making mistakes previously made, or overlooking interventions that have been shown to be effective, it

---

[6]For example, see the website of the American Council on Food and Nutrition, http://www.acfn.org/about/, or the Center for Consumer Freedom, http://www. consumerfreedom. com/.

is prudent to look at other public health experiences when developing strategies to reduce public health problems, such as the prevention of childhood obesity.

In reviewing other public health experiences and determining if there are lessons for preventing childhood obesity, it is useful to compare and contrast the similarities and differences between the other public health problems and the causes of childhood obesity. For example, when one compares the prevention of tobacco use to the prevention of childhood obesity, the first and most obvious difference is that tobacco use, from a public health standpoint, is a behavior to be avoided; it presents a serious health risk and no health benefit. Diet and physical activity, on the other hand, are essentials of life, cannot be avoided, and must be kept in balance to ensure good health. Thus, for tobacco, there is the simple message of avoidance, whereas for diet and physical activity there is the much more complex message that includes concepts such as quality, quantity, frequency, and balance (Mercer et al., 2003; Yach et al., 2003).

In summary, the "environmental classifications" of types of intervention strategies may serve as a useful template to determine the utility of different public health interventions for the prevention of childhood obesity. More broadly, categories such as these may be useful in conceptualizing intervention strategies for various public health problems. To increase the utility of this approach, and determine the relevance of specific public health interventions, it may be useful to further analyze the public health problem in terms of specific criteria to ascertain the similarity of certain problems and the likelihood that an approach that was successful with one public health problem, may be generalizable to another. Possible criteria for comparison could include:

- Description of the behavior (addictiveness, possible health benefits, legal aspects)
- Epidemiologic significance (number of deaths, disease burden)
- Clear understanding of etiology
- Feasibility of change
- Availability of effective interventions
- Level of public interest and awareness
- Extent to which public is affected by problem
- Salience to policy makers
- Nature of relation with product manufacturer
- Role of government
- Degree of product regulation
- International dimensions

CONCLUDING PRINCIPLES AND IMPLICATIONS

Individual Responsibility Versus Collective Action

One of the greatest challenges in our efforts to prevent childhood obesity is to strike the right balance between individual versus structural or environmental efforts. With tobacco control, most observers believe that major progress was not achieved until clinical efforts in smoking cessation were subjugated to policy efforts to change the social environment. This same debate is central to our efforts in preventing childhood obesity (Kersh and Morone, 2002; Zernike, 2003). As with many public health problems, a critical issue is the role of coercion versus individual rights, and striking the appropriate balance between commercial interests and the common good (Gostin, 2000).

Need to Change Social Norms About Food and Physical Activity

Fifty years ago, smoking was the norm. The majority of men smoked, smoking was widely advertised on television and radio, and smoking could occur anywhere, including airplanes, schools, hospitals, and doctor's offices. Today, the situation is reversed, with smoking no longer being normative, and nearly considered, if not a deviant behavior, at least one that is typically done in private. Fifty million Americans have quit smoking and there are more ex-smokers than current smokers. No one could have predicted the magnitude of change in perceptions and public opinion that has occurred with tobacco, but similar changes are possible with respect to food and physical activity. Today, foods are "super-sized" to provide the most food or value for the dollar, but with virtually no consideration for diet or health. While there is nothing wrong in seeking "value," it is not inconceivable that, in the future, health considerations will enter the equation in calculating "value." Similarly, nearly all smokers who quit, enjoyed smoking a great deal, but quit because they were more concerned about their health than they were about the pleasure of smoking. The same can be achieved with food.

Learn from Other Public Health Experiences, But Don't Necessarily Duplicate

Much has been learned from the successes, and continuing challenges, in previous public health experiences. However, there are major differences in these earlier efforts and efforts to prevent childhood obesity. The differences are particularly striking for tobacco control. Most notably, people need to eat, but do not need to smoke. In addition, it is illegal to sell tobacco products to minors, marketing to minors is prohibited, and nonsmokers' rights is a powerful social movement that has changed public norms related to smoking. None of these elements exist for preventing childhood obesity. From a macroperspective, and although progress has taken decades, tobacco control is relatively simple compared to the complexities presented by childhood obesity. Accordingly, childhood obesity prevention strategies should be developed with an appreciation for this complexity.

The Role of the Food Industry Is Critical but Uncertain

Part of the success of the tobacco control movement has been the attacks on and marginalization of the tobacco companies. This was a fairly predictable strategy because of their intransigence over decades and the harm resulting from a product that, when used as intended, kills one out of two lifetime users. While predictable, this strategy has also been effective in changing social norms and focusing youth empowerment against tobacco industry tactics. At this point, it is unclear whether a similar strategy directed against food companies is warranted or would be effective. This question will be partially answered by the extent to which food companies deal honestly and constructively with the obesity epidemic, including a candid assessment of their role in helping to create it (Revill, 2003). To the extent that commercial interests respond, if not lead, on behalf of the public good, they may obviate the need for government action. To the extent that they fail, government action will be demanded (Yach et al., 2003). In either respect, it appears clear to most that the overall environment in which food products are produced, marketed, and sold, must be improved (Ebbeling et al., 2002).

The Problem Is Multifactorial, and So Must Be the Solutions

Based on the experience with many different public health problems (e.g., tobacco control, motor vehicle and firearm injuries), it seems clear that comprehensive and multifactorial approaches are required. At a minimum these approaches should address both the individual behaviors and the social environment in which these behaviors take place, particularly the marketing, price, availability, and accessibility related to both dietary and physical activity behaviors. It is important to avoid glib and simple solutions to complex and poorly understood problems.

Need Evidence on Best Practices and Effective Interventions

The rise in childhood obesity is well documented, but less well understood. The relationships among and relative contribution of dietary factors, the social environment, and physical activity need to be better understood to develop effective interventions (BMJ, 2004). Recent reports by the APA (2004) and the Kaiser Family Foundation (2004) advance the understanding of the role of the media in childhood obesity, but similar analyses are needed for other aspects of childhood obesity prevention, such as the role of fast foods and soft drinks, and how the social environment can be structured to contribute to the prevention of childhood obesity. For tobacco control, we may not know all the answers, but we know enough to make a difference. Research underlies tobacco control guidelines and recommendations, and similar research, recommendations, and guidelines are being developed for preventing childhood obesity. Once the relative effectiveness of various interventions is better known, there needs to be a concerted effort to disseminate and implement approaches that have been found to be effective. The lack of emphasis on the systematic diffusion of effective interventions has plagued multiple public health initiatives.

Need to Consider the Global Dimension

The epidemic of childhood obesity first appeared in the United States, but every indication is that it is beginning to appear in other developed countries, as well as in the developing world. The global implications of our domestic solutions should be considered, so we do not solve our problems by creating a larger one overseas (Yach et al., 2003; WHO, 2004).

REFERENCES

AAP (American Academy of Pediatrics). 2003. Prevention of pediatric overweight and obesity. *Pediatrics* 112(2):424-430.

AAP. 2004. Policy statement: Soft drinks in schools. *Pediatrics* 113(1):152-154.

AHRQ (Agency for Healthcare Research and Quality). 2002. *Guide to Clinical Preventive Services*. [Online]. Available: http://www.ahrq.gov/clinic/cps3dix.htm [accessed February 24, 2004].

APA (American Psychological Association). 2004. *Report of the APA Task Force on Advertising and Children*. [Online]. Available: http://www.apa.org/releases/childrenads.html [accessed February 24, 2004].

APHA (American Public Health Association). 2003. *Food Marketing and Advertising Directed at Children and Adolescents: Implications for Overweight*. Policy # 200317-1. Adopted November 2003. [Online]. Available: http://www.apha.org/legislative/policy/2003/2003-017.pdf [accessed February 24, 2004].

Ashe M, Jernigan D, Kline R, Galaz R. 2003. Land use planning and the control of alcohol, tobacco, firearms, and fast food restaurants. *American Journal of Public Health* 93(9):1404-1408.

Bero L. 2003. Implications of the tobacco industry documents for public health and policy. *Annual Review of Public Health* 24:267-288.

BMJ (British Medical Journal). 2004. Fighting obesity: Evidence of effectiveness will be needed to sustain policies. *British Medical Journal* 328:1327-1328.

Bolen E, Kline R. 2003. *Applying the Legal Tools of Tobacco Control to the Problem of Obesity*. Presented at the annual meeting of the American Public Health Association, San Francisco, November 17, 2003.

Borzekowski DLG, Robinson TN. 2001. The 30-second effect: An experiment revealing the impact of television commercials on food preferences of preschoolers. *Journal of the American Dietetic Association* 101(1):42-46.

Bowen DJ, Beresford SA. 2002. Dietary interventions to prevent disease. *Annual Review of Public Health* 23:255-286.

Bowman SA, Gortmaker SL, Ebbeling CB, Pereira MA, Ludwig DS. 2004. Effects of fast-food consumption on energy intake and diet quality among children in a national household survey. *Pediatrics* 113(1):112-118.

Campaign for Tobacco Free Kids. 2004. *Tobacco Tax Fact Sheets*. [Online]. Available: http://www.tobaccofreekids.org/research/factsheets/pdf/0239.pdf [accessed August 22, 2004].

Campos C. 2004. Suing Mickey D's? Fat chance. *Atlanta Journal Constitution*, February 25, 2004.

CDC (Centers for Disease Control and Prevention). 1994. Guidelines for school health programs to prevent tobacco use and addiction. *MMWR* 43(RR-2):1-24.

CDC. 1996. Guidelines for school health programs to promote lifelong healthy eating. *MMWR* 45(RR-9):1-47.

CDC. 1999a. *Best Practices for Comprehensive Tobacco Control Programs—August 1999*. Atlanta GA: CDC National Center for Chronic Disease Prevention and Health Promotion, Office on Smoking and Health.

CDC. 1999b. Achievements in public health, 1990-1999. *MMWR* 48(50):1141-1147.

CDC. 2000. Declines in lung cancer rates: California—1988-1997. *MMWR* 49(47):1066-1069.

CDC. 2003. *Second National Environmental Exposure Report*. [Online]. Available: http://www.cdc.gov/exposurereport/2nd/pdf/tobaccosmoke.pdf [accessed August 22, 2004].

CDC. 2004a. *The Essential Public Health Services*. [Online]. Available: http://www.phppo.cdc.gov/nphpsp/10EssentialPHServices.asp [accessed August 23, 2004].

CDC. 2004b. *National Public Health Performance Standards Program*. [Online]. Available: http://www.phppo.cdc.gov/nphpsp/index.asp [accessed August 23, 2004].

CDC. 2004c. *The Guide to Community Preventive Services. At-A-Glance*. [Online]. Available: http://www.thecommunityguide.org/overview/at-a-glance.pdf [accessed February 12, 2004].

Day S. 2003. U.S. considers food labels with whole-package data. *New York Times*. November 21, 2003.

Daynard RA. 2003. Lessons from tobacco control for the obesity control movement. *Journal of Public Health Policy* 24(3/4):291-295.

DeJong W, Hingson R. 1998. Strategies to reduce driving under the influence of alcohol. *Annual Review of Public Health* 19:359-378.

DHHS (U. S. Department of Health and Human Services). 1994. *Preventing Tobacco Use Among Young People: A Report of the Surgeon General*, Atlanta, GA: Centers for Disease Control and Prevention, National Center for Chronic Disease Prevention and Health Promotion, Office on Smoking and Health.

DHHS (U.S. Department of Health and Human Services). 2000. *Reducing Tobacco Use: A Report of the Surgeon General*. Atlanta, GA: Centers for Disease Control and Prevention, National Center for Chronic Disease Prevention and Health Promotion, Office on Smoking and Health.

Dietz WH, Gortmaker SL. 2001. Preventing obesity in children and adolescents. *Annual Review of Public Health* 22:337-353.

Ebbeling CB, Pawlak DB, Ludwig DS. 2002. Childhood obesity: Public health crisis, common sense cure. *Lancet* 360(9331):473-482.

Economos CD, Brownson RC, DeAngelis MA, Foerster SB, Foreman CT, Gregson J, Kumanyika SK, Pate RR. 2001. What lessons have been learned from other attempts to guide social change? *Nutrition Reviews* 59(3):S40-S56.

Eriksen MP, Green LW. 2002. Progress and next steps in reducing tobacco use in the United States. In: Scuthfield D, Keck W, eds. *Principles of Public Health Practice*. 2nd edition. Delmar Learning.

Farrelly MC, Pechacek TF, Chaloupka FJ. 2003. The impact of tobacco control program expenditures on aggregate cigarette sales: 1981-2000. *Journal of Health Economics* 22: 843-859.

Fiore MC, Croyle RT, Curry SJ, Cutler CM, Davis RM, Gordon C, Healton C, Koh HK, Orleans CT, Richling D, Satcher D, Seffrin J, Williams C, Williams LN, Keller PA, Baker TB. 2004. Preventing 3 million premature deaths and helping 5 million smokers quit: A national action plan for tobacco cessation. *American Journal of Public Health* 94(2):205-210.

Food Navigator. 2004. *Tax Plans Dismissed as Unworkable*. [Online]. Available: http://www.foodnavigator.com/news/news-NG.asp?id=50054 [accessed February 25, 2004].

Food Standards Agency. 2003. *Does Food Promotion Influence Children? A Systematic Review of the Literature*. Ref R769-36. United Kingdom Food Services Agency, September 25, 2003.

French SA, Story M, Jeffery RW, Snyder P, Eisenberg M, Sidebottom A, Murray D. 1997. Pricing strategy to promote fruit and vegetable purchase in high school cafeterias. *Journal of the American Dietetic Association* 97(9):1008-1010.

French SA, Story M, Neumark-Sztainer D, Fulkerson SA, Hannan P. 2001. Fast food restaurant use among adolescents: Associations with nutrient intake, food choices and behavioral and psychological variables. *International Journal of Obesity* 25(12):1823-1833.

Gamble M, Cotugna N. 1999. A quarter century of TV food advertising targeted at children. *American Journal of Health Behavior* 23(4):261-268.

Gielen AC, Sleet D. 2003. Application of behavior-change theories and methods to injury prevention. *Epidemiologic Reviews* 25:65-76.

Gladwell M. 2000. *The Tipping Point: How Little Things Can Make a Big Difference*. New York: Little Brown and Company.

Glanz K, Rimer BK, Lewis FM, eds. 2002. *Health Behavior and Health Education: Theory, Research and Practice*. 3rd edition. San Francisco, CA: Jossey-Bass.

Goodman RA, Rothstein MA, Hoffman RE, Lopez W, Matthews GW, eds. 2003. *Law in Public Health Practice*. New York: Oxford University Press.

Gostin LO. 2000. Public health law in a new century. Part 1: Law as a tool to advance the community's health. *JAMA* 283 (21): 2837-2841.

Gostin LO. 2003. *Law and Ethics in Population Health*. Keynote address at the Inauguration of the National Centre for Public Health Law of Australia, Melbourne, Australia, July 21, 2003.

Green LW, Kreuter M. 2000. *Health Promotion Planning: An Educational and Ecological Approach*. New York: McGraw-Hill.

Guthrie JF, Lin BH, Frazao E. 2002. Role of food prepared away from home in the American diet, 1977-78 versus 1994-96: Changes and consequences. *Journal of Nutrition Education and Behavior* 34:140-150.

Hahn RA, Bilukha OO, Crosby A, Fullilove MT, Liberman A, Moscicki EK, Snyder S, Tuma F, Briss P, Task Force on Community Preventive Services. 2003. First reports evaluating the effectiveness of strategies for preventing violence: Firearms laws. Findings from the Task Force on Community Preventive Services. *MMWR Recomm Rep* 52(RR-14):11-20.

Hammond D, Fong GT, McDonald PW, Cameron R, Brown KS. 2003. Impact of the graphic Canadian warning labels on adult smoking behaviour. *Tobacco Control* 12:391-395.

Hammond D, Fong GT, McDonald PW, Brown KS, Cameron R. 2004. Graphic Canadian warning labels and adverse outcomes: Evidence from Canadian smokers. *American Journal of Public Health* 94:1442-1445.

Hersey JC, Niederdeppe J, Evans WD, Nonnemaker J, Blahut S, Farrelly MC, Holden D, Messeri P, Haviland ML. 2004. The effects of state counterindustry media campaigns on beliefs, attitudes, and smoking status among teens and young people. *Preventive Medicine* 37(6 Pt 1):544-552.

Higgins M. 2003. Obesity lawsuit curbs sought. *The Washington Times* October 22, 2003.

IOM (Institute of Medicine). 1999. *Reducing the Burden of Injury: Advancing Prevention and Treatment*. Washington, DC: National Academy Press.

IOM. 2002. *Who Will Keep the Public Healthy?* Washington, DC: The National Academies Press.

Ippolito PM, Mathios AD. 1995. Information and advertising: The case of fat consumption in the United States. *The American Economic Review* 85(2):91-95.

Isaacs SL, Schroeder SA. 2001. Where the public good prevailed: Lessons from success stories in health. *The American Prospect* 12(10):26-30.

Jacobson MF, Brownell KD. 2000. Small taxes on soft drinks and snack foods to promote health. *American Journal of Public Health* 90:854-857.

Jacobson PD, Warner KE. 1999. Litigation and public health policy making: The case of tobacco control. *Journal of Health Politics, Policy and Law* 24(4):769-804.

Jago R, Baranowski T. 2004. Non-curricular approaches for increasing physical activity in youth: A review. *Preventive Medicine* 39:157-163.

Kaiser Family Foundation. 2004. *The Role of Media in Childhood Obesity*. Issue Brief, February 2004. [Online]. Available: http://www.kff.org [accessed February 25, 2004].

Kansas Health Institute. 2004. Obesity and public policy: Legislation passed by states—1999-2003. *Interim Report to the Sunflower Foundation*. [Online]. Available: http://www.khi.org/ [accessed August 23, 2004].

Kersh R, Morone J. 2002. The politics of obesity: Seven steps to government action. *Health Affairs* 21(6):142-153.

Kessler D. 2001. *A Question of Intent*. New York: Public Affairs.

Komro KA, Toomey TL. 2002. Strategies to prevent underage drinking. *Alcohol Research and Health* 26(1):5-14.

Kunkel D. 2001. Children and television advertising. In: Singer D, Singer J, eds. *Handbook of Children and the Media*. Thousand Oaks, CA: Sage Publications.

Levine J. 1999. Food industry marketing in elementary schools: Implications for school health professionals. *Journal of School Health* 69(7):290-291.

Matthews AW, McKay B, Ellison S. 2003. FDA re-examines 'serving sizes,' may change misleading labels. *Wall Street Journal*, November 20, 2003.

Mayor S. 2004. Government task force needed to tackle obesity. *British Medical Journal* 328:363.

McQueen DM. 2002. Strengthening the evidence base for health promotion. *Health Promotion International* 16(3):261-268.

Mello MM, Rimm EB, Studdert DM. 2003. The McLawsuit: The fast-food industry and legal accountability for obesity. *Health Affairs* 22(6):207-216.

Mensah GA, Goodman RA, Zaza S, Moulton AD, Kocher PL, Dietz WH, Pechacek TF, Marks JS. 2004. Law as a tool for preventing chronic disease: Expanding the range of effective public health strategies. *Preventing Chronic Disease* 1(1):1-8.

Mercer SL, Green LW, Rosenthal AC, Husten CG, Khan LK, Dietz WH. 2003. Possible lessons from the tobacco experience for obesity control. *American Journal of Clinical Nutrition* 99(Suppl):1073S-1082S.

Muris T. 2004. Don't blame TV. *The Wall Street Journal.* p. A10, June 25, 2004.

New York Times. 2004. The gun's lobby bull's eye. *New York Times.* February 25, 2004.

Nielsen SJ, Popkin BM. 2003. Patterns and trends in food portion sizes, 1977-1998. *JAMA* 289:450-453.

Nielsen SJ, Siega-Riz AM, Popkin BM. 2003. Trends in food locations and sources among adolescents and young adults. *Preventive Medicine* 35:107-113.

NIH (National Institutes of Health). 2004. *School-Based Interventions to Prevent Obesity.* [Online]. Available: http://grants.nih.gov/grants/guide/pa-files/PA-04-145.html [accessed August 22, 2004].

Parmet WE, Daynard RA. 2000. The new public health litigation. *Annual Review of Public Health* 21:437-454.

Revill J. 2003. Food giants join Britain's war on flab. *The Observer.* November 16, 2003.

Schroeder SA. 2004. Tobacco control in the wake of the 1998 Master Settlement Agreement. *New England Journal of Medicine* 350(3):293-301.

Shults RA, Elder RW, Sleet DA, Nichols JL, Alao MO, Carande-Kulis VG, Zaza S, Sosin DM, Thompson RS, Task Force on Community Preventive Services. 2001. Reviews of evidence regarding interventions to reduce alcohol-impaired driving. *American Journal of Preventive Medicine* 21(4S):66-88.

Sowden AJ, Arblaster L. 2004. Mass media interventions for preventing smoking in young people (Cochrane Review). *The Cochrane Library* Issue 3.

Stein R. 2003. Obesity on FDA's plate? *Washington Post.* November 20, 2003.

Strasburger VC, Donnerstein E. 1999. Children, adolescents and the media: Issues and solutions. *Pediatrics* 103(1):129-139.

Vernick JS, Mair JS, Teret SP, Sapsin JW. 2003. Role of litigation in preventing product-related injuries. *Epidemiologic Reviews* 25:90-98.

Warner KE, Jacobsen PD, Kaufman NJ. 2003. Innovative approaches to youth tobacco control: Introduction and overview. *Tobacco Control* 12(June):ii.

Wechsler H, Devereaux RS, Davis M, Collins J. 2000. Using the school environment to promote physical activity and healthy eating. *Preventive Medicine* 31:S121-S137.

WHO (World Health Organization). 2003. *Framework Convention on Tobacco Control.* [Online]. Available: http://www.who.int/tobacco/fctc/en/ [accessed February 25, 2004].

WHO. 2004. *Global Strategy on Diet, Physical Activity and Health.* [Online]. Available: http://www.who.int/gb/ebwha/pdf_files/WHA57/A57_9-en.pdf [accessed August 22, 2004].

Yach D, Hawkes C, Epping-Jordan JE, Galbraith S. 2003. The World Health Organization's Framework Convention on Tobacco Control: Implications for global epidemics of food-related deaths and disease. *Journal of Public Health Policy* 24(3/4):274-290.

Young LR, Nestle M. 2002. The contribution of expanding portion sizes to the US obesity epidemic. *American Journal of Public Health* 92:246-249.

Zernike K. 2003. Is obesity the responsibility of the body politic? *New York Times.* November 9, 2003.

E

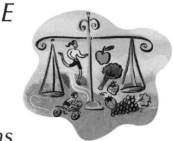

Workshop Programs

STRATEGIES FOR DEVELOPING SCHOOL-BASED POLICIES THAT PROMOTE
NUTRITION AND PHYSICAL ACTIVITY AMONG CHILDREN AND YOUTH

WORKSHOP SPONSORED BY THE
COMMITTEE ON PREVENTION OF OBESITY IN CHILDREN AND YOUTH
INSTITUTE OF MEDICINE

JUNE 16, 2003
1:00 PM—5:30 PM

NATIONAL ACADEMY OF SCIENCES AUDITORIUM
NAS BUILDING
2100 C STREET, NW
WASHINGTON, DC 20418

PROGRAM

1:00 pm **Welcome and Introductions**
*Jeffrey Koplan, M.D., M.P.H., Chair, Committee on
Prevention of Obesity in Children and Youth*

1:10 **Strategies for Developing School-Based Health
Promotion Policies**
*Harold Goldstein, Dr.P.H., California Center for Public
Health Advocacy, Davis, CA*

1:30   Helping Public Schools Meet Expectations: Balancing Obesity
        Prevention and Physical Activity Goals with Fiscal and
        Curriculum Realities
        *Alex Molnar, Ph.D., Education Policy Studies
        Laboratory, Arizona State University, Tempe, AZ*

1:50   Discussion

2:30   Break

2:50   Panel Discussion
        *Mark Vallianatos, J.D., Occidental College,
        Los Angeles, CA
        Judith Young, Ph.D., National Association for Sport
        and Physical Education, Reston, VA
        Jennifer Wilkins, Ph.D., R.D., Division of Nutritional
        Sciences, Cornell University, Ithaca, NY
        Paula Hudson Collins, M.H.D.L., R.H.Ed.,
        North Carolina Department of Public Instruction,
        Raleigh, NC*

3:30   Discussion

4:30   Open Forum
        *Tracy Fox, M.P.H., R.D., Produce for Better Health
        Foundation
        Dianne Ward, M.S., Ed.D., University of North Carolina
        at Chapel Hill
        Margo Wootan, Sc.D., Center for Science in the Public
        Interest
        Kimberly F. Stitzel, M.S., R.D., The American Dietetic
        Association
        Bill Wilkinson, A.I.C.P., National Center for Bicycling
        & Walking
        Alicia Moag-Stahlberg, M.S., R.D., L.D., Action for
        Healthy Kids
        William Potts-Datema, M.S., Harvard School of Public
        Health
        Amy Harris, R.N., National Association of Orthopedic
        Nurses
        Vivian Pilant, M.S., R.D., South Carolina Department of
        Education*

Donna Mazyck, R.N., B.S.N., N.C.S.N., Maryland State Department of Education; National Association of School Nurses
Sandra Hassink, M.D., A.I. duPont Hospital for Children; American Academy of Pediatrics (AAP)

5:30   **Adjourn**

THE PREVENTION OF CHILDHOOD OBESITY:
UNDERSTANDING THE INFLUENCES OF MARKETING,
MEDIA, AND FAMILY DYNAMICS

WORKSHOP SPONSORED BY THE
COMMITTEE ON PREVENTION OF OBESITY IN CHILDREN AND YOUTH
INSTITUTE OF MEDICINE

TUESDAY, DECEMBER 9, 2003
1:00 PM—5:30 PM

KECK CENTER OF THE NATIONAL ACADEMIES
CONFERENCE ROOM 100
500 FIFTH STREET, N.W.
Washington, DC 20001

PROGRAM

1:00 pm   Welcome and Introductions
           *Jeffrey Koplan, M.D., M.P.H., Chair, Committee on
           Prevention of Obesity in Children and Youth*

1:10   Marketing and Media Influences: Identifying
           Challenges and Effective Strategies for the
           Prevention of Childhood Obesity

           1:10 – 1:30 pm
           Neal Baer, M.D., Executive Producer
           University City, CA

           1:30 – 1:50 pm
           Eric Rosenthal, B.B.A., M.S., Marketing Specialist,
           Frankel, Chicago, IL

           1:50 – 2:10 pm
           Mary Engle, Esq., Division of Advertising Practices,
           Federal Trade Commission, Washington, DC

2:10   Discussion Among Presenters and the Committee

3:10   Break

3:30   Family Dynamics: Challenges and Opportunities for
                Preventing Childhood Obesity and Promoting Healthful
                Lifestyles
                Susan McHale, Ph.D., The Pennsylvania State University,
                    University Park, PA

4:00   Discussion

4:45   Open Forum
                Joan Almon, U.S. Alliance for Childhood
                Lilian Cheung, D.Sc., R.D., Harvard School of Public Health
                Jessica Donze, M.P.H., R.D., American Dietetic Association
                Tracy Fox, M.P.H., R.D., Produce for Better Health
                    Foundation
                Lynn Fredericks, B.A., FamilyCook Productions
                Velma LaPoint, Ph.D., Howard University
                David Meyers, M.D., United States Breastfeeding Committee
                Jill Nicholls, Ph.D., National Dairy Council/Dairy
                    Management Inc.
                Anne-Marie Nocton, M.S., M.P.H., R.D., Sports,
                    Cardiovascular, and Wellness Nutritionists
                Robert Pallay, M.D., American Academy of Family
                    Physicians
                Mercedes Rubio, Ph.D., American Sociological Association
                Margo Wootan, Sc.D., Center for Science in the Public
                    Interest

5:30   Adjourn

F

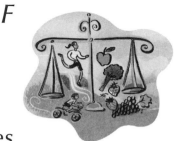

Biographical Sketches

Jeffrey P. Koplan, M.D., M.P.H. *(Chair)*, is the Vice President for Academic Health Affairs at the Woodruff Health Sciences Center at Emory University in Atlanta. He received a B.A. from Yale College, M.D. from Mt. Sinai School of Medicine, and M.P.H. from the Harvard School of Public Health. He is board certified in internal and preventive medicine. From 1998 to 2002, Dr. Koplan served as the Director of the Centers for Disease Control and Prevention (CDC) and Administrator of the Agency for Toxic Substances and Disease Registry. He worked in the area of enhancing the interactions between clinical medicine and public health by leading the Prudential Center for Health Care Research, a nationally recognized health services research organization. Dr. Koplan has worked on a broad range of major public health issues, including infectious diseases such as smallpox and HIV/AIDS, environmental issues such as the Bhopal chemical disaster, and the health toll of tobacco and chronic diseases, both in the United States and globally. Dr. Koplan is a Master of the American College of Physicians, an Honorary Fellow of the Society of Public Health Educators, and a Public Health Hero of the American Public Health Association. He was elected to the Institute of Medicine (IOM) in 1999. He has served on many advisory groups and consultancies on public health issues in the United States and overseas and authored more than 170 scientific papers.

Dennis M. Bier, M.D., is Professor of Pediatrics and the Director of the U.S. Department of Agriculture/Agricultural Research Service (USDA/ARS) Children's Nutrition Research Center at the Baylor College of Medicine in

Houston. Prior to this appointment, he was Co-director of the Pediatric Endocrinology and Metabolism Division and Director of the Pediatric Clinical Research Center at Washington University School of Medicine in St. Louis. Dr. Bier received his B.S. from LeMoyne College and his M.D. from New Jersey College of Medicine. Dr. Bier's primary research interests are focused on the regulation of inter-organ transport of metabolic fuels with a special emphasis on the substrate and hormonal regulation of glucose, lipid, and protein/amino acid fuels. He has expertise in the areas of nutrition in human health and in the prevention and treatment of disease, particularly the role of maternal, fetal, and childhood nutrition on the growth, development, and health of children through adolescence; the long-term consequences of nutrient inadequacy during critical periods of embryonic and fetal life, infancy, and childhood on the pathogenesis of adult chronic diseases; macronutrients; intermediary metabolism; tracer kinetics; and diabetes, obesity, and endocrine disorders. Dr. Bier has served as President of the International Pediatric Research Foundation, Chair of the USDA/ARS Human Studies Review Committee, Councilor for the American Pediatric Society, and as a member of the 1995 USDA/HHS Dietary Guidelines Advisory Committee, the IOM's Food and Nutrition Board (FNB), and the IOM Committee on Implications of Dioxin in the Food Supply. He was elected to the IOM in 1997. He currently serves on the Board of the International Life Sciences Institute (ILSI) North America, and he is a member of the McDonald's Global Advisory Council on Healthy Lifestyles.

Leann L. Birch, Ph.D., is the Distinguished Professor of Human Development and Nutritional Sciences at The Pennsylvania State University in University Park. She holds a Ph.D. in psychology from the University of Michigan. Dr. Birch's research has focused on the development of eating behaviors in infants, children, and adolescents. Her research explores factors shaping food preferences in infants and children, regulation of food intake in children, dieting and problems of energy balance in school-age girls, predictors of maternal child feeding styles, and parental and environmental influences on children's dietary practices. She currently receives research support from the National Institute of Child Health and Human Development (NICHD). Dr. Birch has received national and international recognition for her work including the Lederle Award from the American Society for Nutritional Sciences. She is the author of more than 150 publications.

Ross C. Brownson, Ph.D., is Professor of Epidemiology and the Chair of the Department of Community Health at St. Louis University School of Public Health in Missouri. He was formerly Division Director with the Missouri Department of Health. He received his Ph.D. in environmental health and epidemiology at Colorado State University. Dr. Brownson is a chronic disease epidemiologist whose research has focused on tobacco use prevention, promotion of physical activity, and the evaluation of community-level interventions. He is the principal investigator of a CDC-funded Prevention Research Center that is developing innovative approaches to chronic disease prevention among high-risk rural adults. Dr. Brownson is also developing and testing effective dissemination strategies for CDC designed to increase rates of physical activity among adults. Dr. Brownson receives research support from the National Institutes of Diabetes and Digestive and Kidney Diseases to conduct a diabetes prevention study aimed at promoting walking among high-risk rural adults. Dr. Brownson receives support from the Robert Wood Johnson Foundation (RWJF) to understand the environmental characteristics of activity-friendly communities and to measure the perceptual qualities of urban settings through RWJF's Active Living Research program. He is a member of numerous editorial boards and is associate editor of the *Annual Review of Public Health*. Dr. Brownson is the author or editor of several books including *Chronic Disease Epidemiology and Control, Applied Epidemiology,* and *Evidence-Based Public Health.*

John Cawley, Ph.D., is an Assistant Professor in the Department of Policy Analysis and Management at Cornell University. Dr. Cawley received his undergraduate degree in economics from Harvard University and his Ph.D. in economics from the University of Chicago. Dr. Cawley joined the Cornell faculty in 2001 after spending two years as a Robert Wood Johnson Scholar in Health Policy Research at the University of Michigan. His research focuses on health economics, in particular the economics of obesity. He is currently studying the effect of body weight on labor market outcomes such as wage rates, unemployment, and employment disability; the role of body weight in the decision of adolescents to initiate smoking; the demand for anti-obesity pharmaceuticals; and the extent to which consumption of calories can be considered addictive. His research is conducted with support from the Economic Research Initiative on the Uninsured, the University of Michigan Retirement Research Consortium, J.P. Morgan Private Bank Global Philanthropic Services, RWJF, Merck, and USDA. In addition to his affiliation with Cornell, Dr. Cawley is a Faculty Research Fellow of the National Bureau of Economic Research in the Health Economics and Health Care programs. He also serves on an advisory board to the CDC's Project MOVE: Measurement of the Value of Exercise.

George R. Flores, M.D., M.P.H., is a Senior Program Officer with The California Endowment, a major health foundation, where his focus is on disparities in health status, prevention of childhood obesity, community-based public health, and health policy. Dr. Flores served previously as

Health Officer and Director of Public Health in San Diego and Sonoma Counties, Deputy Health Officer in Santa Barbara County, Assistant Clinical Professor at the University of California San Francisco School of Medicine, and Program Director for Project HOPE in Guatemala. He is a founder and member of the Board of Directors of the Latino Coalition for a Healthy California. Dr. Flores is an alumnus of the University of Utah College of Medicine, the Harvard School of Public Health, the Kennedy School of Government, and the Public Health Leadership Institute. He has served on the IOM Committee on Assuring the Health of the Public in the 21st Century.

Simone A. French, Ph.D., is Professor in the Division of Epidemiology in the School of Public Health at the University of Minnesota in Minneapolis. She received a B.A. in psychology from Macalester College in St. Paul, Minnesota, and a Ph.D. in psychology from the University of Minnesota in Minneapolis. Dr. French's expertise and research focuses broadly on the social and environmental influences on eating and physical activity behaviors, community-based strategies for eating behavior change, and adolescent nutrition and physical activity. Her obesity prevention research has focused on pricing strategies to promote sales of lower fat foods in cafeterias and vending machines, and changing the availability and promotion of healthful foods in school cafeterias to influence student food choices. She has also researched eating disorders, dieting, and other weight management strategies among adolescents and adults. Dr. French presently receives research support that focuses on obesity and nutrition from the National Heart, Lung, and Blood Institute and NICHD. She serves as co-editor of the *International Journal of Behavioral Nutrition and Physical Activity*. Dr. French has authored more than 100 scientific papers in peer-reviewed academic journals.

Susan L. Handy, Ph.D., is an Associate Professor in the Department of Environmental Science and Policy, University of California at Davis. She earned a B.S. in civil engineering from Princeton University, an M.S. in civil engineering from Stanford University, and a Ph.D. in city and regional planning from the University of California at Berkeley. Dr. Handy's research focuses on the relationships between transportation and land use, including the impact of land use on travel behavior, and the impact of transportation investments on land development patterns. Her work is directed toward developing strategies to enhance accessibility and reduce automobile dependence, including land use policies and telecommunications services. She is the Chair of the Committee on Telecommunications and Travel Behavior and a member of the Committee on Transportation and Land Development of the Transportation Research Board. She is also a co-principal investigator on a project funded by The RWJF's Active Living and Environmental Studies Program.

Robert C. Hornik, Ph.D., is the Wilbur Schramm Professor of Communication and Health Policy at the Annenberg School for Communication, University of Pennsylvania in Philadelphia. He has a wide range of experience in mass-media communication evaluations, ranging from breastfeeding promotion, AIDS education, immunization and child survival projects, to anti-drug and domestic violence media campaigns at the community, national, and international levels. Dr. Hornik has served as a member of the IOM Committee on International Nutrition Programs, the National Research Council (NRC) Committee on Communication for Behavior Change in the 21st Century: Improving the Health of Diverse Populations, and the NRC Committee to Develop a Strategy to Prevent and Reduce Underage Drinking. He has received the Andreasen Scholar award in social marketing, and the Fisher Mentorship award from the International Communication Association. He has also been a consultant to other agencies such as the U.S. Agency for International Development, UNICEF, CDC, and the World Bank. Dr. Hornik serves on the editorial boards of several journals, including *Social Marketing Quarterly* and the *Journal of Health Communication*. Dr. Hornik was the scientific director for the evaluation of the Office of National Drug Control Policy's National Youth Anti-Drug Media Campaign and he is currently the director of the University of Pennsylvania's National Cancer Institute-funded Center of Excellence in Cancer Communication Research. He most recently edited *Public Health Communication* and was the author of *Development Communication*, and co-author of *Educational Reform with Television: The El Salvador Experience*, and *Toward Reform of Program Evaluation*.

Douglas B. Kamerow, M.D., M.P.H., is the Chief Scientist for Health, Social, and Economics Research at RTI International where he focuses on health-related behaviors, evidence-based care, and improving the quality of health care. Among his responsibilities is serving as principal investigator on an evaluation of the RWJF's National Diabetes Program. He is also a Clinical Professor of Family Medicine at Georgetown University. A family physician who is also board certified in preventive medicine, Dr. Kamerow received his A.B. from Harvard College, M.D. from the University of Rochester, and M.P.H. from Johns Hopkins University. While a Commissioned Officer in the U.S. Public Health Service, he served as Director of the Center for Practice and Technology Assessment, Agency for Healthcare Research and Quality, Department of Health and Human Services and Director of the Clinical Preventive Services staff of the Public Health Service Office of Disease Prevention and Health Promotion. He conceived and supervised the creation of the Evidence-based Practice Centers Program and the National Guideline Clearinghouse, was managing editor of the first and second editions of the U.S. Preventive Services Task Force *Guide to Clinical Preventive Services*, and led the development of the *Put Prevention into Practice* campaign, which sought to incorporate clinical preventive services, including nutrition counseling, into routine medical practice.

Shiriki K. Kumanyika, Ph.D., M.P.H., R.D., is Professor of Epidemiology in the Department of Biostatistics and Epidemiology, Associate Dean for Health Promotion and Disease Prevention, and the Director of the Graduate Program in Public Health Studies at the University of Pennsylvania School of Medicine. She received her B.A. from Syracuse University, M.S.W. from Columbia University, Ph.D. in human nutrition from Cornell University, and M.P.H. from Johns Hopkins University. The main themes in Dr. Kumanyika's research concern the role of nutritional factors in the primary and secondary prevention of chronic diseases with a particular focus on obesity, sodium reduction, and related health problems such as hypertension and diabetes. She directs a National Institutes of Health (NIH)-funded EXPORT (Excellence in Partnerships for Community Outreach, Research, and Training) Center that focuses on reduction of obesity-related health disparities. Dr. Kumanyika is the lead investigator or a collaborator on several federally-funded studies of obesity prevention and treatment in adults and children, of which some focus specifically on African Americans. She has served on a number of expert panels, including the 1995 and 2000 U.S. Dietary Guidelines Advisory Committees, and she served on the NIH Advisory Committee for the National Children's Study in 2002-2003. She was vice-chair of the Joint WHO/FAO Expert Consultation on Diet, Nutrition and the Prevention of Chronic Diseases in 2002, and also chaired the 2002 WHO Expert Consultation on Appropriate BMI Standards for Asian Populations. Dr. Kumanyika's current activities include serving on the IOM's FNB, the NIH Clinical Obesity Research Panel, and the Prevention Group of the International Obesity Task Force. She was elected to the IOM in 2003.

Barbara J. Moore, Ph.D., is the President and Chief Executive Officer of Shape Up America!, a national initiative to promote healthy weight and increased physical activity in America. She earned an undergraduate degree in philosophy from Skidmore College, received her M.S. and Ph.D. in nutrition from Columbia University, and served as a Postdoctoral Fellow in nutrition and physiology at the University of California at Davis. Previous positions include service as Deputy Director in the Division of Nutrition Research Coordination at the NIH, Acting Assistant Director of Social and

Behavioral Sciences at the White House Office of Science and Technology Policy, Chief Nutritionist of Weight Watchers International, and Assistant Professor of Nutrition at Rutgers University. Dr. Moore has conducted research on animal models of obesity and on addressing the public health and socioeconomic implications of obesity in the United States. She has served on the IOM Subcommittee on Military Weight Management.

Arie L. Nettles, Ph.D., is an Assistant Professor and Assistant Research Scientist of Education, and previously served as Clinical Assistant Professor of Pediatrics and Communicable Diseases at the University of Michigan. Her research focuses on the study of academic achievement and the impact of sickle cell disease on children and equity issues in educational assessment. Prior to her appointment at the University of Michigan, she was an Assistant Professor of School Psychology at the University of Tennessee. Other faculty appointments include Tennessee State University, Fisk University, and Trenton State College. Dr. Nettles has been a public school teacher in Iowa and Tennessee and a practicing school psychologist in Kentucky and New Jersey. She is a licensed psychologist in Tennessee and Michigan, and nationally certified in school psychology, endorsed by the National Association of School Psychology. She has a B.S. in social science education and M.S. in education administration from the University of Tennessee at Knoxville. She received a Ph.D. in psychology from Vanderbilt University specializing in clinical and school psychology. Dr. Nettles has served on the NRC Committee on Goals 2000 and the Inclusion of Students with Disabilities.

Russell R. Pate, Ph.D., is the Associate Dean for Research and a Professor at the Norman J. Arnold School of Public Health, University of South Carolina in Columbia. He received a B.S. in physical education from Springfield College, and M.S. and Ph.D. in exercise physiology from the University of Oregon. Dr. Pate's research interest and expertise focuses on physical activity measurement, determinants, and promotion in children and youth. He also directs a national postgraduate course aimed at developing research competencies related to physical activity and public health. Dr. Pate is also involved in the CDC-funded Prevention Research Center at the University of South Carolina. His research includes studies on preschoolers' physical activity levels and how schools can influence these levels and multi-center trials on the promotion of physical activity among middle and high school-age girls. Dr. Pate serves as an investigator for the RWJF Active for Life program that encourages physical activity among seniors. He is a Past-President of both the American College of Sports Medicine and the National Coalition on Promoting Physical Activity.

John C. Peters, Ph.D., is the Associate Director of Food and Beverage Technology and Director of the Nutrition Science Institute at Procter & Gamble Company in Cincinnati. He received his B.S. in biochemistry from the University of California at Davis and his Ph.D. in biochemistry and nutrition from the University of Wisconsin at Madison. Dr. Peters' research has focused on amino acid metabolism and dietary intake, triglycerides and lipid levels in humans, effects of weight cycling on susceptibility to obesity, and effects of fat replacements on energy, fat intake, and micronutrient metabolism. He has served on the scientific advisory board of the Arkansas Children's Hospital Research Institute; on the planning committee of the Cincinnati Health Improvement Collaborative; as Vice Chair of the scientific advisory board of the ILSI Center for Health Promotion; and Treasurer of the public-private Partnership for Healthy Eating and Active Living. Dr. Peters is currently President of the ILSI Center for Health Promotion.

Thomas N. Robinson, M.D., M.P.H., is an Associate Professor of Pediatrics and of Medicine in the Division of General Pediatrics and Stanford Prevention Research Center, Stanford University School of Medicine. Dr. Robinson received both his B.S. and M.D. from Stanford University and M.P.H. in maternal and child health from the University of California at Berkeley. He completed his internship and residency in pediatrics at Children's Hospital in Boston and at Harvard Medical School, and then returned to Stanford for postdoctoral training as a Robert Wood Johnson Clinical Scholar. Dr. Robinson's community-, school-, and family-based health behavior change research has focused on nutrition, physical activity, and smoking behavior in children and adolescents; the effects of television viewing on health-related behaviors; childhood obesity prevention and treatment; and using interactive communication technologies to promote health behavior change. Dr. Robinson was an RWJF Generalist Physician Faculty Scholar awardee during his participation on this committee. Dr. Robinson is board certified in pediatrics, a Fellow of the American Academy of Pediatrics, and practices general pediatrics and directs the Center for Healthy Weight at the Lucile Packard Children's Hospital at Stanford.

Charles Royer, B.S., is a Senior Lecturer at the University of Washington with appointments in the School of Public Health and Community Medicine and in the Evans School of Public Affairs. He is also National Program Director of the Urban Health Initiative, an effort to improve the health and safety of children across five regions. He holds a B.S. from the University of Oregon. From 1990 to 1994, Mr. Royer was Director of the Institute of Politics at Harvard University and Lecturer at the Kennedy School of Government. Prior to this, Mr. Royer served as Mayor of Seattle from 1978 to 1989, following a career in newspaper and television journalism. He has served as President of the National League of Cities and as a member of the National Commission on State and Local Public Service, the Democratic National Committee, and the President's Commission on White House Fellowships. He was named one of the top 20 American mayors in 1988 and received the 1989 Distinguished Urban Mayor Award from the National Urban Coalition.

Shirley R. Watkins, M.Ed., is an Educational and Nutrition Services Consultant. From 1997 to 2001, she was Under Secretary for Food, Nutrition, and Consumer Services at USDA, the first African-American woman to hold that position. In that capacity she oversaw USDA's food assistance programs and its dietary guidance promotion efforts. She also served USDA as Deputy Assistant Secretary for Marketing and Regulatory Programs and Deputy Under Secretary for Food, Nutrition, and Consumer Services. Before joining USDA in 1993, Ms. Watkins was Director of Nutrition Services for Memphis, Tennessee city schools. Previous positions included food-service supervisor, home economics teacher, elementary school teacher, and a home demonstration agent with the University of Arkansas Extension Service. She is a past president of the American School Food Services Association. She received a B.S. in home economics from the University of Arkansas at Pine Bluff and an M.Ed. from the University of Memphis.

Robert C. Whitaker, M.D., M.P.H., is a Senior Fellow at Mathematica Policy Research, Inc., in Princeton, New Jersey. Before joining Mathematica he was a Visiting Senior Research Scholar at the Center for Health and Wellbeing at the Woodrow Wilson School of Public and International Affairs at Princeton University, and was an Associate Professor of Pediatrics at the University of Cincinnati College of Medicine and Cincinnati Children's Hospital Medical Center. His research has focused on the childhood antecedents of adult chronic disease. This has included studies on school nutrition, obesity prevention strategies in preschool children, parent-child feeding interaction, the epidemiology of childhood obesity, and the determinants of social and emotional well-being in children. He served on the IOM Committee on Dietary Risk Assessment in the WIC Program. Dr. Whitaker received a B.A. in chemistry from Williams College, an M.D. from The Johns Hopkins University School of Medicine, and an M.P.H. from the University of Washington School of Public Health and Community Medicine. Dr. Whitaker completed his residency and fellowship in pediatrics at the University of Washington School of Medicine, and he received postdoctoral training as a Robert Wood Johnson Clinical Scholar.

IOM Staff

Tazima A. Davis is a Research Associate in the FNB at the IOM and has been with the FNB since September 2000. Prior to joining the National Academies, she worked as a Quality Control Supervisor with Kraft Foods and Bestfoods Foodservice. Ms. Davis earned a B.S. in food science from the University of Illinois at Urbana-Champaign (UIUC). During her undergraduate years at UIUC, she participated in research internships including ice cream ingredient development in Chicago; applied food microbiology research in Boslwart, Netherlands; and carotenoid research in Urbana, Illinois.

Vivica I. Kraak, M.S., R.D., is a Senior Program Officer in the IOM's FNB. In addition to working on the Prevention of Obesity in Children and Youth Study, she directs the international activities within FNB. She received her B.S. in nutritional sciences from Cornell University and completed a coordinated M.S. in nutrition and dietetic internship at Case Western Reserve University and the University Hospitals of Cleveland. Prior to joining the IOM in 2002, she worked as a Clinical Dietitian at Columbia-Presbyterian Medical Center and as a Public Health Nutritionist specializing in HIV disease in New York City. From 1994 to 2000, she was a Research Nutritionist in the Division of Nutritional Sciences at Cornell University, where she collaborated on several domestic and international food policy and community nutrition research initiatives. She has co-authored a variety of publications related to food security and community food systems, nutrition and HIV/AIDS, international food aid and food security, viewpoints about genetically engineered foods, use of dietary supplements, and the influence of commercialism on the food and nutrition-related decisions and behaviors of children and youth.

Catharyn T. Liverman, M.L.S., is a Senior Program Officer in the FNB and the Board on Health Sciences Policy at the IOM. She served as study director for this study. In 12 years at IOM, she has worked on projects addressing a number of topics, including veterans' health, drug abuse, injury prevention, and clinical trials of testosterone therapy. IOM reports she has co-edited include *Testosterone and Aging: Clinical Research Directions; Gulf War and Health, Vol. 1; Reducing the Burden of Injury; Toxicology and Environmental Health Information Resources;* and *The Development of Medications for the Treatment of Opiate and Cocaine Addiction.* Her background is in medical library science, with previous jobs at the National Agricultural Library and the Naval War College Library. She received her B.A. from Wake Forest University and her M.L.S. from the University of Maryland.

Rose Marie Martinez, Sc.D., is the Director of the IOM's Board on Health Promotion and Disease Prevention . Prior to joining the IOM, Dr. Martinez was a Senior Health Researcher at Mathematica Policy Research from 1995 to 1999 where she conducted research on the impact of health system change on the public health infrastructure, access to care for vulnerable populations, managed care, and the health-care workforce. Dr. Martinez is a former Assistant Director for Health Financing and Policy with the U.S. General Accounting Office where she directed evaluations and policy analysis in the area of national and public health issues. She also served as Chief of Health Studies at the Regional Institute for Health and Social Welfare, the research arm of the Regional Ministry of Health in Madrid, Spain. Dr. Martinez received her B.A. from the University of Southern California and her Doctor of Science from the Johns Hopkins School of Hygiene and Public Health.

Linda D. Meyers, Ph.D., is the Director of the IOM's FNB. She has also served as FNB Deputy Director and as a Senior Program Officer. Prior to joining the IOM in 2001, she worked for 15 years in the Office of Disease Prevention and Health Promotion in the U.S. Department of Health and Human Services where she was a Senior Nutrition Advisor, Deputy Director, and Acting Director. Dr. Meyers has received a number of awards for her contributions to public health, including the Secretary's Distinguished Service Award for *Healthy People 2010* and the Surgeon General's Medallion. Dr. Meyers has a B.A. in health and physical education from Goshen College in Indiana, M.S. in food and nutrition from Colorado State University, and Ph.D. in nutritional sciences from Cornell University.

Janice Rice Okita, Ph.D., R.D., is a Senior Program Officer in the IOM's FNB. Since joining the IOM in 2002, she has worked on projects involving evaluation of the safety of dietary supplements for the Food and Drug Administration, and reviewing the food packages used in the USDA Special Supplemental Food Program for Women, Infants, and Children. Dr. Okita participated in biomedical research in the Department of Pharmaceutical Sciences, College of Pharmacy, Washington State University in Pullman from 1990-2001; the Department of Biochemistry, Medical College of Wisconsin in Milwaukee from 1988-1990; and the Platelet Biochemistry Laboratory, Blood Center of Southeastern Wisconsin in Milwaukee from 1982-1988. Dr. Okita earned a B.S. in human food and nutrition from Florida State University in Tallahassee, and Ph.D. in biochemistry from the University of Texas Health Science Center at Dallas. She is a Registered Dietitian and practiced clinical dietetics in Dallas from 1972 to 1974.

Shannon L. Ruddy is a Senior Program Assistant in the FNB at the IOM. She has also worked with the NRC where she worked on several reports, including *Partnerships for Reducing Landslide Risk, Fair Weather: Effective Partnerships in Weather and Climate Services, Government Data Centers: Meeting Increasing Demands, Resolving Conflicts Arising from the Privatization of Environmental Data, Review of EarthScope Integrated Science,* and *National Spatial Data Infrastructure Partnership Programs: Rethinking the Focus.* She has been with the National Academies since 2001. She holds a B.A. in environmental science from LaSalle University in Philadelphia. Previously, she worked as a Researcher for Booz-Allen & Hamilton in the Environmental Protection Agency's Region 3 CERCLA/ Superfund Records Center.

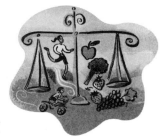

Index

A

Abdominal obesity, 69, 70
Academic performance, 105, 215, 252, 253
Action plan for prevention
    clinical medicine approach, 107-108,
        109
    contexts for, 25-44
    definitions and terminology, 79-83
    developing recommendations, 16, 111-
        115, 323
    energy balance, 3, 90-106
    evidence-based strategies, 3, 16, 107-
        115, 322-323
    framework, 83-85
    goals, 4-5, 86-90, 115
    public health approach, 108-110, 115,
        127, 129
Active Living by Design, 206
Added caloric sweeteners, 31, 145-146, 290
Adolescents. See Children and adolescent
        obesity; Older Children and Youth
Adopted children, studies, 93
Adults
    diabetes, 68
    energy balance, 90, 160
    obesity, 5, 22, 43-44, 63-65, 68
    overweight, 80
    physical activity, 29, 35, 179

prevention goals, 88
    treatment for obesity, 108
    TV viewing time, 160-161
Advertising and marketing
    alcoholic beverages, 175
    bans and restrictions on, 174-175, 178,
        268, 353, 362, 363
    codes and monitoring mechanisms, 176-
        177
    and eating behavior, 169-170, 172-173
    energy density of advertised foods, 172
    and energy imbalance, 172, 173, 174,
        355
    ethnic groups targeted by, 106
    evidence of effects of, 353-354, 355
    expenditures, 172
    exposure time for children, 171, 174
    First Amendment rights, 174-175, 353,
        362
    health and nutrient claims, 169-170, 176
    litigation, 354
    packaging, 172, 356
    prevention through, 128, 268, 353, 367;
        see also Public education
    quantity and nature of commercials, 172
    recommendations, 9, 177
    research needs, 177, 268
    in schools, 176, 251, 265-269
    self-regulation by industry, 175, 354